AF324120

Radiation Medicine Rounds

Charles R. Thomas, Jr., MD

Editor-in-Chief

Professor and Chair
Department of Radiation Medicine
Professor, Division of Hematology/Oncology
Department of Medicine
Knight Cancer Institute
Oregon Health & Science University Cancer Institute
Portland, Oregon

Radiation Medicine Rounds

VOLUME 3, ISSUE 3

Hematologic Malignancies

Guest Editors

Michael B. Tomblyn, MD, MS
Assistant Member
Radiation Oncology
Moffitt Cancer Center and Research Institute
Tampa, Florida

Karen M. Winkfield, MD, PhD
Director
Hematologic Malignancy Service
Department of Radiation Oncology
Massachusetts General Hospital Cancer Center
Boston, Massachusetts

Bouthaina S. Dabaja, MD
Associate Professor and Section Chief Lymphoma
Department of Radiation Oncology
The University of Texas MD Anderson Cancer Center
Houston, Texas

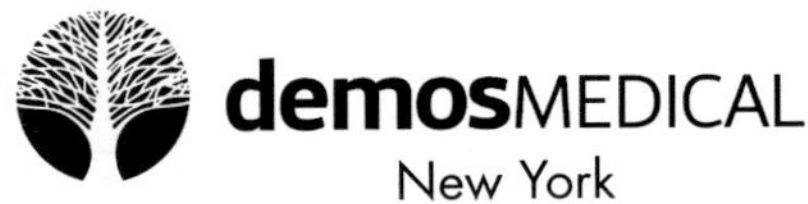

demosMEDICAL
New York

Acquisitions Editor: Richard Winters
Cover Design: Joe Tenerelli
Compositor: Newgen Imaging
Printer: Hamilton

Visit our website at www.demosmedpub.com

Radiation Medicine Rounds is published three times a year by Demos Medical Publishing.

Business Office. All business correspondence including subscriptions, renewals, and address changes should be sent to Demos Medical Publishing, 11 West 42nd Street, 15th Floor, New York, NY, 10036.

The ideas and opinions expressed in *Radiation Medicine Rounds* do not necessarily reflect those of the Publisher. The Publisher does not assume any responsibility for any injury and/or damage to persons or property arising out of or related to any use of the material contained in this periodical. The reader is advised to check the appropriate medical literature and the product information currently provided by the manufacturer of each drug to be administered to verify the dosage, the method and duration of administration, or contraindications. It is the responsibility of the treating physician or other health care professional relying on independent experience and knowledge of the patient, to determine drug dosages and the best treatment for the patient. Mention of any product in this issue should not be construed as endorsement by the contributors, editors, or the Publisher of the product or manufacturer's claims.

ISSN: 2151-4208
ISBN: 978-1-936287-77-2
E-ISBN: 978-1-617051-49-4

Library of Congress Cataloging-in-Publication Data

Hematologic malignancies / guest editors, Michael Tomblyn, Karen M. Winkfield, Bouthaina Dabaja.
     p.; cm.—(Radiation medicine rounds, ISSN 2151-4208; v. 3, issue 3)
  Includes bibliographical references and index.
  ISBN 978-1-936287-77-2—ISBN 978-1-61705-149-4 (e-ISBN)
  I. Tomblyn, Michael. II. Winkfield, Karen Marie, 1970- III. Dabaja, Bouthaina. IV. Series: Radiation medicine rounds; v. 3, issue 3. 2151-4208
  [DNLM: 1. Hematologic Neoplasms. 2. Hodgkin Disease. 3. Lymphoma, Non-Hodgkin. W1 RA162HD v.3 no.3 2012 / WH 525]

  616.99418—dc23

                                                                                        2012041753

Printed in the United States of America
12 13 14 15   5 4 3 2 1

Contents

Foreword

■ FROM THE EDITOR-IN-CHIEF

This latest issue of *Radiation Medicine Rounds* is dedicated to the topic of *Hematologic Malignancies.* On behalf of the editorial board, I am very delighted that we were able to secure commitments from three of the top emerging thought leaders to serve as Guest Editors: Drs. Michael Tomblyn, Karen Winkfield, and Bouthaina Dabaja. They have gathered a stellar ensemble of insightful investigators who understand the role of radiotherapy in the management of hematologic cancers. They are to be congratulated for delivering a timely educational, research, and clinically applicable product that covers the state of the art on this timely topic. We congratulate Drs. Tomblyn, Winkfield, and Dabaja for putting together an outstanding volume that will be useful to colleagues who are involved in the delivery of clinical care to patients with hematologic tumors.

Dr. Charles R. Thomas, Jr.
Series Editor-in-Chief
Radiation Medicine Rounds
Portland, Oregon

Preface

With over 100,000 new diagnoses of lymphoma and plasma cell dyscrasias in the United States each year, these hematologic malignancies represent a significant burden of disease. Unlike most solid tumor sites with only a few discrete histologic entities, there are literally dozens of distinct lymphoma subtypes, each with its own unique molecular and clinical features. While systemic cytotoxic and targeted therapies for hematologic malignancies have improved dramatically over the past several decades, radiation therapy continues to represent an important modality for optimal clinical outcomes.

Recent advances in radiotherapy for hematologic malignancies have allowed for maintenance of excellent local control with improvements in toxicity through reductions in field sizes, in dose delivered, and with increasingly conformal delivery techniques. Perhaps no lymphoma subtype better represents this paradigm shift than does Hodgkin lymphoma. Drs. Terezakis and Hoppe provide an excellent review of the dramatic changes in the radiotherapeutic approach to the disease and offer insights on the potential role for highly conformal delivery of therapy using modern techniques.

Mature B-cell non-Hodgkin lymphomas represent the most common subtypes seen by radiation oncologists. The approach to these lymphomas has also undergone a dramatic shift over the past two decades. Dr. Dabaja offers an update on the management of diffuse large B-cell lymphoma. Drs. Barnes and Winkfield provide the latest information on radiotherapy for follicular lymphoma. Drs. Pinnix and Dabaja review the role of radiotherapy for marginal zone lymphomas. Drs. Bhavsar and Tomblyn present management recommendations for patients with mantle cell lymphoma and other aggressive B-cell subtypes.

T-cell and NK-cell lymphomas, although less common in clinical practice, represent areas for radiation oncologists to take lead roles in the therapy of hematologic malignancies. Dr. Dabaja reviews the radiotherapy techniques for the treatment of mycosis fungoides, and Drs. Mitin and Winkfield share their insights on the modern management of natural killer cell lymphomas.

Other hematologic malignancies relevant to the radiation oncologist are covered as well. Drs. Pinnix and Dabaja discuss radiotherapy approaches to the patient with leukemia. Drs. Yee, Winkfield, and Raje review the role of radiotherapy in the management of plasma cell dyscrasias.

Finally, novel approaches to radiotherapy for hematologic malignancies are considered. Drs. Abramson and Muse offer an excellent review of the role of FDG-PET in the management and treatment planning for lymphoma. Dr. Tomblyn provides a comprehensive review of radioimmunotherapy for non-Hodgkin lymphomas. Drs. Tomblyn and Tomblyn discuss the many uses for radiotherapy before, during, and following hematopoietic stem cell transplantation for patients with hematologic malignancies.

This issue is dedicated to the many patients with hematologic malignancies for whom we have had the privilege to care for over the years.

Michael B. Tomblyn, MD, MS
Karen M. Winkfield, MD, PhD
Bouthaina S. Dabaja, MD

Contributors

Jeremy S. Abramson, MD, MMSc
Director
Center for Lymphoma
Massachusetts General Hospital Cancer Center
Boston, MA

Jeffrey Barnes, MD, PhD
Assistant Physician
Center for Lymphoma
Massachusetts General Hospital Cancer Center
Boston, MA

Shripal Bhavsar, MD, MBA
Clinical Assistant Instructor
Department of Radiation Oncology
SUNY-Upstate Medical University
Syracuse, NY

Bouthaina S. Dabaja, MD
Associate Professor and Section Chief Lymphoma
Department of Radiation Oncology
The University of Texas MD Anderson
    Cancer Center
Houston, TX

Bradford S. Hoppe, MD, MPH
Assistant Professor
Department of Radiation Oncology
University of Florida
Jacksonville, FL

Timur Mitin, MD, PhD
Instructor
Department of Radiation Oncology
Massachusetts General Hospital
Boston, MA

Victorine V. Muse, MD
Associate Radiologist
Department of Radiology
Massachusetts General Hospital
Boston, MA

Chelsea C. Pinnix, MD
Assistant Professor
Department of Radiation Oncology
The University of Texas MD Anderson
    Cancer Center
Houston, TX

Noopur S. Raje, MD
Director
Center for Multiple Myeloma
Department of Hematology/Oncology
Massachusetts General Hospital Cancer Center
Boston, MA

Stephanie A. Terezakis, MD
Assistant Professor
Residency Program Director
Department of Radiation Oncology and Molecular
    Radiation Sciences
Sidney Kimmel Comprehensive Cancer Center at
    Johns Hopkins
Baltimore, MD

Marcie Tomblyn, MD, MS
Associate Member
Department of Blood and Marrow Transplantation
H. Lee Moffitt Cancer Center and Research
    Institute
Tampa, FL

Michael B. Tomblyn, MD, MS
Assistant Member
Department of Radiation Oncology
H. Lee Moffitt Cancer Center and Research
    Institute
Tampa, FL

Karen M. Winkfield, MD, PhD
Director
Hematologic Malignancy Service
Department of Radiation Oncology
Massachusetts General Hospital Cancer Center
Boston, MA

Andrew J. Yee, MD
Assistant in Medicine
Center for Multiple Myeloma,
    Department of Hematology/Oncology
Massachusetts General Hospital Cancer Center
Boston, MA

Radiation Medicine Rounds

VOLUME 3, ISSUE 3

Hematologic Malignancies

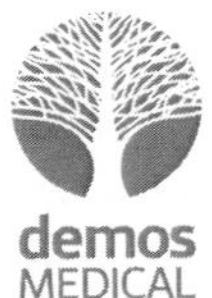

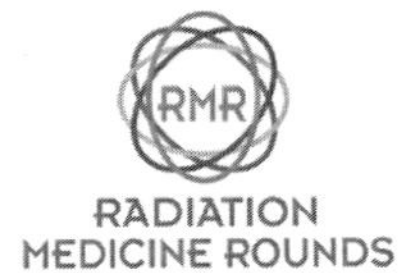

Advances in Radiation Treatment of Hodgkin Lymphoma

Stephanie A. Terezakis*[1] and Bradford S. Hoppe[2]

[1]*Sidney Kimmel Comprehensive Cancer Center at Johns Hopkins, Baltimore, MD*
[2]*University of Florida Proton Therapy Institute, Jacksonville, FL*

■ ABSTRACT

Treatment paradigms for Hodgkin lymphoma (HL) that incorporate radiotherapy (RT) have markedly changed during the last several decades. Modern reduced-volume treatment fields and reduced treatment doses avoid normal tissue exposure and reduce the risk of long-term toxicity while avoiding in-field or marginal failures. Advanced RT techniques, such as three-dimensional conformal RT, intensity-modulated RT (IMRT), and proton therapy (PT), further enhance the radiation oncologist's ability to develop an individualized RT plan based on the risks and benefits of treatment. Further refinements in tailored treatment regimens, incorporating risk stratification and response-based assessment, are currently being evaluated in an effort to optimize the incorporation of RT and determine which subsets of patients benefit most from RT.

Keywords: Hodgkin lymphoma, IFRT, INRT

■ INTRODUCTION

Before the development of effective chemotherapy regimens for Hodgkin lymphoma (HL), radiotherapy (RT) was used alone as a curative paradigm; however, this approach necessitated large treatment fields that exposed large volumes of normal tissue to high radiation doses. Thus, despite the effectiveness of RT, the incidence of late toxicities was substantial such that late effects, including cardiovascular disease and secondary malignancies, contributed to the cause of death in HL survivors. The advent of combined modality therapy has significantly changed the approach to RT for HL, allowing for the delivery of smaller treatment fields and the use of lower doses while still maintaining effectiveness. RT delivery has also drastically changed in the modern era using advanced imaging techniques and sophisticated planning and delivery systems that allow further reduction in the exposure of normal structures to radiation. The use of RT in the curative paradigm of HL remains controversial because of the persistent concern of late effects. Thus, modern-day approaches to HL treatment seek to optimize the therapeutic ratio by determining the proper selection of patients who may benefit most from RT and by taking advantage

*Corresponding author, Residency Program Director, Department of Radiation Oncology and Molecular Radiation Sciences, Sidney Kimmel Comprehensive Cancer Center at Johns Hopkins, 401 N. Broadway, Suite 1440, Baltimore, MD

E-mail address: stereza1@jhmi.edu

Radiation Medicine Rounds 3:3 (2012) 367–380.

DOI: 10.5003/2151–4208.3.3.367

of state-of-the-art technology to improve the quality of RT delivered.

■ COMBINED MODALITY THERAPY VERSUS CHEMOTHERAPY ALONE

The role of RT in the treatment of HL is controversial despite evidence supporting that a higher risk of relapse is associated with its omission (1–3). The primary concern with RT is that any impact on overall survival (OS), due to the improvement in progression-free survival (PFS), may be potentially outweighed by the many treatment-related deaths occurring decades after RT from late effects, such as cardiovascular complications and secondary malignancies. Nevertheless, the magnitude of RT's benefit differs by patient based on risk stratification (favorable stage I/II, unfavorable stage I/II, and stage III/IV), bulky disease, or early response to chemotherapy. Furthermore, modern RT uses lower doses and smaller fields, which results in less normal tissue irradiation, and is likely to lower the risk of late effects expected from RT.

Despite the clear benefit conferred by RT in relapse-risk reduction, prospective studies comparing chemotherapy to combined modality therapy using modern chemotherapy regimens and RT techniques and fields have not clearly demonstrated a statistically significant OS advantage (1,4,5), in part due to the high salvage rate in patients who relapse and the development of treatment-related late complications requiring longer follow-up of at least a decade (Table 1).

The European Organization for Research and Treatment of Cancer (EORTC)–Group d'Etude des Lymphomes d'Adulte (GELA) H9-F trial studied early, favorable HL and investigated the reduction or omission of involved-field RT (IFRT) after complete remission to six cycles of epirubicin, bleomycin, vinblastine, and prednisone (EBVP). There were no differences seen between 20 and 36 Gy of radiation on interim analysis (2). Nonetheless, the no-RT arm was closed due to excess relapses identified (2). The 4-year failure-free survival was only 69% with EBVP alone despite patients achieving complete remission, with some researchers suggesting that excess treatment failures may be related to ineffective chemotherapy.

Laskar et al. (6) published a randomized study investigating "modern" chemotherapy that evaluated six cycles of adriamycin (doxorubicin), bleomycin, vinblastine, and dacarbazine (ABVD) chemotherapy with or without RT and demonstrated a survival benefit to RT. Eight-year event-free survival (EFS) and OS in the chemotherapy-alone arm

TABLE 1   Select studies of early stage HL comparing chemoradiation and chemotherapy alone

Study	Cohort	Evaluable Patients	Chemotherapy	Radiation	FFS or EFS	OS
NCIC-ECOG HD6 (1,7)	Nonbulky, IA–IIA	203	None (for low risk) or ABVD × 2	STNI	80% (12 years)	87% (12 years)
		196	ABVD × 4–6	None	85%	94%
EORTC-GELA H9-F, interim analysis (2)	Early favorable I–II, with CR only	239	EBVP × 6	IRFT 36 Gy	88% (4 years)	98% (4 years)
		209	EBVP × 6	IFRT 20 Gy	85%	100%
		130	EBVP × 6	None	69%	98%
Straus et al. (4)	Nonbulky I–II, or nonbulky IIIA	76	ABVD × 6	IFRT or modified EFRT	—	97% (5 years)
		76	ABVD × 6	None	—	90%

ABVD = doxorubicin, bleomycin, vinblastine, dacarbazine; CR = complete response; EBVP = epirubicin, bleomycin, vinblastine, prednisone; EFRT = extended-field radiation therapy; IFRT = involved-field radiation therapy; EFS = event-free survival; EORTC-GELA = European Organization for Research and Treatment of Cancer–Groupe d'Études des Lymphomes de l'Adulte; FFS = failure-free survival; NCIC-ECOG = National Cancer Institute of Canada–Eastern Cooperative Oncology Group; OS = overall survival; STNI = subtotal nodal irradiation.

were 76% and 89%, respectively, compared to 88% and 100% in the combined modality arm (P = .01 and .006, respectively). Unfortunately, this study had some limitations, including short-term follow-up and heterogeneity in stage, disease bulk (15% bulky), mediastinal involvement (72% uninvolved), age (46% younger than age 15 years), and histology (11% lymphocyte-predominant and mostly mixed cellularity).

A randomized study conducted at the Memorial Sloan-Kettering Cancer Center (MSKCC, New York, NY) (4) compared six cycles of ABVD followed by RT versus six cycles of ABVD without RT for nonbulky, mostly limited-stage disease (Table 1). No significant difference in 5-year freedom from progression (FFP) was observed, although the study had significant limitations in that it was powered to detect only a 20% difference. There was a tendency toward better 5-year OS in the RT arm (97% vs 90%; P = .08), although longer follow-up would be required to capture the impact of late effects.

The recently published National Cancer Institute of Canada–Eastern Cooperative Oncology Group HD6 trial (1,7) analyzed patients with non-bulky, stages IA–IIA HL. Patients were randomized to four to six cycles of ABVD alone compared to subtotal nodal irradiation (STNI) with or without two cycles of ABVD, depending on favorable risk factors. With an 11-year median follow-up, there was a trend toward improved 12-year FFP in the RT arm (P = 0.05), but a statistically significantly inferior OS as compared to the no-RT arm (7). In the subgroup of patients with poorer-risk disease, there was significantly improved disease control but inferior OS compared to patients treated with chemotherapy alone. In patients with favorable-risk features, there was no difference in disease control or OS between the two arms. Inferior OS in the RT arm was attributed to deaths from causes other than lymphoma or early toxicity. It is crucial to note that the HD6 trial used much more extensive, nearly antiquated RT than would be routinely delivered today. The routine use of STNI has long been abandoned, particularly in the patient population studied in this trial. STNI is associated with well-known risks of late side effects that accompany extensive RT volumes that are treated with relatively high doses. Thus, this trial does not give us insight into the comparison of chemotherapy alone versus chemoradiation using modern HD radiation techniques, fields, and doses. Importantly, in a separate analysis of treatment failures from the study, there was a significant increased failure rate within

the expected extended-field RT (EFRT) field in the chemotherapy-alone arm (20/23 vs 3/10; P = .002) and within what would have been an IFRT field (16/23 vs 2/10; P = .02). These results highlight the predictable pattern of relapse in chemotherapy-alone patients (8). The trial also reported that in patients treated with ABVD alone, the 5-year FFP was significantly better in those who had achieved a complete response (CR) or unconfirmed CR on computed tomography (CT) after two cycles of ABVD (95% at 5 years vs 81% in those who did not achieve a CR or unconfirmed CR; P = 0.007) (1). This finding suggests that consolidative RT may be most beneficial in the subset of patients who do not achieve an early response to chemotherapy.

It must be emphasized that patients with bulky disease were excluded from these randomized studies of chemotherapy alone. Combined modality therapy remains the standard of care in bulky, limited stage HL. In a randomized study by Aviles et al. (9), patients with bulky early stage HL were randomized to six cycles of ABVD, a combined modality arm involving ABVD with RT, or EFRT alone. After a median follow-up duration of 11.4 years, a significant tumor control and OS advantage to combined modality therapy was seen. Patients on the combined modality arm had an OS of 88% compared to 53% in patients who received RT alone and 59% who received chemotherapy alone.

A recent meta-analysis evaluated unconfounded trials of combined modality therapy compared to chemotherapy alone for early stage HD (3). In this analysis, the impact of RT was assessed among five randomized controlled studies in which the only difference in the arms was the use of RT. The studies included were Mexico B2H031, a study of 201 patients treated with six cycles of ABVD ± RT; Cancer and Leukemia Group B (CALGB) 7751, a study of 37 patients treated with six cycles of CVPP ± RT; EORTC-GELA H9F, a study of 568 patients treated with six cycles of EBVP ± RT (20 and 36 Gy); Argentine Group for Acute Leukemia Treatment (GATLA) 9H77, a study of 277 patients treated with six cycles of CVPP ± RT; and MSKCC 90–44, a study of 152 patients treated with six cycles of ABVD ± RT. In total, 1245 patients made up the cohort and the hazard ratio (HR) demonstrated an improvement in tumor control with the addition of RT to chemotherapy (HR, 0.41; confidence interval [CI], 0.25–0.66) and in OS (HR, 0.4; CI, 0.27–0.61) over chemotherapy alone. However, a weakness in this meta-analysis was the limited follow-up, which averaged approximately 60 months.

In advanced-stage HL, the role of RT is less defined (10–13); however, studies have variably supported and refuted the integration of RT into the treatment of advanced HL. For example, a recently reported retrospective study suggested both a PFS and an OS advantage to consolidative RT for advanced HL, despite the presence of more adverse prognostic features in the irradiated patients (11). A meta-analysis (12) investigating the addition of RT to chemotherapy in patients with stage III/IV disease demonstrated an improvement in PFS of 11% at 10 years (CI, 4%–18%) with the addition of RT. Yet there was no benefit in OS with the addition of RT ($P = .6$). Given the more advanced disease in this second study and the use of larger RT fields (total nodal irradiation and EFRT), it has been hypothesized that in patients with advanced-stage disease, the benefit in PFS from RT may be limited due to late RT toxicities, specifically cardiovascular and secondary malignancies. Thus, the use of RT in patients with advanced disease might be limited to those who present with one or two sites of bulky disease. It is crucial to point out that those patients undergoing Stanford V treatment for stage III/IV disease are required to receive RT to sites of initial bulky disease.

There are clear subsets of patients who benefit from the addition of RT, but more accurate identification of such patients is required to understand how to balance the risks and benefits. The use of interim ^{18}F-fluorodeoxyglucose (FDG) positron emission tomography (PET) to stratify patients based on early response to treatment is the subject of several ongoing trials and may help elucidate which patients may benefit most from RT (Table 2).

■ RESPONSE-BASED THERAPY

The results of ^{18}F-FDG PET, when performed after only two or three cycles of chemotherapy have been shown to be prognostically significant in classical HL whether in the frontline (14–22) or relapsed (23,24) setting. A negative midtreatment PET scan has been associated with favorable outcomes. Although outcomes for HL patients who have a positive midtreatment PET scan are generally worse, they have been quite variable, likely due in part to the small number of PET-positive patients represented in these series. Recently, clinical trials have used end-of-chemotherapy PET to guide whether and which sites to irradiate. For

example, PET performed after completion of bleomycin sulfate, etoposide phosphate, adriamycin, cyclophosphamide, oncovin, procarbazine hydrochloride, and prednisone (BEACOPP) has been used to restrict RT to residually FDG-avid masses, with encouraging outcomes in advanced HL (25,26). In the German Hodgkin Study Group (GHSG) HD18 trial for advanced HL, patients achieving a negative PET after two cycles of escalated BEACOPP do not receive RT (27).

The effectiveness of adding RT to sites of residual PET-positive disease, however, is not fully defined. Unfortunately, tumors that are resistant to chemotherapy, reflected by a positive postchemotherapy PET, are theoretically resistant to radiation (28,29). However, most early stage HL patients with positive postchemotherapy PET scans achieve durable remissions after RT (30), and thus, RT may be the appropriate salvage approach in these instances. In a study by Sher et al. (30), 13 of 73 patients who had completed ABVD chemotherapy to manage their HL had residual PET activity. All 13 patients received RT, and the 2-year FFS was 69%, indicating that most patients can still be cured with RT despite residual PET-positive activity at the completion of chemotherapy.

In early HL, several large, randomized clinical trials are evaluating response-based determination of therapy based on PET performed after 2 or 3 cycles of first-line chemotherapy (31–33). These trials seek to determine when to escalate a patient's therapy and when to omit RT based on a negative interim PET scan. Although this approach may be valid, caution is advised, as it is not yet clear whether the excellent cure rates already achievable in such patients will be maintained with de-escalation of therapy. This principle has already been demonstrated in the EORTC-GELA H10 trial for patients with early favorable or unfavorable HL (31). In this ongoing study, the experimental arm in which patients with negative PET after two cycles of ABVD receive one or two additional cycles of ABVD without RT was closed early due to excess treatment failure. RT has since been added to this arm after ABVD completion.

In the pediatric population, interim PET is being actively used to guide therapy. In the recently completed Children's Oncology Group (COG) AHOD 0031 study, patients received two cycles of ABVE-PC followed by response assessment; patients with rapid early response (RER) received two additional cycles of ABVE-PC followed by a second response assessment. Those with a CR were randomized to 21 Gy IFRT or no further therapy. Patients with an RER who did

TABLE 2 Selected studies that use interim PET to guide radiation treatment

Study	Timing of Interim PET	Treatment	Characteristics
		Interim PET in early stage HL	
RAPID trial (32)	After ABVD × 3	PET–, randomize to RT vs no further therapy	Stage IA or IIA, nonbulky disease
		PET+, further ABVD + IFRT	
GHSG HD16 (33)	After ABVD × 2	Standard arm: IFRT (20 Gy)	Early favorable disease
		Experimental: PET–, no further therapy	
		Experimental: PET+, IFRT (20 Gy)	
EORTC-GELA H10 (31)	After ABVD × 2	Standard arm: complete ABVD + INRT (30 Gy) regardless of interim PET	Favorable and unfavorable, including bulky, HL
		Experimental: PET–, complete ABVD without RT	Arm closed after interim analysis
		Experimental: PET–, complete ABVD + INRT (30 Gy)	New arm since interim analysis
		Experimental: PET+, BEACOPPesc + INRT (30 Gy)	
		Interim PET in advanced HL	
GHSG HD18 (27)	After BEACOPPesc × 2	PET–, randomize to 2 vs 6 more cycles (no RT)	
		PET+, randomize to BEACOPPesc with vs without rituximab	RT restricted to residual PET+ sites >2.5 cm
RATHL, from UK NCRI (75)	After ABVD × 2	PET–, randomize to ABVD vs AVD (no RT)	
		PET+, BEACOPP-14 or BEACOPPesc	RT optional in patients with persistent PET+ disease
		Interim and posttreatment PET to guide RT	
HD0607 for advanced HL, from GITIL (76)	After ABVD × 2	PET–, complete ABVD; if still PET–, randomize to IFRT (30 Gy) vs no RT	RT is to initially bulky and/or residual disease
		PET+, randomize to BEACOPPesc with vs without rituximab	No RT planned
HD0801 (77) for advanced HL, from IIL	After ABVD × 2	PET–, complete ABVD; if still PET–, randomize to IFRT (30 Gy) vs no RT	RT is to initially bulky sites
		PET+, high-dose therapy with autologous SCT	

ABVD = doxorubicin, bleomycin, vinblastine, dacarbazine; PET = positron emission tomography; HL = Hodgkin lymphoma; IFRT = involved-field RT; RAPID = a Randomized Phase III Trial to determine the role of FDG-PET imaging in clinical stages IA/IIA of Hodgkin disease; GHSG = German Hodgkin Study Group; EORTC-GELA = European Organization for Research and Treatment of Cancer–Groupe d'Études des Lymphomes de l'Adulte; BEACOPPesc, bleomycin sulfate, etoposide phosphate, adriamycin, cyclophosphamide, oncovin, procarbazine hydrochloride, prednisone; RATHL, = a randomised phase III trial to assess response adapted therapy using FDG-PET imaging in patients with newly diagnosed advanced Hodgkin lymphoma; NCRI = National Cancer Research Institute; GITIL = Gruppo Italiano Terapie Innovative Nei Linfomi.

Source: Adapted from Ref (78).

not have a CR were all assigned to receive IFRT. Slow early responders (SER) were all randomized to either two additional cycles of ABVE-PC or dexamethasone, etoposide, cisplatin, and cytarabine (DECA) followed by an additional two cycles of ABVE-PC. All SER patients received 21 Gy IFRT after chemotherapy. Three-year EFS rates were 87.1% for RER patients versus 77.8% for SER patients (P = .0001). The 3-year OS rate for RER patients was 98.7% versus 96.9% for SER patients (P = .02). The 3-year EFS rate was 87.9% for RER/CR patients randomized to receive IFRT versus 85.4% for those randomized to no IFRT (P = .07). These results suggest that early response to chemotherapy defined by early reduction (60%) in tumor size based on CT after two cycles can be a powerful predictor of outcome and help optimize subsequent treatment. A secondary analysis of PET response after two cycles of ABVE-PC demonstrated that PET may further assist with treatment optimization (34).

Because the role of interim PET in guiding lymphoma treatment is still under investigation, treatment decisions on this basis in the adult setting are best made in the context of clinical trials. Furthermore, the limitations of PET scanning must be considered, including the risk of false-positives and false-negatives, the uncertainty with regard to the definition of an adequate metabolic response, and issues with the reproducibility and interpretation of the scan (29).

■ RADIATION FIELD SIZE

EFRT, which delivers RT to both involved and uninvolved lymph node regions, is now rarely used for HL. The effectiveness of chemotherapy to address microscopic disease has permitted reduction in the radiation delivered both in terms of field size and dose, without compromise of outcome (35,36) (Figure 1). IFRT, in which the RT field is limited to the site of the clinically involved lymph node group or groups, is now considered standard of care in the context of combined modality therapy (37). The prechemotherapy extent of disease is used for the design of RT fields while taking into account the anatomic displacement of normal structures that may return to their original position after the shrinkage of lymph nodes after chemotherapy. In the mediastinum, the postchemotherapy transverse extent of disease is used to delineate the RT field. In this case, the size of enlarged mediastinal lymph nodes may decrease, allowing normal lung tissue to re-expand in the medial direction. In an effort to spare lung tissue,

the postchemotherapy volume is used to dictate the transverse extent of the RT field (37). In limited cases where patients cannot receive chemotherapy, an EFRT field may be more appropriate than IFRT due to limitations in PET/CT imaging, which may not identify all subclinical disease that would have been addressed by systemic therapy.

IFRT is standard in the context of combined modality treatment regardless of risk category. For instance, in the EORTC-GELA H8U trial randomizing patients with unfavorable HL to four cycles of MOPP/ABV (mechlorethamine, oncovin [vincristine], procarbazine, and prednisone/adriamycin [doxorubicin], bleomycin, vinblastine plus 36 to 40 Gy IFRT or 36 to 40 Gy STNI, no difference was detected with the reduced field size (35). In the GHSG HD8 study, patients with unfavorable features were randomized between the standard arm of two cycles of cyclophosphamide, oncovin (vincristine), procarbazine, and prednisone–ABVD and 30 Gy EFRT (+10 Gy for bulky disease) versus 2 cycles of cyclophosphamide, vincristine, procarbazine, and prednisone–ABVD and 30 Gy IFRT (+10 Gy for bulky disease); there were no significant differences in disease control outcomes (38). Compared with IFRT, however, EFRT had a statistically significant increased rate of nausea (62.5% vs 29.1%, P < .001), pharyngitis (49.1% vs 40.5%, P = .001), leucopenia (49.1 vs 33.3%, P < .001), thrombocytopenia (16.7% vs 5.5%, P < .001), and gastrointestinal toxicity (17.5% and 4.1%, P < .001) without any significant improvement in freedom from treatment failure or OS for the entire cohort because of the efficacy of four cycles of chemotherapy for controlling subclinical disease. In a subgroup analysis of 89 patients who were 60 years old or older, the World Health Organization grades 3 and 4 toxicity was remarkably higher with EFRT compared with IFRT (26.5% vs 8.6%). In particular, secondary cancers, grades 3 and 4 leucopenia and nausea, and grades 1 and 2 esophagitis and pharyngitis were considerably increased in the EFRT arm (39). Lastly, in a meta-analysis evaluating the risk of secondary cancers in randomized controlled studies of patients with HL, there was a significantly higher risk of developing breast cancer after EFRT (odds ratio [OR]= 3.25; P = .04) compared with IFRT (40). This risk is due to the omission of the axillary fields in patients for whom the axilla was uninvolved, resulting in the reduction of a large component of breast dose from the mantle field.

Patients with early stage HL treated with chemotherapy alone have an elevated risk for relapse in the initially involved lymph nodes (1,41). Given the desire to reduce treatment field size, the EORTC-GELA recently introduced the concept of involved-node radiotherapy (INRT), which includes treatment of only the initially involved macroscopic disease. For INRT, it is essential to use all available clinical information, including prechemotherapy and postchemotherapy imaging with CT and ^{18}F-FDG PET scan to define the treatment field according to the original extent of disease. Per EORTC-GELA guidelines, the clinical target volume should include only the site of originally involved lymph nodes identified before chemotherapy (42). In a study of early stage HL, 36% of patients had suspicious lymph nodes on ^{18}F-FDG PET that were occult on CT (43). Therefore, when using an INRT approach, prechemotherapy evaluation with PET is required to help delineate the extent of disease (43). Controversy exists regarding the optimal margins to be used in INRT field design, with groups using different definitions (44–46). The appropriate design of INRT fields is an open question, with North American and European protocols allowing variable designations of the radiation field that INRT should encompass (42,45,46). Therefore, it is important to delineate the INRT field according to the specific protocol being followed.

Studies demonstrating the feasibility of INRT are still limited with short follow-up and small numbers, although early clinical data are emerging. Paumier et al. (47) recently reported the clinical outcomes of 50 HL patients who received INRT per EORTC-GELA guidelines. Nearly all had early stage disease and received six cycles of ABVD. With a median follow-up of 53 months, four relapses (including two in-field) were identified. The EORTC-GELA is now investigating INRT in early favorable and early unfavorable HL (31).

Providing further insight into the potential role for reduced treatment field size, Campbell et al. (45) analyzed the outcomes of 325 patients with limited-stage HL treated with combined modality therapy from 1989 to 2005. EFRT was used until 2006 (39% of patients), IFRT was used between 1996 and 2001 (30% of patients), and treatment fields described as INRT + 5 cm were used from 2001 onward (31% of patients). The INRT fields used in this study were designed with a margin of up to 5 cm, and radiation was delivered using conventional treatment planning. Ninety-five percent of patients received two cycles of chemotherapy. After a median follow-up of 80 months, 12 relapses were identified: 4 after EFRT (3%), 5 after IFRT (5%), and 3 after INRT (3%) (P = 0.9) (45). Although no marginal recurrences were identified in patients who underwent

INRT, the margins for INRT used in this study were tantamount to a reduced IFRT field. INRT as defined by the EORTC-GELA and GHSG uses significantly smaller margins (42,46) and encompasses the initially involved volume with a margin for uncertainty. Conformal RT is also routinely used in the application of INRT as defined by the EORTC. Until further clinical data are obtained, INRT is best performed on a protocol where the radiation field definition is standardized in the context of the risk category and chemotherapy regimen.

Radiation Dose Effects

The data that informs us on the potential for radiation late effects is largely based on studies in which patients who received RT were young and received radiation doses and fields sufficient for cure without the use of chemotherapy. Thus, the radiation fields in these studies were overall more extensive, and the radiation doses higher than is typically used in combined modality regimens in the modern era. Secondary malignancy development and cardiovascular disease are the two most commonly reported late effects that have a significant impact on longevity and quality of life in survivors (48). The most common secondary malignancies in HL survivors include lung cancer, breast cancer (for women), gastrointestinal cancer, and thyroid cancer (49), although rare cancers such as bone sarcoma and mesothelioma have also been reported (50,51). During the last decade, several studies have attempted to quantify the risk for developing cancer based on the radiation dose and the use of chemotherapy, specifically nested case–control studies of HL survivors who developed or did not develop the second malignancy of interest. In a study evaluating the risk of breast cancer, Travis et al. (52) demonstrated that increasing the radiation dose more than 4 Gy to the breast was associated with an increased risk of subsequent breast cancer compared to patients who had not received RT. The relative risk (RR) of developing breast cancer in patients who received RT was 1.8 for doses of 4 to 7 Gy and 8 for doses of 40 to 60 Gy compared to patients who did not receive RT. In a separate study, evaluating the risk of secondary lung cancer, Travis et al. (53) reported an increasing risk with increased radiation doses to the lung of 5 Gy or more. The RR for developing lung cancer was 4.1 for doses of 5 to 15 Gy and 8.6 for doses of 30 Gy or more. In a third study, assessing the risk of secondary gastric cancer, the RR for developing a subsequent gastric cancer was 9.9 when patients received a mean stomach dose of 20 Gy or higher compared to those who received doses less than 11 Gy (54). In an analysis from the Childhood Cancer Survivor Study evaluating the development of secondary thyroid cancers among pediatric cancer survivors, there was a linear relationship when radiation dose was increased to 20 Gy, although the RR of developing thyroid cancer subsequently decreased in doses beyond 20 Gy (55).

Mediastinal RT in combination with cumulative anthracycline dose has been implicated in the etiology of late cardiac sequelae in HL survivors. Cardiomyopathy, coronary artery disease, valvular disease, and pericarditis specifically have been associated with increased RT dose to the heart. In the Childhood Cancer Survivor Study, Mulrooney et al. (56) evaluated cardiac complications among the patients with a minimum follow-up of 10 years and found increased HRs for congestive heart failure (2.2), myocardial infarction (2.4), and valvular disease (3.3) with mean cardiac doses of 15 Gy and higher when compared with patients who did not receive RT. This study also showed that even the lowest anthracycline doses were associated with an increased risk of congestive heart failure, including an HR of 2.4 for doses less than 250 mg/m^2 compared with those not receiving anthracyclines, and an HR of 5.2 for doses of 250 mg/m^2 or higher.

Multiple studies have now suggested that a lower RT dose should translate into a reduction in late effects when used judiciously (48,51,57–59). It has also been demonstrated that a reduction in the volume of normal tissue treated can translate into a reduction in late effects (51). This finding is particularly important because most late effects data are derived from a period when EFRT alone was the primary curative treatment for HL. It is therefore to be expected that the risks of these serious late radiation-related toxicities could be reduced or eliminated by reducing the radiation dose to nontargeted critical structures, such as the heart, thyroid, breasts, and lung.

Radiation Dose

The advent of combined modality therapy has enabled a reduction in radiation field size and radiation dose compared to the era when radiation treatment was used alone for cure. Lower radiation dose delivered to the target results in lower dose delivered to in-field nontargeted normal tissue. Therefore, reduced toxicity would be expected with modern RT

delivered with a combined modality strategy relative to the histolrical treatment paradigm of radiation alone. The recent GHSG HD10 study for patients with favorable-risk stage I/II HL demonstrated that in conjunction with two cycles of ABVD, IFRT delivered to 20 Gy was equivalent to 30 Gy with no significant differences in rates of freedom from treatment failure and OS. In addition, severe acute toxicity (grade 3 or 4) and number of adverse events were greater in patients who received 30 Gy compared to 20 Gy (60). Unfavorable-risk stage I/II patients were evaluated in the GHSG HD11 study, which was a four-arm study comparing two radiation dose levels (20 vs 30 Gy) and two chemotherapy regimens (four cycles of ABVD vs. BEACOPP) (61). Again similar rates of freedom from treatment failure, OS, and PFS were observed with 20 and 30 Gy in patients receiving BEACOPP chemotherapy; however, grades 3 and 4 toxicity rate was reduced with the lower dose of RT from 12% to 5.7%. Furthermore, inferiority of 20 Gy compared to 30 Gy could not be excluded after four cycles of ABVD were used. Thus, radiation dose is contingent upon the chemotherapy regimen used.

Metabolic Imaging for Radiation Planning

^{18}F-FDG PET contributes complementary information to anatomic information derived from CT scans and can aid in delineating anatomic areas at risk in the design of the radiation treatment field (Figure 2). Therefore, PET can be integrated into RT planning and contributes functional information to the design of the tumor volume. The addition of PET can potentially alter the volume should additional suspected sites be identified (62,63).

Multiple studies have now demonstrated that PET/CT treatment planning can affect tumor-volume definition and management in lymphoma patients (43,62–66). For example, Hutchings et al. (62) studied 30 patients with early stage HL who received a staging PET/CT and short-course ABVD followed by RT. The integration of PET information in IFRT planning would have resulted in an increase in the treated volume in seven patients and a decrease in the treated volume in two patients. Pommier et al. (66) performed a prospective multicenter study reporting on the effect of obtaining a pre-RT PET scan in 137 early stage HL patients. Using the information derived from the pre-RT PET scan, RT was cancelled in 4.8% of patients, and the treatment plan was modified in 13%. Overall, the concordance

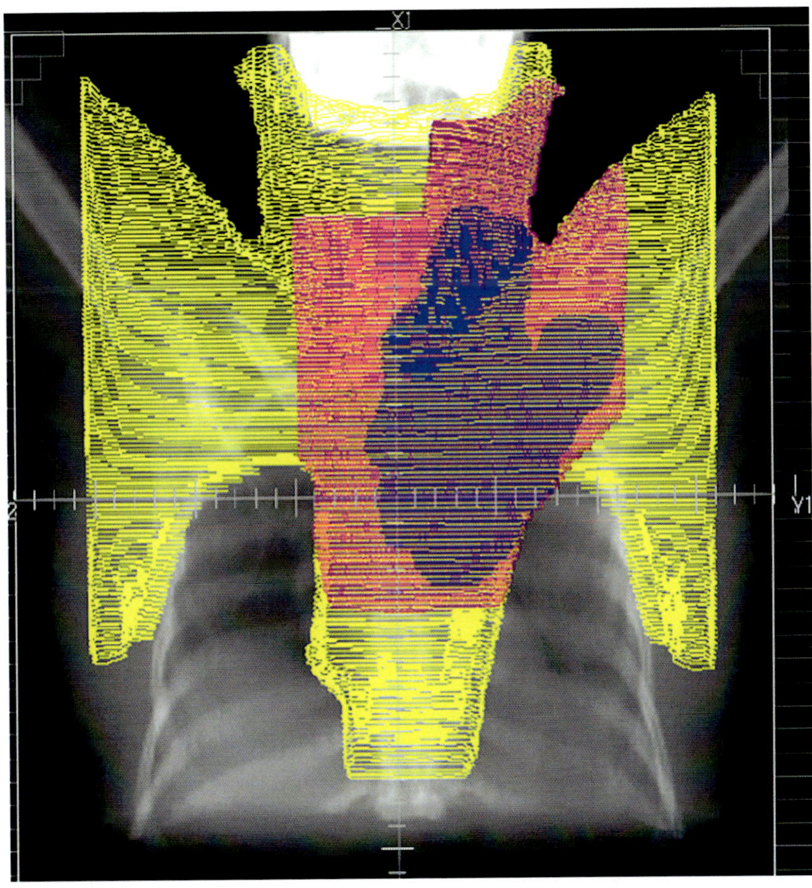

FIGURE 1 Mantle field (extended-field RT) is represented in yellow, IFRT is represented in pink, and involved node field RT is represented in blue.

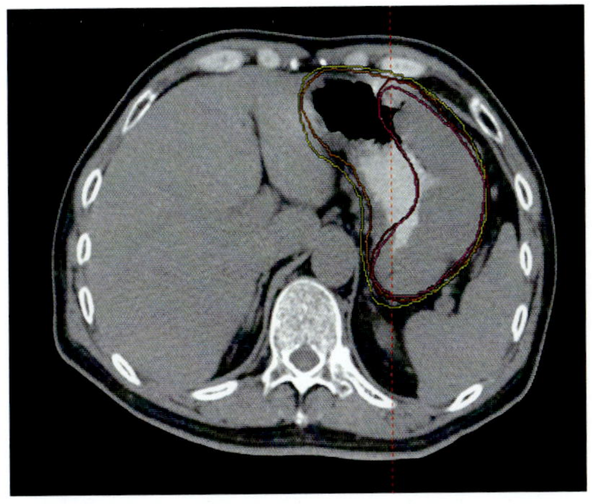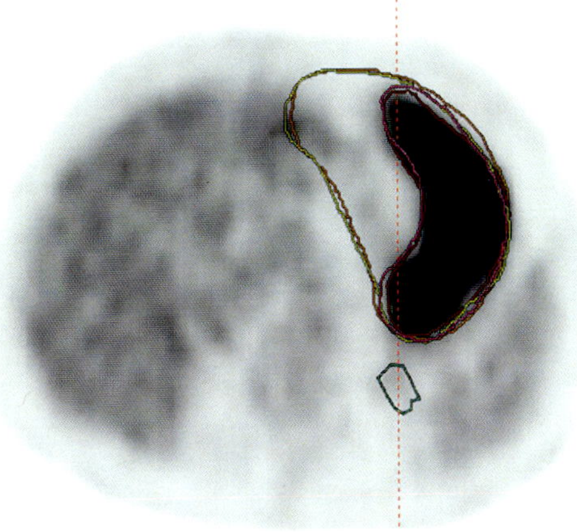

FIGURE 2 Demonstration of the utility of using positron emission tomography (PET) to define the site of gross disease. The pink contour represents the gross tumor volume (GTV) of an extranodal lymphoma clearly depicted on [18]FDG-PET (right), which is otherwise difficult to precisely define using computed tomography (CT) alone (left). The yellow contour represents the stomach.

in treatment strategy with or without pre-RT PET was 82%. Because the use of PET/CT for radiation planning may at times result in an increase in treatment volume, PET for fusion in RT planning must be cautiously applied as concerns for late effects are paramount.

Advanced Radiation Treatment Techniques

Intensity-modulated RT (IMRT) is a sophisticated RT technique that uses multiple radiation beams aimed at a target from different directions, with the beams varying in size, shape, and intensity that create a three-dimensional dose distribution conforming to the target volume. IMRT succeeds in increasing dose conformality to the actual target volume compared to simpler, conventional RT techniques that were historically used in the treatment of HL. However, the dose is "spread out" using IMRT such that a larger volume receives a low dose compared to conventional techniques. Several studies have been published comparing the dose distributions of conventional three-dimensional conformal RT (3DCRT) plans with IMRT in patients with HL. In one of the first studies, investigators compared IMRT with 3DCRT and demonstrated a reduction in mean lung dose by 12% with IMRT (67). In another study by Girinsky and Ghalibafi [63], IMRT could protect the heart and coronary arteries better compared with 3DCRT, but there was additional concern regarding the increased volume of normal tissue receiving "low doses" of RT compared with 3DCRT. More recently, Weber et al. (68) reported that in a nonlinear model for development of secondary malignancies, IMRT increased the risk of breast, lung and thyroid cancers compared with 3DCRT. This modeling predicts increased second cancers because of this redistribution of dose with IMRT that leads to an increased volume of normal tissue receiving low doses of RT relative to 3DCRT techniques. Similarly, a recent study (69) from the GHSG demonstrated reduced dose to the heart and spinal cord using IMRT but increased dose to the lung and breasts compared with 3DCRT.

Clinical studies using modern radiation techniques are only beginning to emerge. Paumier et al. (47) reported on 32 patients treated with an INRT field with IMRT after chemotherapy and demonstrated a 5-year PFS and OS of 92% and 94%, respectively, comparable with standard techniques. Only two patients developed an in-field relapse and only one patient developed grade 3 pneumonitis.

Unlike x-rays, protons are charged particles with mass and travel a finite distance. The actual range of protons in tissue can be controlled, thereby eliminating the "exit" dose to nontargeted tissues. In addition, protons deposit most of their radiation dose in tissue near the end of their range in a striking pattern called the Bragg peak, with relatively little dose deposited along the "entrance" path.

Dosimetric studies evaluating the use of proton therapy (PT) in HL date back to 1974 (70); however, more sophisticated treatment planning studies have since been published. In a prospective phase II study of INRT in patients with mediastinal HL (71), the first 10 patients enrolled underwent treatment planning with 3DCRT (AP/PA), IMRT, and PT plans and were offered treatment with the plan that best spared the organs at risk while maintaining appropriate target coverage. In all 10 cases, PT was associated with the best plan and all patients were offered treatment with PT (Figure 3).

Using modern RT techniques for the treatment of HL, radiation oncologists must balance the risks and benefits of RT modalities. Although secondary cancers are considered the greatest concern in HL survivors that have received RT, heart-related late effects are responsible for more deaths than any other organ-specific malignancy. In a prospective study from the University of Florida (UF; Jacksonville, FL) of 10 patients with HL (71), the mean dose to the heart was 19.4 Gy with 3DCRT, 12.2 Gy with IMRT, and 8.9 Gy (relative biological effectiveness [RBE]) with PT. With PT, the dose was reduced by more than 5 Gy in 9 of 10 patients when compared with 3DCRT and in 4 of 10 patients when compared with IMRT. In a study from M.D. Anderson Cancer Center (Houston, TX), PT similarly reduced the mean heart dose of 10 patients with mediastinal lymphoma (72). In the UF study (71), the mean lung dose was 13.2 Gy for 3DCRT, 10.6 Gy for IMRT, and 7.1 Gy (RBE) for PT. In particular, PT reduced the dose to the lungs by greater than 5 Gy in six patients when compared with 3DCRT and in two patients when compared with IMRT. Similarly, MDACC demonstrated a reduction in mean lung dose by 3.3 Gy with PT compared to 3DCRT (72). Because of the tissue density in the lung, however, the dose might be slightly underestimated for the PT plans.

In the UF study (71), the mean breast dose was not substantially reduced because of the limited treatment field, which resulted in mean breast doses that averaged 5.4 Gy for 3DCRT, 5.5 Gy for IMRT, and 4.6 Gy for PT. However, in two patients with residual bulky disease extending posterior to

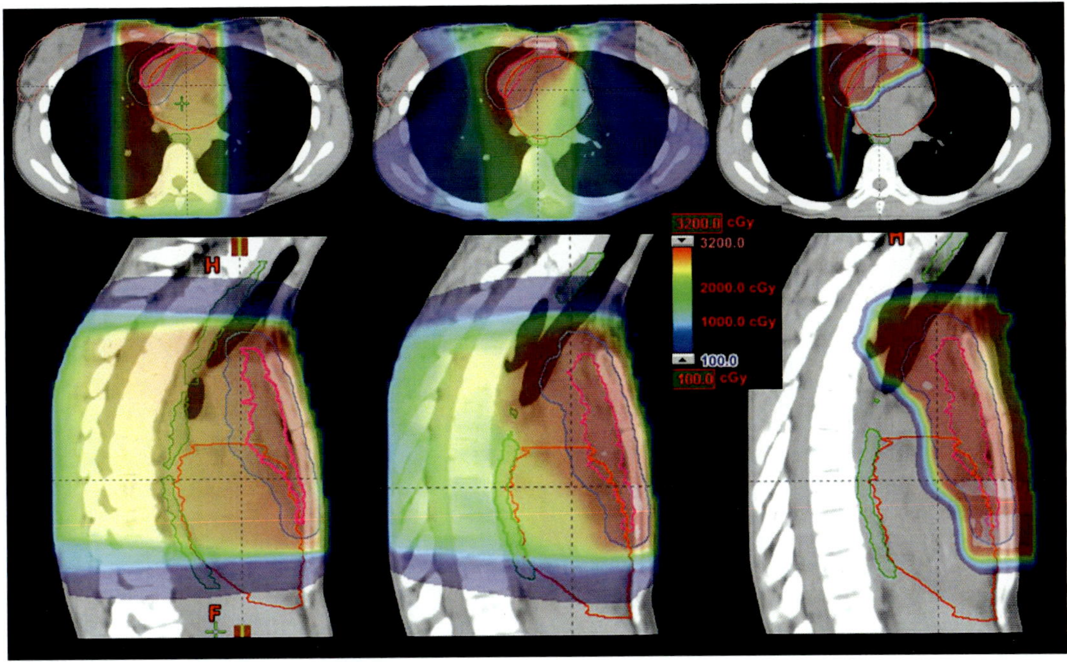

FIGURE 3   Comparison of 3DCRT versus IMRT vs proton RT plans demonstrating representative differences in dose distributions with each technique.

the breast, PT was able to reduce the mean breast dose by more than 5 Gy compared with 3DCRT or IMRT. In a study by Andolino et al. (73), however, PT reduced the mean dose to the breasts when treating mantle fields from 4.7 to 1 Gy compared with 3DCRT. Because this study chose a posterior treatment approach with the beam entering the anterior mediastinum through the posterior chest and heart, the heart received a higher mean dose (17 Gy) with PT compared with 3DCRT (14 Gy), highlighting the occasional trade-off between sparing anterior or posterior structures with central tumors. These trade-offs exist for many cases involving the use of advanced treatment technologies. Using IMRT, one may spare the heart while greater volumes of breast tissue receive a low radiation dose due to the spreading of dose with IMRT.

PT treatment planning is more complex than with x-ray treatment planning. The depth that protons will travel in tissue depends on their energy and the composition of their pathway. Minor variations in daily patient positioning may result in minor variations in the proton path length that must be accounted for in the treatment planning process. Improved treatment planning and delivery systems will reduce this uncertainty and minimize adjustments necessary in the treatment planning process.

Although concerns have been raised about the uncertainty of secondary neutron scatter in patients receiving double-scatter PT, these effects are minimal compared to the reduction in dose relative to x-ray treatment. Clinical experience with current follow-up has not demonstrated an increase in the risk of second malignancy with PT (74).

■ CONCLUSION

RT is an incredibly powerful tool in the treatment of HL. Judicious use of RT is necessary to balance its potential to enhance long-term disease control and survival with its ability to cause long-term toxicities. Factors such as age, female gender, family history of malignancies such as breast cancer or cardiac disease, and smoking history should all be used to individualize the care of the patient when having discussions of the risks and benefits of RT. Similarly, clinical trade-offs exist in the use of different RT techniques, such as IMRT and PT compared to conventional techniques, and one cannot assume that all patients will benefit from the same approach. Ongoing trials focused on risk stratification using response-based approaches have the potential to provide further insight into the development of individually tailored treatment regimens that incorporate RT in the most advantageous manner. Ultimately, further study on the selective integration of RT is needed to optimize the therapeutic ratio.

■ REFERENCES

1. Meyer RM, Gospodarowicz MK, Connors JM, et al. Randomized comparison of ABVD chemotherapy with a strategy that includes radiation therapy in patients with limited-stage Hodgkin's lymphoma: National Cancer Institute of Canada Clinical Trials Group and the Eastern Cooperative Oncology Group. *J Clin Oncol.* 2005;23:4634–4642.

2. Eghbali H, Brice P, Creemers G-Y, et al. Comparison of three radiation dose levels after EBVP regimen in favorable supradiaphragmatic clinical stages (CS) I–II Hodgkin's lymphoma (HL): preliminary results of the EORTC-GELA H9-F trial. *Blood.* 2005;106:Abstract 814.

3. Herbst C, Rehan FA, Skoetz N, et al. Chemotherapy alone versus chemotherapy plus radiotherapy for early stage Hodgkin lymphoma. *Cochrane Database Syst Rev.* 2011;CD007110.

4. Straus DJ, Portlock CS, Qin J, et al. Results of a prospective randomized clinical trial of doxorubicin, bleomycin, vinblastine, and dacarbazine (ABVD) followed by radiation therapy (RT) versus ABVD alone for stages I, II, and IIIA nonbulky Hodgkin disease. *Blood.* 2004;104:3483–3489.

5. Kung FH, Schwartz CL, Ferree CR, *et al.* POG 8625: a randomized trial comparing chemotherapy with chemoradiotherapy for children and adolescents with stages I, IIA, IIIA1 Hodgkin disease: a report from the Children's Oncology Group. *J Pediatr Hematol Oncol.* 2006;28:362–368.

6. Laskar S, Gupta T, Vimal S, et al. Consolidation radiation after complete remission in Hodgkin's disease following six cycles of doxorubicin, bleomycin, vinblastine, and dacarbazine chemotherapy: is there a need? *J Clin Oncol.* 2004;22:62–68.

7. Meyer RM, Gospodarowicz MK, Connors JM, et al. ABVD alone versus radiation-based therapy in limited-stage Hodgkin's lymphoma. *N Engl J Med.* 2012;366:399–408.

8. Macdonald DA, Ding K, Gospodarowicz MK, et al. Patterns of disease progression and outcomes in a randomized trial testing ABVD alone for patients with limited-stage Hodgkin lymphoma. *Ann Oncol.* 2007;18:1680–1684.

9. Aviles A, Delgado S. A prospective clinical trial comparing chemotherapy, radiotherapy and combined therapy in the treatment of early stage Hodgkin's disease with bulky disease. *Clin Lab Haematol.* 1998;20:95–99.

10. Aleman BM, Raemaekers JM, Tirelli U, et al. Involved-field radiotherapy for advanced Hodgkin's lymphoma. *N Engl J Med.* 2003;348:2396–2406.

11. Johnson PW, Sydes MR, Hancock BW, et al. Consolidation radiotherapy in patients with advanced Hodgkin's lymphoma: survival data from the UKLG LY09 randomized controlled trial (ISRCTN97144519). *J Clin Oncol.* 2010;28:3352–3359.

12. Loeffler M, Brosteanu O, Hasenclever D, et al. Meta-analysis of chemotherapy versus combined modality treatment trials in Hodgkin's disease. International Database on Hodgkin's Disease Overview Study Group. *J Clin Oncol.* 1998;16:818–829.

13. Fabian CJ, Mansfield CM, Dahlberg S, et al. Low-dose involved field radiation after chemotherapy in advanced Hodgkin disease. A Southwest Oncology Group randomized study. *Ann Intern Med.* 1994;120:903–912.

14. Friedberg JW, Fischman A, Neuberg D, et al. FDG-PET is superior to gallium scintigraphy in staging and more sensitive in the follow-up of patients with de novo Hodgkin lymphoma: a blinded comparison. *Leuk Lymphoma.* 2004;45:85–92.

15. Gallamini A, Hutchings M, Rigacci L, et al. Early interim 2-[18F]fluoro-2-deoxy-d-glucose positron emission tomography is prognostically superior to international prognostic score in advanced-stage Hodgkin's lymphoma: a report from a joint Italian-Danish study. *J Clin Oncol.* 2007;25:3746–3752.

16. Gallamini A, Rigacci L, Merli F, et al. The predictive value of positron emission tomography scanning performed after two courses of standard therapy on treatment outcome in advanced stage Hodgkin's disease. *Haematologica.* 2006;91:475–481.

17. Hutchings M, Loft A, Hansen M, et al. FDG-PET after two cycles of chemotherapy predicts treatment failure and progression-free survival in Hodgkin lymphoma. *Blood.* 2006;107:52–59.

18. Zinzani PL, Tani M, Fanti S, et al. Early positron emission tomography (PET) restaging: a predictive final response in Hodgkin's disease patients. *Ann Oncol.* 2006;17:1296–1300.

19. Furth C, Steffen IG, Amthauer H, et al. Early and late therapy response assessment with [18F]fluorodeoxyglucose positron emission tomography in pediatric Hodgkin's lymphoma: analysis of a prospective multicenter trial. *J Clin Oncol.* 2009;27:4385–4391.

20. Cerci JJ, Pracchia LF, Linardi CC, et al. 18F-FDG PET after 2 cycles of ABVD predicts event-free survival in early and advanced Hodgkin lymphoma. *J Nucl Med.* 2010;51:1337–1343.

21. Straus DJ, Johnson JL, LaCasce AS, et al. Doxorubicin, vinblastine, and gemcitabine (CALGB 50203) for stage I/II nonbulky Hodgkin lymphoma: pretreatment prognostic factors and interim PET. *Blood.* 2011;117:5314–5320.

22. Hutchings M, Mikhaeel NG, Fields PA, et al. Prognostic value of interim FDG-PET after two or three cycles of chemotherapy in Hodgkin lymphoma. *Ann Oncol.* 2005;16:1160–1168.

23. Moskowitz CH, Yahalom J, Zelenetz AD, et al. High-dose chemo-radiotherapy for relapsed or refractory Hodgkin

lymphoma and the significance of pre-transplant functional imaging. *Br J Haematol.* 2010;148:890–897.

24. Jabbour E, Hosing C, Ayers G, et al. Pretransplant positive positron emission tomography/gallium scans predict poor outcome in patients with recurrent/refractory Hodgkin lymphoma. *Cancer.* 2007;109:2481–2489.

25. Kobe C, Dietlein M, Franklin J, et al. Positron emission tomography has a high negative predictive value for progression or early relapse for patients with residual disease after first-line chemotherapy in advanced-stage Hodgkin lymphoma. *Blood.* 2008;112:3989–3994.

26. Engert A, Haverkamp H, Kobe C, et al. Reduced intensity of chemotherapy and PET-guided radiotherapy in patients with advanced stage Hodgkin lymphoma: the GHSG HD15 final results. *Blood.* 2011;118:Abstract 589.

27. ClinicalTrials.gov. *HD18 for advanced stages in Hodgkins lymphoma.* Available at: http://www.clinicaltrials.gov/ct2/show/NCT00515554. Accessed July 1, 2010.

28. Kasamon YL, Jones RJ, Wahl RL. Integrating PET and PET/CT into the risk-adapted therapy of lymphoma. *J Nucl Med.* 2007;48:19S–27S.

29. Kasamon YL. Prognostication and risk-adapted therapy of Hodgkin's lymphoma using positron emission tomography. *Adv Hematol.* 2011;2011:271595.

30. Sher DJ, Mauch PM, Van Den Abbeele A, et al. Prognostic significance of mid- and post-ABVD PET imaging in Hodgkin's lymphoma: the importance of involved-field radiotherapy. *Ann Oncol.* 2009;20:1848–1853.

31. ClinicalTrials.gov. *Fludeoxyglucose F 18 PET scan-guided therapy or standard therapy in treating patients with previously untreated stage I or stage II Hodgkin's lymphoma.* Available at: http://www.clinicaltrials.gov/ct2/show/NCT00433433. Accessed August 1, 2011.

32. ClinicalTrials.gov. *PET scan in planning treatment in patients undergoing combination chemotherapy for stage IA or stage IIA Hodgkin lymphoma.* Available at: http://www.clinicaltrials.gov/ct2/show/NCT00943423. Accessed July 1, 2010.

33. ClinicalTrials.gov. *HD16 for early stage Hodgkin lymphoma.* Available at: http://www.clinicaltrials.gov/ct2/show/NCT00736320. Accessed July 1, 2010.

34. Friedman DL, Wolden S, Constine L, et al. AHOD0031: a phase III study of dose-intensive therapy for intermediate risk Hodgkin lymphoma: A report from the Children's Oncology GroupClinically Relevant Abstract 53rd ASH Annual Meeting and Exposition. Vol 766. Orange County Convention Center: American Society of Hematology; 2010.

35. Ferme C, Eghbali H, Meerwaldt JH, et al. Chemotherapy plus involved-field radiation in early-stage Hodgkin's disease. *N Engl J Med.* 2007;357:1916–1927.

36. Bonadonna G, Bonfante V, Viviani S, et al. ABVD plus subtotal nodal versus involved-field radiotherapy in early-stage Hodgkin's disease: long-term results. *J Clin Oncol.* 2004;22:2835–2841.

37. Yahalom J, Mauch P. The involved field is back: issues in delineating the radiation field in Hodgkin's disease. *Ann Oncol.* 2002;13:79–83.

38. Engert A, Schiller P, Josting A, et al. Involved-field radiotherapy is equally effective and less toxic compared with extended-field radiotherapy after four cycles of chemotherapy in patients with early-stage unfavorable Hodgkin's lymphoma: results of the HD8 trial of the German Hodgkin's Lymphoma Study Group. *J Clin Oncol.* 2003;21:3601–3608.

39. Klimm B, Eich HT, Haverkamp H, et al. Poorer outcome of elderly patients treated with extended-field radiotherapy compared with involved-field radiotherapy after chemotherapy for Hodgkin's lymphoma: an analysis from the German Hodgkin Study Group. *Ann Oncol.* 2007;18:357–363.

40. Franklin J, Pluetschow A, Paus M, et al. Second malignancy risk associated with treatment of Hodgkin's lymphoma: meta-analysis of the randomised trials. *Ann Oncol.* 2006;17:1749–1760.

41. Shahidi M, Kamangari N, Ashley S, et al. Site of relapse after chemotherapy alone for stage I and II Hodgkin's disease. *Radiother Oncol.* 2006;78:1–5.

42. Girinsky T, van der Maazen R, Specht L, et al. Involved-node radiotherapy (INRT) in patients with early Hodgkin lymphoma: concepts and guidelines. *Radiother Oncol.* 2006;79:270–277.

43. Girinsky T, Ghalibafian M, Bonniaud G, et al. Is FDG-PET scan in patients with early stage Hodgkin lymphoma of any value in the implementation of the involved-node radiotherapy concept and dose painting? *Radiother Oncol.* 2007;85:178–186.

44. Girinsky T, Specht L, Ghalibafian M, et al. The conundrum of Hodgkin lymphoma nodes: to be or not to be included in the involved node radiation fields. The EORTC-GELA lymphoma group guidelines. *Radiother Oncol.* 2008;88:202–210.

45. Campbell BA, Voss N, Pickles T, et al. Involved-nodal radiation therapy as a component of combination therapy for limited-stage Hodgkin's lymphoma: a question of field size. *J Clin Oncol.* 2008;26:5170–5174.

46. Eich HT, Muller RP, Engenhart-Cabillic R, et al. Involved-node radiotherapy in early-stage Hodgkin's lymphoma. Definition and guidelines of the German Hodgkin Study Group (GHSG). *Strahlenther Onkol.* 2008;184:406–410.

47. Paumier A, Ghalibafian M, Beaudre A, et al. Involved-node radiotherapy and modern radiation treatment techniques in patients with Hodgkin lymphoma. *Int J Radiat Oncol Biol Phys.* 2011;80:199–205.

48. Ng AK, Bernardo MP, Weller E, et al. Long-term survival and competing causes of death in patients with early-stage Hodgkin's disease treated at age 50 or younger. *J Clin Oncol.* 2002;20:2101–2108.

49. Hodgson DC, Gilbert ES, Dores GM, et al. Long-term solid cancer risk among 5-year survivors of Hodgkin's lymphoma. *J Clin Oncol.* 2007;25:1489–1497.

50. Smith J. Postradiation sarcoma of bone in Hodgkin disease. *Skeletal Radiol.* 1987;16:524–532.

51. De Bruin ML, Burgers JA, Baas P, et al. Malignant mesothelioma after radiation treatment for Hodgkin lymphoma. *Blood.* 2009;113:3679–3681.

52. Travis LB, Hill DA, Dores GM, et al. Breast cancer following radiotherapy and chemotherapy among young women with Hodgkin disease. *JAMA.* 2003;290:465–475.

53. Travis LB, Gospodarowicz M, Curtis RE, et al. Lung cancer following chemotherapy and radiotherapy for Hodgkin's disease. *J Natl Cancer Inst.* 2002;94:182–192.

54. van den Belt-Dusebout AW, Aleman BM, Besseling G, et al. Roles of radiation dose and chemotherapy in the etiology of stomach cancer as a second malignancy. *Int J Radiat Oncol Biol Phys.* 2009;75:1420–1429.

55. Bhatti P, Veiga LH, Ronckers CM, et al. Risk of second primary thyroid cancer after radiotherapy for a childhood cancer in a large cohort study: an update from the childhood cancer survivor study. *Radiat Res.* 2010;174:741–752.

56. Mulrooney DA, Yeazel MW, Kawashima T, et al. Cardiac outcomes in a cohort of adult survivors of childhood and adolescent cancer: retrospective analysis of the Childhood Cancer Survivor Study cohort. *BMJ.* 2009;339:b4606.

57. Travis LB, Rabkin CS, Brown LM, et al. Cancer survivorship—genetic susceptibility and second primary cancers: research strategies and recommendations. *J Natl Cancer Inst.* 2006;98:15–25.

58. Arakelyan N, Jais JP, Delwail V, et al. Reduced versus full doses of irradiation after 3 cycles of combined doxorubicin, bleomycin, vinblastine, and dacarbazine in early stage Hodgkin lymphomas: results of a randomized trial. *Cancer.* 2010;116:4054–4062.

59. van Leeuwen FE, Klokman WJ, Stovall M, et al. Roles of radiation dose, chemotherapy, and hormonal factors in breast cancer following Hodgkin's disease. *J Natl Cancer Inst.* 2003;95:971–980.

60. Engert A, Plutschow A, Eich HT, et al. Reduced treatment intensity in patients with early-stage Hodgkin's lymphoma. *N Engl J Med.* 2010;363:640–652.

61. Eich HT, Diehl V, Gorgen H, et al. Intensified chemotherapy and dose-reduced involved-field radiotherapy in patients with early unfavorable Hodgkin's lymphoma: final analysis of the German Hodgkin Study Group HD11 trial. *J Clin Oncol.* 2010;28:4199–4206.

62. Hutchings M, Loft A, Hansen M, et al. Clinical impact of FDG-PET/CT in the planning of radiotherapy for early-stage Hodgkin lymphoma. *Eur J Haematol.* 2007;78:206–212.

63. Girinsky T, Ghalibafian M. Radiotherapy of hodgkin lymphoma: indications, new fields, and techniques. *Semin Radiat Oncol.* 2007;17:206–222.

64. Terezakis SA, Hunt MA, Kowalski A, et al. [(1)F]FDG-positron emission tomography coregistration with computed tomography scans for radiation treatment planning of lymphoma and hematologic malignancies. *Int J Radiat Oncol Biol Phys.* 2011;81:615–622.

65. Lee YK, Cook G, Flower MA, et al. Addition of 18F-FDG-PET scans to radiotherapy planning of thoracic lymphoma. *Radiother Oncol.* 2004;73:277–283.

66. Pommier P, Dussart S, Girinsky T, et al. Impact of 18F-fluoro-2-deoxyglucose positron emission tomography on treatment strategy and radiotherapy planning for stage I-II Hodgkin disease: a prospective multicenter study. *Int J Radiat Oncol Biol Phys.* 2011;79:823–828.

67. Goodman KA, Toner S, Hunt M, et al. Intensity-modulated radiotherapy for lymphoma involving the mediastinum. *Int J Radiat Oncol Biol Phys.* 2005;62:198–206.

68. Weber DC, Johanson S, Peguret N, et al. Predicted risk of radiation-induced cancers after involved field and involved node radiotherapy with or without intensity modulation for early-stage Hodgkin lymphoma in female patients. *Int J Radiat Oncol Biol Phys.* 2011;81:490–497.

69. Koeck J, Abo-Madyan Y, Lohr F, et al. Radiotherapy for early mediastinal Hodgkin lymphoma according to the German Hodgkin Study Group (GHSG): the roles of intensity-modulated radiotherapy and involved-node radiotherapy. *Int J Radiat Oncol Biol Phys.* 2012;83:268–276.

70. Archambeau JO, Bennett GW, Levine GS, et al. Proton radiation therapy. *Radiology.* 1974;110:445–457.

71. Hoppe BS, Flampouri S, Su Z, et al. Consolidative involved-node proton therapy for stage IA–IIIB mediastinal Hodgkin lymphoma: preliminary dosimetric outcomes from a phase II study. *Int J Radiat Oncol Biol Phys.* 2012;83:260–267

72. Li J, Dabaja B, Reed V, et al. Rationale for and preliminary results of proton beam therapy for mediastinal lymphoma. *Int J Radiat Oncol Biol Phys.* 2011;81:167–174.

73. Andolino DL, Hoene T, Xiao L, et al. Dosimetric comparison of involved-field three-dimensional conformal photon radiotherapy and breast-sparing proton therapy for the treatment of Hodgkin's lymphoma in female pediatric patients. *Int J Radiat Oncol Biol Phys.* 2011;81:e667–671.

74. Chung CS, Keating N, Yock T, et al. Comparative analysis of second malignancy risk in patients treated with proton therapy versus conventional photon therapy. *Int J Radiat Oncol Biol Phys.* 2008;72:S8.

75. ClinicalTrials.gov. *Fludeoxyglucose F 18-PET/CT imaging in assessing response to chemotherapy in patients with newly diagnosed stage II, stage III, or stage IV Hodgkin lymphoma.* Available at: http://www.clinicaltrials.gov/ct2/show/NCT00678327. Accessed July 1, 2010.

76. ClinicalTrials.gov. *Positron emission tomography (PET)–adapted chemotherapy in advanced Hodgkin lymphoma (HL) (HD0607).* Available at: http://www.clinicaltrials.gov/ct2/show/NCT00795613. Accessed on July 1, 2010.

77. ClinicalTrials.gov. *High-dose chemotherapy and stem cell transplantation, in patients PET-2 positive, after 2 courses of ABVD and comparison of RT versus no RT in PET-2 negative patients (HD0801).* Available at: http://www.clinical-trials.gov/ct2/show/NCT00784537. Accessed on July 1, 2010.

78. Kasamon YL. Prognostication and risk-adapted therapy of Hodgkin's lymphoma using positron emission tomography. *Adv Hematol.* 2011;2011:271595.

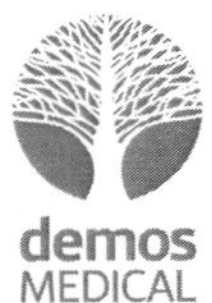

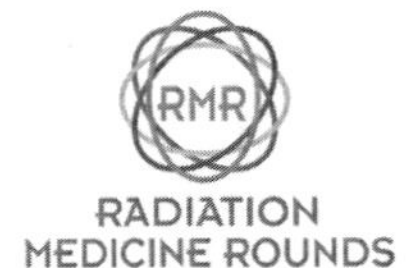

Diffuse Large B-Cell Lymphoma: Nodal and Extranodal Including Primary Mediastinal Lymphoma

Bouthaina S. Dabaja*

The University of Texas MD Anderson Cancer, Houston, TX

■ ABSTRACT

Aggressive B-cell lymphoma, as defined by the 2008 World Health Organization (WHO) classification, is a complex group (1). Major advances that have occurred in the past two decades in the ability to diagnose the different histopathologic subtypes will address the implication of immunohistochemistry, morphologic, cytogenetic, and clinical presentation and will show how they helped to stratify patients into different risk groups. We will discuss the different treatment modalities including different chemotherapy regimens. We will also address the incorporation of the imaging advance namely PET/CT in the treatment decision. The role of radiation therapy as a consolidation and the literature to support it will be discussed.

Keywords: diffuse large cell lymphoma, large cell, primary mediastinal lymphoma, radiation, non-Hodgkin lymphoma, aggressive lymphoma

■ INTRODUCTION

The treatment of diffuse large B-cell lymphoma (DLBCL) has to take into consideration the complexity of the disease and the prognostic factors represented by clinical, pathological, laboratory, and cytogenetic features. For each patient, once these factors are determined, then, the type, number of cycles, and intensity of chemotherapy as well as the need for consolidation radiation therapy will be recommended. Series of studies performed defined our current knowledge about the risk model and treatment strategy regarding chemotherapy and radiation will be addressed.

■ PATHOLOGY AND DIAGNOSIS

DLBCL is a heterogenous disease with a variable clinical presentation. Its variability is tightly related to the immune-phenotyping, cytogenetic features, and site of presentation, which subsequently determine the clinical outcome, response to therapy and survival. Aggressive presentation is characterized by a short clinical presentation and the association with the following factors: (a) B symptoms including fever (temperature >38ºC), drenching night sweats, and/or unexplained loss of more than 10% of body weight within 6 months preceding diagnosis; (b) low performance status; (c) advanced stage III/ IV; (d) bulky disease; (e) above normal level of LDH. The International Prognostic Index (IPI) developed as a method to predict survival and tailor therapy in patients with aggressive non-Hodgkin's

*Corresponding author, The University of Texas MD Anderson Cancer Center, 1515 Holcombe Boulevard, Houston, TX

E-mail address: ccpinnix@mdanderson.org

Radiation Medicine Rounds 3:3 (2012) 381–392.

DOI: 10.5003/2151–4208.3.3.381

TABLE 1 International Prognostic Index

Adverse factor	Risk group	Number of factors	5 year DFS (%)	5 year OS (%)
Age >60 years	Low	0–1	70	73
PS ≥ 2	Low/Intermediate	2	50	51
LDH > normal	High/Intermediate	3	49	43
Extranodal sites ≥2	High	4–5	40	26
Stage III–IV				

lymphoma (Table 1). The model included stage, age, LDH level, performance status, and extranodal involvement. IPI score predicted disease-free survival and overall survival based on four prognostic groups (2).

Recently, stage and IPI were considered insufficient to predict outcome of patients with DLBCL. To further understand the complexity and variability of the clinical outcome, studies focused on pathways of transformation and molecular alterations as a way to further sub classify these tumors into more relevant subgroups. Three venues are worth mentioning:

1. Gene-expression profile (GEP) showing that there are three major groups of DLBCL, Germinal center B cells associated with a better outcome compared to activated B cells with poorer outcome, although not confirmed yet in the Rituximab era, the third subtype includes primary mediastinal lymphoma (PML) or entities that can not be included in either. Germinal center B-cell-like subtype is derived from germinal center B-cells and maintains the GCB differentiation program, while the ABC subtype arises from the B-cells that are arrested in their differentiation towards plasma cells. Furthermore, patients in the GCB subgroup had significantly better survival than patients in the ABC subgroup (3–7)
2. Immunohistochemical profiles proposed as surrogates of the GEP, the classic Hans algorithm uses BCL6, CD10, and MUM 1/IRF4. In recent studies, the correlation with GEP was variable (8,9). Ideally GCB are CD10+, BCL6+, IRF4/MUM1–, whereas non-GCB are CD10– BCL6—with variability in MUM1
3. Morphologic features, immunoblastic has more ABC profile, whereas centroblastic has more GCB profile. However, since it is not a reproducible method it has a limited diagnostic value.

In conclusion, the typical immunophenotyping is CD20+, CD45+, CD3–; the panel, however, should include CD10, CD5, BCL2, BCL6, and IRF4/

MUM1. Other markers include CD138 (to rule out plasmacytic origin), cyclin D1 to rule out mantle cell lymphoma, and ALK1 to rule out anaplastic origin.

A direct application of how important it is to get an immunophenotyping is the recognition of Double hit lymphoma as a new entity associated with an aggressive B cell with MYC breakpoint, located at chromosome band 8q24. Encoding for a variety of cellular processes can occur in 7% to 10% of DLBCL, and associated with an adverse prognosis, when associated with IGH-BCL-2 called "double hit lymphoma," which has a poor outcome with a high proliferation index (average 80%) (10).

Etiology of Diffuse Large Cell Lymphoma

Many risk factors have been implicated in the etiology, most commonly:

1. HIV infection causing low CD4 counts is associated with systemic non-Hodgkin's lymphomas with the most frequent being DLBCL. In recent years there has been a decline in the risk of DLBCL with use of highly active antiretroviral therapy (11–14)
2. Although the major determinant genetic risk of lymphomas is unknown, some work suggested an inherited genetic variation in patients with DLBCL suggesting a genetic risk factor (15). In particular, a combination of polymorphisms in four genes was found including IL A, IL 8RB, IL4R, and tumor necrosis factor
3. Host exposure to long-term immunosuppression therapy leads to lympho-proliferative disorders, the use of methotrexate for autoimmune disease, infliximab for patients with Crohn's disease, or Interferon alpha antagonists has been described to increase the risk of a variety of lymphomas, in particular methotrexate use was linked to DLBCL (16)
4. Inflammatory microenvironment includes abnormal accumulation of cells and or growth -promoting cytokines. IL 6 is a cytokine associated with

inflammation and poorer prognosis in NHL (17). Two separate gene expression signatures derived from nonmalignant cells named stromal 1 and 2 were associated in survival with better outcome for stromal 1 while poor outcome for stromal 2

■ CLINICAL PRESENTATION AND WORKUP

Age at presentation is 6th decade, with the one-third of the patients presenting with stage I/ II. There is slight male-to-female predilection: one-third presents with bulky disease (>10 cm), and 40% extranodal sites are more common, and up to 20% presents with bone marrow involvement (18). The staging workup will help to determine all sites of disease and the IPI score. Blood work with CBC, platelets, LDH, kidney and liver function tests, b2 microglobulin, unilateral bone marrow aspirate and biopsy. Lumbar puncture is indicated in patients with one or more of the following sites: paranasal sinus, testicular, epidural, or bone marrow involvement, it also indicated with patients presenting with presenting with more than two extranodal sites or HIV associated lymphoma. Diagnostic contrast enhanced CT of the neck, chest, abdomen, and pelvis, and PET CT is now recognized as a standard staging workup.

Use of PET scan in staging FDG–PET uses a target glucose metabolism. Combined with CT, it has become an important tool in pretreatment staging of patients. Nevertheless the frequency with which the stage is changed with PET compared to CT is low and the likelihood of a change in treatment even lower with no data to support an improvement in outcome (19,20).

CECT is still considered the standard of care in addition to PET CT for staging workup. It is worth a reminder that the Ann Arbor staging as of now is CT based.

Treatment Approach

Determining the stage, IPI score (that include the stage), presence of B symptoms, and bulk of the disease is essential to determine therapy. Recently, gene expression profile and immunohistochemistry are taken into consideration.

The use of CHOP (cyclophosphamide, Adriamycin, vincristine, and prednisone) was determined as the standard of care based on a randomized study comparing different regimens and CHOP was less toxic and equally effective (21). Coiffier et al. showed that adding Rituximab in elderly patients >60 years of age provided a statistically significant increase in the relapse-free survival and overall survival compared to patients treated with CHOP alone (22). Eventually, the results were reinforced in patients less than 60 years of age in the Mabthera International Trial randomizing patients to 6 cycles of CHOP-like therapy with and without Rituximab and with a follow up of 3 years the event-free survival rates as well the overall survival rates were significantly in favor of the Rituximab arm (23).

Although RCHOP has been established as the standard of care, there are three regimens that are worth mentioning and that can be considered in patients considered to have aggressive disease.

1. DA-EPOCH: The National Cancer Institute developed a regimen based on the concept of overcoming drug resistance by exposing the cells to continuous low dose drug exposure. Dose-adjusted EPOCH regimen contains doxorubicin, vincristine, and etoposide all infused over 96 hours and adjusted based on neutrophil nadir, while etoposide and cyclophosphamide are administered on a bolus schedule. Sixtynine patients with stages II–IV DLBCL received DA-EPOCH-R; CR rate was 84%. With a median follow up of 5 years, the event-free survival and overall survival was 75% and 84%, respectively. The time to treatment progression specifically in high IPI scores was 54%. Seven percent developed grade 4 hematological toxicity and 14% developed neuropathy. The conclusion was that this regimen provides a durable remission and that head-to-head comparison with RCHOP is needed (24).

2. ACVBP regimen (adriamycin, cyclophosphamide, vindesine, bleomycin, and prednisone) that includes CNS prophylaxis and was compared to 8 CHOP in a randomized trial conducted by the GELA group (25,26). In the said regimen, 635 patients were eligible, while both regimen were equivalent with a rate of complete remission at 58% in ACVBP group and 56% in the CHOP group (P =.05), ACVBP had a higher treatment-related death (13%) compared to 7% for CHOP. At 5years, the overall survival rate was in favor of ACVBP (46% vs. 38%; P = .036). This trial was repeated in low intermediate risk IPI score patients and published in 2011. This

time, adding Rituximab to both arms, RACVBP had a better progression-free survival and overall survival (87% and 92% compared to 73% and 84%, respectively, for RCHOP) but serious side events were substantially higher with RACVBP (27) (42% vs. 15%).

3. CHOP given at a different schedule: the German high-grade NHL study group compare CHOP 14 to CHOP 21 and CHOEP 14 to CHOEP 21. In both patients less than 60 and >60 there was a benefit for the 14-day schedule for OS (85% and 53%; P =.004; vs. 58% and 41% $P <$ .001). No benefit was seen for the addition of etoposide for the older group, and only a benefit in the progression-free survival was observed for patients less than 60 years of age (28,29). In a recently reported phase III trial study on 1080 patients treated with Rituximab added, mostly stage III/ IV (63%: 62%, B symptoms 44%, bulky disease 51%: 48%). The overall survival as reported in the ASCO meeting 2011 was not significant between the two arms, no cohort showed a benefit when death, relapse or progression were examined.

Treatment of Limited Stages I and II

The number of cycles of chemotherapy and the addition of consolidation in limited stage is the subject of debate. The common practice is to add radiation when using an abbreviated course of three to four cycles of RCHOP for patients with low risk IPI disease. With the emerging knowledge (as discussed above) that IPI score is not enough to predict the risks of failure, this approach has to be used with caution.

To date, there are four randomized trials, all of them were conducted in the pre-Rituximab era and tried to address the issue of radiation (Table 2). On the other hand in the Rituximab era, most studies are retrospective in design.

The four trials can be summarized as follows:

1. The Southwest Oncology Group (SWOG) 8736 (30) trial published originally in 1998, in 401 patients with intermediate or high grade stage I (bulky), nonbulky stage II and II E (only one extranodal site was allowed), 75% had diffuse large B cell other subtypes included diffuse small cleaved, mixed small and large, and small non cleaved. The study compared three cycles of CHOP+ radiation (dose of 4000 cGy to 5500 cGy) to eight cycles of CHOP. Radiation with three CHOP significantly improved the progression-free survival (77% vs. 64%; P = .03) and overall survival (82% vs. 72%; P = .02). Progression-free survival was higher for patients with 0 or 1 IPI score compared to those with 3 risk factors (77% vs. 34%). There were more life-threatening events including ventricular dysfunction and

TABLE 2 Different regimens of chemotherapy results from trials

Chemotherapy regimen/ trial/year of publication	ACVBP compared to 8 CHOP/ GELA/2003	ACVBP compared to 8 RCHOP/ LNH03–2B/2011	DA-REPOCH/ NCI/phase II	CHOP14 compared to CHOP21±VR16 / DSHNHLB2/2004	CHOP14 compared to CHOP21±VR16/ DSHNHL/2004
Number of patients/risk group	635/at least one risk factor (poor risk)	380/age adjusted IPI, 92%–96% = IPI 1, majority non bulky	69/stage II–IV	689 and older than 60	710/younger than 61 years
Outcome	5-year OS: 46% vs. 38% in favor of ACVBP	3-year OS 92% vs. 84% in favor of ACVBP	84% low IPI, 54% for high IPI score	5-year OS 53% vs. 40% and 58% vs. 41% in favor of 14	CHOP14(+-VP16) improved OS in multivariate analysis
Treatment related death/side effects	13% vs.7% in favor of CHOP	Grade 2–4 toxicity 38% vs. 9% in favor of RCHOP		Infection and mucositis 24% and 14% CHOEP 14 compared to 8 and 0% CHOP21	Infection and mucositis 6.9% and 5.2% CHOEP 14 compared to 2.9 and 1.8% CHOP21; 20 second malignancies not correlated with any regimen

cardiac deaths. In patient's receiving eight cycles of CHOP, 40% had had life-threatening toxic effects in the CHOP-alone arm compared to 30% in the CHOP RT arm (7 CHF in the CHOP alone versus none in the CHOP RT). Updated results in an abstract form showed that OS curves cross at 9 years and FFS curves cross at 7 years with 15 relapses and deaths due to lymphoma in the IFRT arm between 5 and 10 years compared to 8 in chemotherapy-alone arm. The OS for stage modified IPI favorable group with no adverse factors was 94% dropping to 71% for 1 risk factor and 50% for 3 adverse risk factors. The authors concluded that a more intense regimen of chemotherapy given to patients with worse adverse factors may be optimal to overcome the late relapses occurring in the abbreviated chemotherapy arm (31). One can also conclude that radiation cannot compensate for inadequate chemotherapy, therefore, patients who are selected for abbreviated chemotherapy has to be chosen very carefully in terms of risk factors and not based on the fact that they are getting radiation afterwards.

2. Using eight cycles of CHOP, ECOG (32) compared the outcome with and without radiation, this time with less favorable group stage I bulky with mediastinal and retroperitoneal disease and more than 2/3 of the study population had stage II disease and almost half with extranodal involvement (166/352). Patients who achieved CR were randomly assigned to 30 Gy or observation whereas those with PR received 40 Gy. At 6 years the DFS was significantly greater for CR patients who received RT (73% vs. 56%; *P* = .05). In the as-treated analysis, the 6 year FFS was 75% for RT and 56% for observation. The TTP estimates for RT and observed patients at 5, 10, and 15 years were 82%, 78%, and 78%, compared with 71%, 67%, and 64%, respectively. Although not significant, the OS tend to be better for those who received RT in the as-treated analysis. At 5, 10, and 15 years, the estimated OS rates were 87%, 68%, and 60% for CR patients consolidated with RT, versus 73%, 65%, and 44% for CR patients who were observed (two-sided *P* = .24). Among the 215 CR patients, 26% of observation patients and 18% of RT patients died with progressive disease (*P* = .15). In the as-treated population, treatment failed in 17 RT patients and 31 observed patients. Only three patients treated with RT progressed in previously involved sites, compared with 15 observed patients (*P* = .06).

Obviously, with the trial designed to detect 20% improvement in 2 year DFS and more bulky disease in the RT arm, there was still a benefit seen for the RT arm and worth to mention that patients in PR enjoyed a 6-year DFS and OS of 63% and 69% comparable to those with CR.

3. GELA LNH 93–01 conducted in a similar population stages I–II mostly low-risk compared the three CHOP and radiation to a more aggressive chemotherapy than eight CHOP, ACVBP a dose intensified doxorubicin, cyclophosphamide, vindesine, bleomycin, and prednisone, followed sequentially by methotrexate, etoposide, ifosphamide, and cytarabine. Since this regimen is even more aggressive than eight CHOP, the results were not surprising to show that it is superior to three CHOP and radiation, the 5 year estimates of EFS (82% vs. 74%) and OS (90% vs. 81%) were superior for ACVBP (the toxicity of this regimen, on the other hand, is high) (33).

4. GELA used four cycles of CHOP with and without radiation in patients older than 60 years. Stages I and II have no adverse factors, 65% of patients were stage I, 95% had IPI score of 0, only 8% had bulky disease, and 50% had extranodal disease. With a median follow-up of 7 years, there was no difference in the EFS or OS. The 5-year EFS and OS were 61% and 72%, respectively, for chemotherapy alone and 64% and 68%, respectively, for chemotherapy +RT. It is curious that although the patient population in this trial had the lowest risk factors, the event-free survival was relatively low, like what we have seen in the previous trials, therefore, the implications from this trial were limited (34).

Based on the above four trials we can conclude the following:

1. Drawing a clear recommendation based on these trials is difficult in view of the heterogeneity of the patient characteristics and treatment given.
2. These trials did not include Rituximab, which its addition to CHOP is currently the standard of care.
3. The addition of radiation did influence the outcome when CHOP is considered; more intensive chemotherapy, although it minimized the role of radiation, was at the expense of more toxicities, so no gain was achieved.
4. The decision of abbreviated versus full-course chemotherapy should depend on patient's characteristics independently from the decision of using radiation as a consolidation.

5. The dose, field, and technique of radiation used in these trials are outdated. This reality has to be taken into consideration. Currently, a true involved field, with a dose of 30 to 36 Gy, using available modern technologies including 3D conformal, intensity modulated radiation therapy, and breath-hold techniques can potentially avoid some of the side effects observed in these trials.

For the argument that the addition of R negate the benefit of radiation here are 2 trials defeating that argument. A retrospective study from MD Anderson Cancer Center showed that the addition of radiation improved both OS and PFS. The benefit was seen across all stages; the majority of patients receive six or more cycles of RCHOP. The 5-year OS and PFS were 90 and 91, respectively, for those who received radiation compared to 75% and 83%, respectively, for no radiation group ($P < .001$). A matched pair analysis done based on stage and taking into account number of cycles of RCHOP, radiation, IPI score, tumor response to therapy, bulk of the disease, confirmed the benefit of radiation with longer OS and PFS in favor of radiation (OS and PFS HR of 0.52 and 0.45 for those who did receive radiation).

The Mint trial was undertaken to assess the effect of maximum tumor diameter in the presence or absence of rituximab. Rituximab decreased but did not eliminate the adverse prognostic effect of tumor bulk on outcome (35).

Dose and Field of Radiation

The dose of radiation to be used can be 30–36 Gy depending on the bulk of the disease. Many investigators have shown no benefit of radiation dose higher than 32.5 Gy (36,37). Involved field radiation addressing the initially involved disease/site is the current standard of care. Fields should target the initial site of disease based on the prechemotherapy imaging including PET/CT and CECT as well as the postchemotherapy residual mass seen on CECT even if it is not FDG avid. While planning, it is important to take into consideration the surrounding critical organs (examples 1 and 2; see the Figures 1–4). Modern technology should be considered including intensity modulated radiation therapy, 4D CT simulation, CT on rail, and breath-hold. These techniques will have the ability to minimize the collateral radiation dose to the critical organs in the vicinity of the target.

Role of PET Scan in Risk Adapted Therapy

The use of PET scan mid-treatment and its implication is of current interest for many groups. So far, there is contradictory evidence, while at the largest series, Haioun et al. (38) and Safar et al. (39) showed that interim PET can predict outcome, whereas Pregno et al. (40) failed to detect a different outcome according to the mid-term PET (16).

In a unique study from Memorial Sloan Kettering, the interim PET was evaluated by obtaining a biopsy. The biopsy showed persistent disease in only 5 of 37 patients with positive scans; progression-free survival was identical for patients with positive interim PET and negative biopsy results and those with negative interim PET scans (41). A study from MD Anderson Cancer Center looking at the effect of midterm positive PET scan on the outcome, 296 patients were included, while the positive midterm PET scan was predictive of lower outcome all patients and patients who received chemotherapy alone (5-year PFS and OS were 71% and 78%, respectively, for negative mid-term PET versus 52% and 50% for positive midterm PET ($P = .02$ and .004, respectively). However, it lost its significance in patients who received consolidation RT (PFS and OS, 85% and 90%, respectively, for negative mid-term PET; P =.87 vs. 82% and 81%, respectively for positive midterm PET; P= .38) (42).

The presence of residual mass with negative PET scan at the end of therapy has been emerging lately as a risk for relapse and a reason to give consolidation radiation. In a study presented at the ASH meeting 2011, the presence of >2 cm mass with a negative PET scan did significantly affect the disease-free survival and overall survival in patients treated with chemotherapy alone (43). Until further studies are out to confirm the aforementioned, this is still an investigational approach and should not have a bearing on clinical decisions.

Advanced Stage and Relapse

The largest trial that addressed the role of radiation in advanced stage is by Aviles et al. (44). This is a prospective controlled clinical trial that evaluated the impact of radiation on EFS and OS of patients with stage IV disease. Three hundred and forty-one patients were enrolled; the EFS and OS were better in the radiated patients (82% and 87% compared

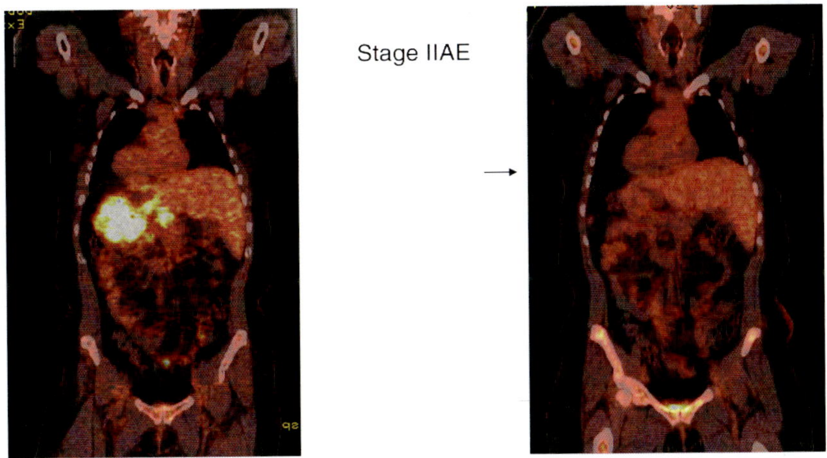

FIGURE 1   Patient with DLBCL of the stomach (left), after 6 cycles of RCHOP with CR (right).

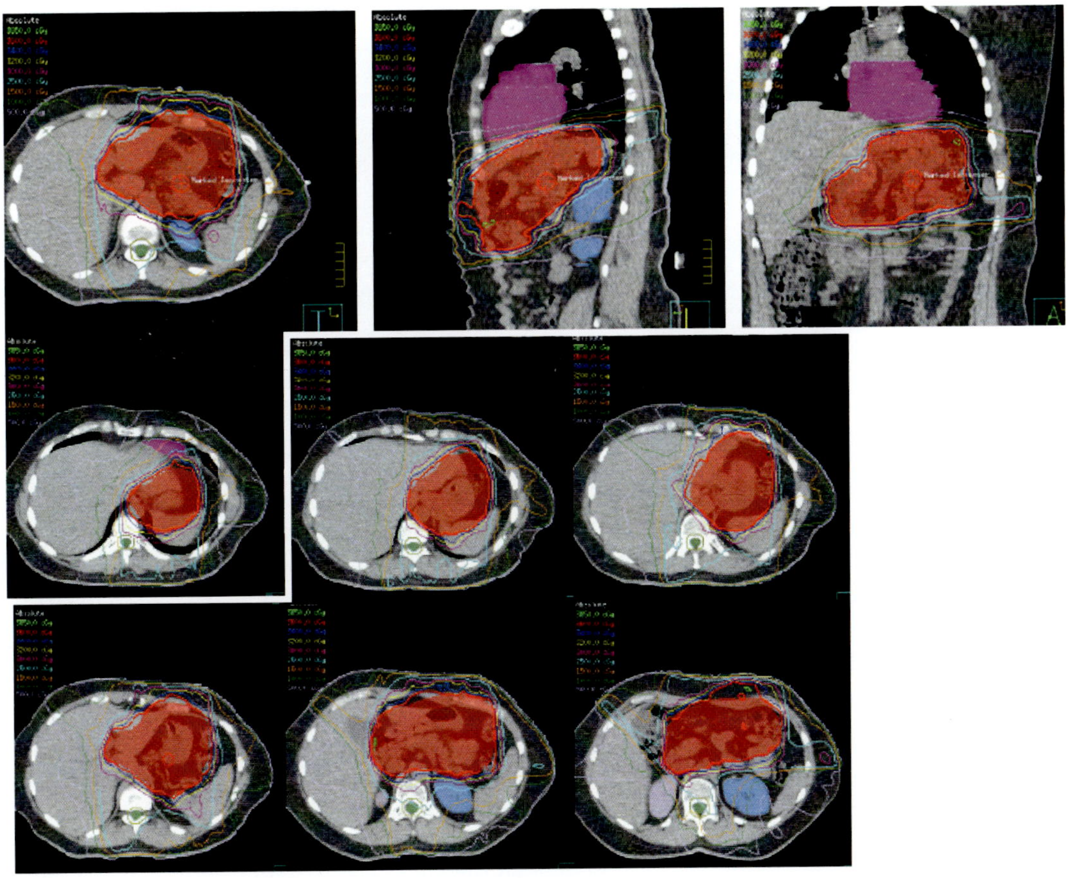

FIGURE 2   Planning done using intensity modulated radiation therapy.

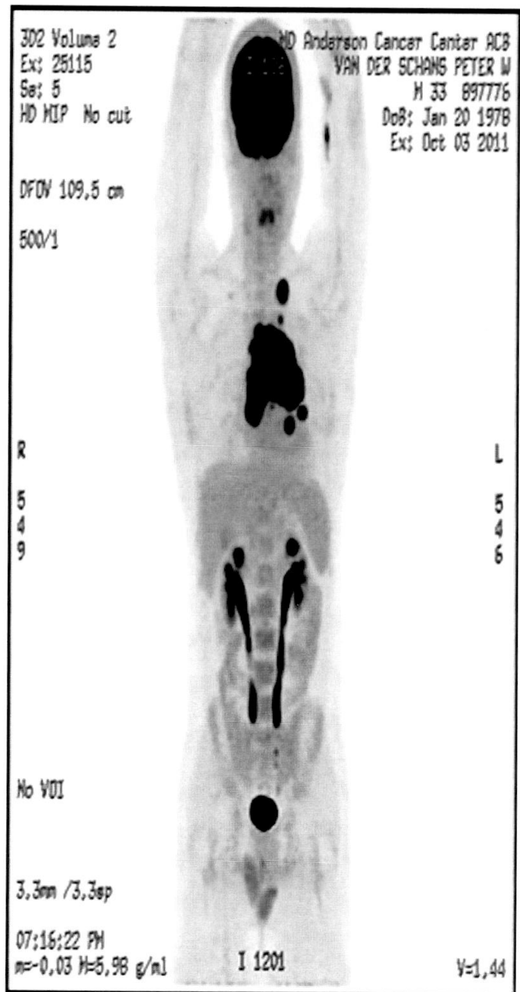

FIGURE 3   Initial presentation with primary mediastinal lymphoma.

to 55% and 66%, respectively; $P < .001$ and $P < .01$, respectively).

A number of randomized trials have been conducted to compare chemotherapy versus high-dose chemotherapy in both untreated and relapsed patients (Table 3). Although the approach has a merit in relapsed patients, it is of unproven efficacy in upfront approach according to a meta-analysis using 3079 patients (45).

Conclusions: Patients with limited stage DLBCL with an IPI score of 0 or 1 can be treated with abbreviated course of RCHOP (three to four cycles) followed by involved-field radiation. Abbreviated chemotherapy has to be used with caution in the presence of other factors known to affect the outcome beside stage and IPI score as discussed above, including: bulky disease and or aggressive pathology features. In that case, six RCHOP should be considered followed by involved-field radiation. The choice of more aggressive chemotherapy depending on the initial presentation cannot be used to deny the benefit of radiation.

Primary Mediastinal Lymphoma

Considered as a separate entity in the WHO classification, PML is believed to be of thymic B cell origin, the presence of thymic lobules as well as Hassall's corpuscles will help to indicate the thymic origin. Cells are usually medium to large size, with strands of fibrosis present in the background. Expression of surface or cytoplasmic immunoglobulin is often absent. CD21 expression is also typically absent while CD30 is sometimes present in addition to CD19, 20, and 45. Chromosome 9p24 amplification can be present in up to 50%. The typical clinical presentation is the mediastinum, and young age and histopathologic features usually help to confirm the diagnosis.

It often presents with a rapidly growing invasive tumor with contiguous spread. Chest pain, cough, and dyspnea, pleural, and pericardial effusion are also common.

The treatment consists of chemotherapy, multiple chemotherapy regimens have been used including: CHOP, CHOP R, MACOP-B, VACOP-P, ProMACE CytaBOM, or high-dose chemotherapy. The use of CHOP or CHOP-like regimens led to the early impression that PML has a worse prognosis. With the application of more aggressive combination chemotherapy programs, better CR, RFS, and OS rates were obtained. The best results so far have been seen with MACOP-B followed by radiation (46). The use of radiation has been adopted by many centers; the most compelling evidence in favor of using radiation is from a multicenter Italian study in which a large proportion converted the Gallium positive disease to negative after the use of consolidation radiation of 30 to 36 Gy. Lazzarino et al. (47) and Kirn et al. (48) also reported similar results with a higher rate of intrathoracic recurrences in patients who did not

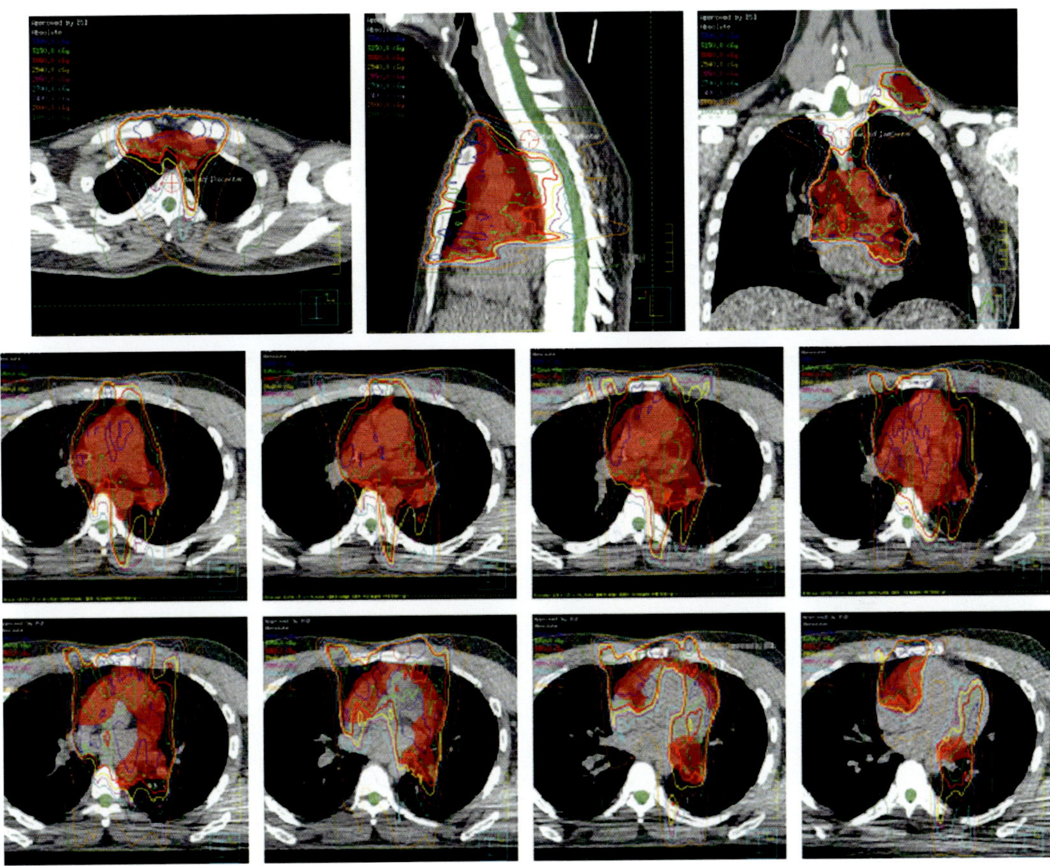

FIGURE 4 Radiation plan delivered after chemotherapy using intensity modulated radiation therapy. Breath hold and daily CT on rail are used to ensure reproducibility of the set-up.

receive radiation. Recent data from NCI, published only in an abstract form, reported a high control rate using DA-EPOCH-R. Patients were highly selective with PML excluding gray zone cases and no radiation was allowed. These results challenged the role of radiation, but until the final publication is out, radiation therapy has been shown to play a role to consolidate and improve the local control in primary mediastinal lymphoma. The radiation therapy to be used should aim at targeting the mediastinum and positive neck lymph nodes if present, in effort to avoid the critical organs in the vicinity namely the heart and lung is essential, therefore modern technology should be considered including intensity modulated radiation therapy, breath-hold, and imaging on board. The accepted dose of radiation is 36 Gy, and the inclusion of originally involved pericardial and pleural effusion is not advised in fear of excess toxicity to the heart. Finally, until randomized studies are carried, combined modality should be considered in this disease.

■ CONCLUSIONS

In conclusion combined modality still has a merit in the treatment of diffuse large B-cell lymphoma until further studies are out to demonstrate a different approach. Characterizing the disease is essential and this best done by considering other important factors in addition to the IPI score, including the bulk of the disease, immunophenogenotyping profiling, as well as the response to therapy including early response and type of response based on the PET/CT findings as well as CECT findings.

TABLE 3 Randomized trials characteristics

Trial (year) patients /treatment arms	Stage (%)	Extra-nodal/ number of risk factors	Bulky> 10cm	Histology	Initial site recurrence in field of radiation	Survival estimates	Toxicity
SWOG 8736 (1998)/401 patients/8 CHOP vs. 3 CHOP+40–55 Gy RT	Stage I (67%), bulky allowed; stage Ii (33%) non bulky	37%/0 orl (71–74%)	Not reported	24% follicular	Not available	5-year PFS 77% CHOP-RT vs. 64% CHOP; 5-year OS 82% CHOP-RT vs. CHOP	Decreased LV 0% CHOP RT vs. 7% CHOP; G4 neutropenia & 54% CHOP-RT vs. 71% CHOP
ECOG 1484 (2004)/ (352 patients/ 8 CHOP with and without 30 Gy RT (40 Gy for PR patients)	Stage II (2/3) No IPI	50%	31%> 10 cm	> 80% DLBCL Follicular and Burkitt excluded	Patients with CR: failure 17/79 in Rt and 31/93 in observed. Only 3 failure in initial sties in RT group vs. 15 in observed.	5-y-TTP 82% CHOP- RT vs. 71% CHOP; 5-y-OS 87% CHOP- RT vs. 73% CHOP. PR patients converted to CR with RT had similar survival to CR patients	4 treated related death, 2 congestive heart failure and 32% G4 toxicity related to CHOP of the whole cohort.
GELA <60 (2005)/630 patients/ ACVBP vs. 3 CHOP +40 Gy RT	I (67%)	57–63%	10%–12%	7% NK/ anaplastic	Initial site: 23% in field and 41% out of field; out of field: 38% for chemo-RT and 72% for chemo alone	5-year EFS 82% vs. 74%; 5-year OS 90% ACVBP vs. 81% CHOP RT	16 deaths, 7 in ACVBP.
GELA >60(2007)/ 576 patients/$ CHOP vs. 4 CHOP + 40Gy RT.	I (65%)	50%	8%	80% aggressive	21 % infield in CHOP-RT and 47% initial site in CHOP alone	5-year EFS 61% in observed (NS); 5-year OS 72% in observed vs. 68% in RT group (NS)	5 deaths related to chemotherapy, G3 infection occurred in 3% in both groups

TTP = time to treatment failure, EFS = event-free survival, OS= overall survival

■ REFERENCES

1. Jaffe ES, Harris NL, Stein H, et al. Classification of lymphoid neoplasms: the microscope as a tool for disease discovery. *Blood*. 2008;112(12):4384–4399.

2. A predictive model for aggressive non-Hodgkin's lymphoma. The International Non-Hodgkin's Lymphoma Prognostic Factors Project. *N Engl J Med*. 1993;329(14):987–994.

3. Alizadeh AA, Eisen MB, Davis RE, et al. Distinct types of diffuse large B-cell lymphoma identified by gene expression profiling. *Nature*. 2000;403(6769):503–511.

4. Wright G, Tan B, Rosenwald A, et al. A gene expression-based method to diagnose clinically distinct subgroups of diffuse large B cell lymphoma. *Proc Natl Acad Sci U S A*. 2003;100(17):9991–9996.

5. Rosenwald A, Wright G, Leroy K, et al. Molecular diagnosis of primary mediastinal B cell lymphoma identifies a clinically favorable subgroup of diffuse large B cell lymphoma related to Hodgkin lymphoma. *J Exp Med*. 2003;198(6):851–862.

6. Savage KJ, Monti S, Kutok JL, et al. The molecular signature of mediastinal large B-cell lymphoma differs from that of other diffuse large B-cell lymphomas and shares features with classical Hodgkin lymphoma. *Blood*. 2003;102(12):3871–3879.

7. Hans CP, Weisenburger DD, Greiner TC, et al. Confirmation of the molecular classification of diffuse large B-cell lymphoma by immunohistochemistry using a tissue microarray. *Blood*. 2004;103(1):275–282.

8. Meyer PN, Fu K, Greiner TC, et al. Immunohistochemical methods for predicting cell of origin and survival in patients with diffuse large B-cell lymphoma treated with Rituximab. *J Clin Oncol*. 2011;29(2):200–207.

9. Nyman H, Jerkeman M, Karjalainen-Lindsberg ML, et al. Prognostic impact of activated B-cell focused classification in diffuse large B-cell lymphoma patients treated with R-CHOP. *Mod Pathol*. 2009;22(8):1094–1101.

10. Aukema SM, Siebert R, Schuuring E, et al. Double-hit B-cell lymphomas. *Blood*. 2011;117(8):2319–2331.

11. Dal Maso L, Polesel J, Serraino D, et al. Pattern of cancer risk in persons with AIDS in Italy in the HAART era. *Br J Cancer*. 2009;100(5):840–847.

12. Franceschi S, Lise M, Clifford GM, et al. Changing patterns of cancer incidence in the early- and late-HAART periods: the Swiss HIV Cohort Study. *Br J Cancer*. 2010;103(3):416–422.

13. van Leeuwen MT, Vajdic CM, Middleton MG, et al. Continuing declines in some but not all HIV-associated cancers in Australia after widespread use of antiretroviral therapy. AIDS. 2009;23(16):2183–2190.

14. Geh JI, Spittle MF. Oncological problems in AIDS—a review of the clinical features and management. *Ann Acad Med Singapore*. 1996;25(3):380–391.

15. Habermann TM, Wang SS, Maurer MJ, et al. Host immune gene polymorphisms in combination with clinical and demographic factors predict late survival in diffuse large B-cell lymphoma patients in the pre-Rituximab era. *Blood*. 2008;112(7):2694–2702.

16. Safar V DJ, Jardin F, et al. Early 18 fluourodeoxyglucos PET scan as a prognostic tool in diffuse large B-cell lymphma patiens treated wtih an anthracycline-based chemotherapy plus Rituximab. *Blood*. 2009;114(45).

17. Niitsu N, Okamato M, Nakamine H, et al. Simultaneous elevation of the serum concentrations of vascular endothelial growth factor and interleukin-6 as independent predictors of prognosis in aggressive non-Hodgkin's lymphoma. *Eur J Haematol*. 2002;68(2):91–100.

18. Harris NL, Jaffe ES, Stein H, et al. A revised European-American classification of lymphoid neoplasms: a proposal from the International Lymphoma Study Group. *Blood*. 1994;84(5):1361–1392.

19. Schaefer NG, Hany TF, Taverna C, et al. Non-Hodgkin lymphoma and Hodgkin disease: coregistered FDG PET and CT at staging and restaging–do we need contrast-enhanced CT? *Radiology*. 2004;232(3):823–829.

20. Hutchings M, Loft A, Hansen M, et al. Position emission tomography with or without computed tomography in the primary staging of Hodgkin's lymphoma. *Haematologica*. 2006;91(4):482–489.

21. Fisher RI, Gaynor ER, Dahlberg S, et al. Comparison of a standard regimen (CHOP) with three intensive chemotherapy regimens for advanced non-Hodgkin's lymphoma. *N Engl J Med*. 1993;328(14):1002–1006.

22. Coiffier B, Lepage E, Briere J, et al. CHOP chemotherapy plus Rituximab compared with CHOP alone in elderly patients with diffuse large-B-cell lymphoma. *N Engl J Med*. 2002;346(4):235–242.

23. Pfreundschuh M, Trumper L, Osterborg A, et al. CHOP-like chemotherapy plus Rituximab versus CHOP-like chemotherapy alone in young patients with good-prognosis diffuse large-B-cell lymphoma: a randomised controlled trial by the MabThera International Trial (MInT) Group. *Lancet Oncol*. 2006;7(5):379–391.

24. Wilson WH, Dunleavy K, Pittaluga S, et al. Phase II study of dose-adjusted EPOCH and Rituximab in untreated diffuse large B-cell lymphoma with analysis of germinal center and post-germinal center biomarkers. *J Clin Oncol*. 2008;26(16):2717–2724.

25. Tilly H, Lepage E, Coiffier B, et al. Intensive conventional chemotherapy (ACVBP regimen) compared with standard CHOP for poor-prognosis aggressive non-Hodgkin lymphoma. *Blood*. 2003;102(13):4284–4289.

26. Andre M, Mounier N, Leleu X, et al. Second cancers and late toxicities after treatment of aggressive non-Hodgkin lymphoma with the ACVBP regimen: a GELA cohort study on 2837 patients. *Blood*. 2004;103(4):1222–1228.

27. Recher C, Coiffier B, Haioun C, et al. Intensified chemotherapy with ACVBP plus Rituximab versus standard CHOP plus Rituximab for the treatment of diffuse large B-cell lymphoma (LNH03–2B): an open-label randomised phase 3 trial. *Lancet*. 2011;378(9806):1858–1867.

28. Pfreundschuh M, Trumper L, Kloess M, et al. Two-weekly or 3-weekly CHOP chemotherapy with or

without etoposide for the treatment of young patients with good-prognosis (normal LDH) aggressive lymphomas: results of the NHL-B1 trial of the DSHNHL. *Blood.* 2004;104(3):626–633.

29. Pfreundschuh M, Trumper L, Kloess M, et al. Two-weekly or 3-weekly CHOP chemotherapy with or without etoposide for the treatment of elderly patients with aggressive lymphomas: results of the NHL-B2 trial of the DSHNHL. *Blood.* 2004;104(3):634–641.

30. Miller TP, Dahlberg S, Cassady JR, et al. Chemotherapy alone compared with chemotherapy plus radiotherapy for localized intermediate- and high-grade non-Hodgkin's lymphoma. *N Engl J Med.* 1998;339(1):21–26.

31. Fisher RI MT, O'Connor O. CHOP Alone Compared to CHOP Plus Radiotherapy for Early Stage Aggressive Non-Hodgkin's Lymphomas: Update of the Southwest Oncology Group (SWOG) Randomized Trial. *Blood.* 2004:221–236.

32. Horning SJ, Weller E, Kim K, et al. Chemotherapy with or without radiotherapy in limited-stage diffuse aggressive non-Hodgkin's lymphoma: Eastern Cooperative Oncology Group study 1484. *J Clin Oncol.* 2004;22(15):3032–3038.

33. Reyes F, Lepage E, Ganem G, et al. ACVBP versus CHOP plus radiotherapy for localized aggressive lymphoma. *N Engl J Med.* 2005;352(12):1197–1205.

34. Bonnet C, Fillet G, Mounier N, et al. CHOP alone compared with CHOP plus radiotherapy for localized aggressive lymphoma in elderly patients: a study by the Groupe d'Etude des Lymphomes de l'Adulte. *J Clin Oncol.* 2007;25(7):787–792.

35. Pfreundschuh M, Ho AD, Cavallin-Stahl E, et al. Prognostic significance of maximum tumour (bulk) diameter in young patients with good-prognosis diffuse large-B-cell lymphoma treated with CHOP-like chemotherapy with or without Rituximab: an exploratory analysis of the MabThera International Trial Group (MInT) study. *Lancet Oncol.* 2008;9(5):435–444.

36. Mendenhall NP, Rodrigue LL, Moore-Higgs GJ, et al. The optimal dose of radiation in Hodgkin's disease: an analysis of clinical and treatment factors affecting in-field disease control. *Int J Radiat Oncol Biol Phys.* 1999;44(3):551–561.

37. Schewe KL, Reavis J, Kun LE, et al. Total dose, fraction size, and tumor volume in the local control of Hodgkin's disease. Int *J Radiat Oncol Biol Phys.* 1988;15(1):25–28.

38. Haioun C, Itti E, Rahmouni A, et al. [18F]fluoro-2-deoxy-D-glucose positron emission tomography (FDG-PET) in aggressive lymphoma: an early prognostic tool for predicting patient outcome. *Blood.* 2005; 106(4): 1376–1381.

39. Safar V, Dupuis J, Itti E, et al. Interim [18F] Fluorodeoxyglucose positron emission tomography scan in diffuse large B-cell lymphoma treated with anthracycline-based chemotherapy plus rituximab. *J Clin Oncol.* 2012; 30(2): 184–190.

40. Pregno P, Chiappella A, Bello M, et al. Interim 18-FDG-PET/CT failed to predict the outcome in diffuse large B-cell lymphoma patients treated at the diagnosis with Rituximab-CHOP. *Blood.* 2012;119(9):2066–2073.

41. Moskowitz CH, Schoder H, Teruya-Feldstein J, et al. Risk-adapted dose-dense immunochemotherapy determined by interim FDG-PET in Advanced-stage diffuse large B-Cell lymphoma. *J Clin Oncol.* 2010;28(11):1896–1903.

42. Dabaja FL, Shihadeh F, Etzel C, et al. Mid-Therapy PET Scan Significantly Predict Outcome in Patients with Diffuse Large B-Cell Lymphoma (DLBCL) Treated with Chemotherapy alone but not when Consolidation Radiation is added. *Am Soc Ther Radiat Oncol.* 2012.

43. Dabaja BS, Phan J, Medeiros LJ, et al. Clinical Implications of Residual mass on CT scan with Negative PET at Completion of Chemotherapy in Patients with DLBCL. *Am Soc Hematol.* 2011.

44. Aviles A, Fernandez R, Perez F, et al. Adjuvant radiotherapy in stage IV diffuse large cell lymphoma improves outcome. *Leuk Lymphoma.* 2004;45(7):1385–1389.

45. Greb A, Bohlius J, Schiefer D, et al. High-dose chemotherapy with autologous stem cell transplantation in the first line treatment of aggressive non-Hodgkin lymphoma (NHL) in adults. *Cochrane database of systematic reviews.* 2008(1):CD004024.

46. Zinzani PL, Martelli M, Bertini M, et al. Induction chemotherapy strategies for primary mediastinal large B-cell lymphoma with sclerosis: a retrospective multinational study on 426 previously untreated patients. *Haematologica.* 2002;87(12):1258–1264.

47. Lazzarino M, Orlandi E, Paulli M, et al. Treatment outcome and prognostic factors for primary mediastinal (thymic) B-cell lymphoma: a multicenter study of 106 patients. *J Clin Oncol.* 1997;15(4):1646–1653.

48. Kirn D, Mauch P, Shaffer K, et al. Large-cell and immunoblastic lymphoma of the mediastinum: prognostic features and treatment outcome in 57 patients. *J Clin Oncol.* 1993;11(7):1336–1343.

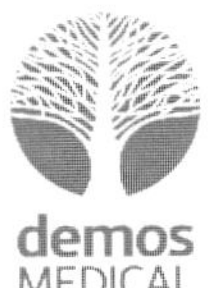

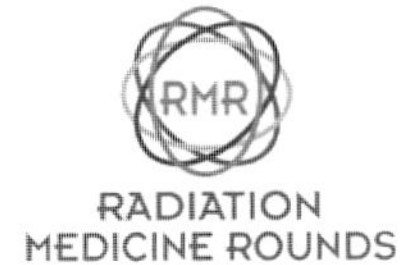

Follicular Lymphoma

Jeffrey Barnes[1,*] and Karen M. Winkfield[2]

[1]*Center for Lymphoma, Massachusetts General Hospital Cancer Center, Boston, MA*

[2]*Hematologic Malignancy Service, Department of Radiation Oncology, Massachusetts General Hospital Cancer Center, Boston, MA*

■ ABSTRACT

Follicular lymphoma is the most common type of indolent non-Hodgkin lymphoma seen in the United States. It frequently presents as asymptomatic adenopathy. Lymph node biopsy shows effacement of the lymph node architecture by closely packed follicles harboring the translocation t(14:18), bringing the immunoglobulin heavy chain regulatory region on chromosome 14 in proximity to the antiapoptotic gene BCL2 on chromosome 18. Patients with limited-stage disease, defined as involvement of nodes limited to one side of the diaphragm, are candidates for curative radiation therapy. Patients with advanced stage disease may be observed until symptomatic progression, at which time a variety of treatment options are available including monoclonal antibodies, chemoimmunotherapy, radioimmunotherapy, and stem cell transplantation.

Keywords: follicular lymphoma, radioimmunotherapy, rituximab, bendamustine, RCHOP

■ EPIDEMIOLOGY

In 2012, there will be an estimated 70,130 new cases of non-Hodgkin lymphoma (NHL) in the United States with approximately 18,940 deaths (1). Follicular lymphoma (FL) is the most common indolent lymphoma in North America and Western Europe, accounting for approximately one-third of all NHLs with a slightly lower incidence in Eastern Europe and Asia (2). The median age at diagnosis is 59 years, with a slight female predominance 1.4:1 (3). There is a slight increased risk in first degree family members of affected individuals (RR = 4.0; 95%CI: 1.6–9.5) (4).

■ PATHOLOGY

FL is a germinal center–derived B-cell neoplasm characterized by the translocation t(14:18) bringing the immunoglobulin heavy chain regulatory region on chromosome 14 in proximity to the antiapoptotic gene BCL2 on chromosome 18 (5). The typical appearance is of closely packed follicles that efface the nodal architecture, as shown in Figure 1. These follicles lack the normal polarization of germinal centers with distinct areas of centrocytes and centroblasts seen in reactive follicles. The typical immunophenotype includes positivity for surface immunoglobulin and the B cell–associated antigens CD19, CD20,

*Corresponding author, Center for Lymphoma, Massachusetts General Hospital Cancer Center, Boston, MA

E-mail address: jabarnes@partners.org

Radiation Medicine Rounds 3:3 (2012) 393–406.

DOI: 10.5003/2151–4208.3.3.393

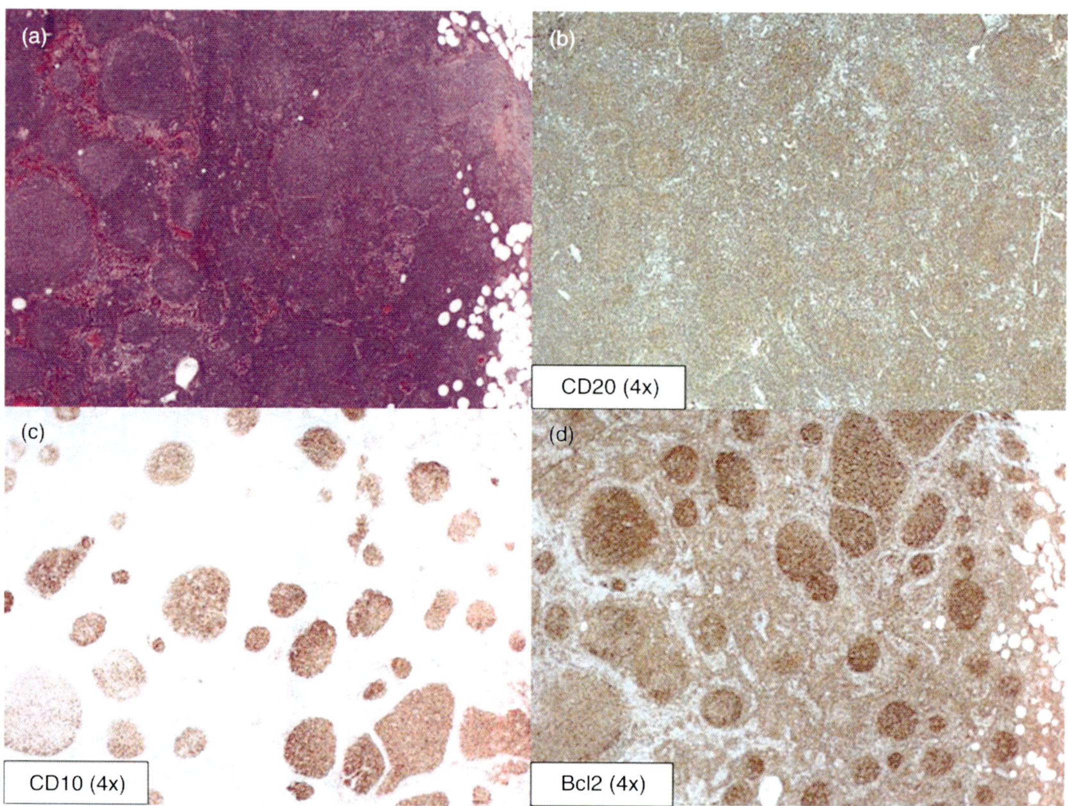

FIGURE 1   (a) Typical appearance of FL with a predominant follicular pattern of closely packed follicles causing effacement of the lymph node architecture, with expression of (b) CD20, (c) CD10, (d) BCL-2.

Source: Courtesy of Dr. Abner Louissaint.

CD22, and CD79a. There is also expression of CD10, BCL2, and BCL6 with lack of expression of CD5 and CD43. FL is frequently found in the bone marrow and has a distinctive paratrabecular pattern of involvement. The proliferation index as measured by Ki67 staining is usually <20%, although there is some suggestion that FL with a higher proliferation index may behave in a more aggressive manner (6).

FL is graded according to the number of centroblasts per high-powered field (hpf). Grade 1 (defined as 0–5 centroblasts per hpf) and Grade 2 (defined as 6–15 centroblasts per hpf) are most common, representing 80% of cases, and are typically reported together as low grade 1 to 2, because there is no clinically relevant difference between the two. Grade 3 represents the remaining 20% of cases and is defined as >15 centroblasts per hpf, with a further subclassification of grade 3a having centrocytes remaining and grade 3b being composed entirely of centroblasts.

There are significant clinical implications to FL grade with grade 1 to 2 and 3a having a median overall survival (OS) of 12.4 and 12.2 years, respectively, and grade 3b with a median OS of only 4.4 years (7). Because of this significant difference, patients with grade 3b are often treated more aggressively with notable plateaus on survival curves, suggesting that there may be cures with the use of anthracycline containing chemotherapy (5).

■ CLINICAL FEATURES

FL is an indolent B-cell non-Hodgkin lymphoma that may be present for months to years before a diagnosis is made. A majority of patients present with palpable asymptomatic adenopathy that may have waxed and waned for a prolonged period of time. Only a minority of patients (~10%–20%) presents with systemic

TABLE 1 Incidence of follicular lymphoma by stage

Stage	Description	% of cases
I	Involvement of a single lymph node region or of a single extralymphatic organ or site (IE)*	17
II	Involvement of two or more lymph node regions or lymphatic structures on the same side of the diaphragm alone or with involvement of limited, contiguous extralymphatic organ or tissue (IIE)*	15
III	Involvement of lymph node regions on both sides of the diaphragm which may include the spleen (IIIS) or limited, contiguous extralymphatic organ or site (IIIE) or both (IIIES)	30
IV	Diffuse or disseminated foci of involvement of one or more extralymphatic organs or tissues, with or without associated lymphatic involvement	37

* The designation "E" in stages IE and IIE is used when a single site of extranodal disease can be encompassed within a radiation portal.

Source: Adapted from Ref (48).

"B" symptoms such as fever, night sweats, or weight loss (8). Common sites of involvement include both central and peripheral LNs, bone marrow, spleen, peripheral blood, and gastrointestinal tract (5,8,9). Patients are staged according to the Ann Arbor criteria; most patients present with stage III or IV disease (see Table 1) (10)

Given the variability in patient outcomes, with many patients enjoying decades without progression and others who experience a much more aggressive course, there have been several attempts to develop a prognostic index. The Follicular Lymphoma International Prognostic Index (FLIPI) is one such index that stratifies patients based on the following five factors:

- Age ≥60 years
- Ann Arbor stage ≥III
- Number of nodal sites >4
- Serum lactate dehydrogenase (LDH) level greater than the upper limit of normal
- Hemoglobin <12 g/dl (9)

One point is given for each of these characteristics, resulting in a score ranging from zero to five. Table 2 shows the three distinct risk groups that the FLIPI score defines, each with its projected 10 year survival rate. At diagnosis, 36% of patients fall in the low-risk group, 37% in the intermediate risk group, and 27% in the high-risk group.

■ TRANSFORMATION

All indolent NHLs have the ability to transform into a more aggressive histology, most commonly diffuse

TABLE 2 Risk group and overall survival based on follicular lymphoma international prognostic index (FLIPI)

FLIPI Score	Risk Group	10-year OS
0–1	Low risk	70.7%
2	Intermediate risk	50.9%
3 or more	High risk	35.5%

Adapted from Ref (9).

large B-cell lymphoma (DLBCL). The risk of transformation is 1% to 4% per year or 17% to 22% at 5 years and 28% to 31% at 10 years (11,12). Factors that suggest a high risk of transformation include lack of a complete remission to initial therapy, low serum albumin <3.5g/dL, elevated levels of beta 2 microglobulin >3mg/L, elevated LDH, and high-risk FLIPI score. Histologic transformation is associated with an inferior survival, with a median survival from transformation of 7 to 14 months. Clinical factors that would suggest a transformation event include rapid onset of B symptoms, sudden rise in LDH, and rapid progression of adenopathy, or involvement of unusual extranodal sites such as the CNS and should prompt consideration of rebiopsy.

■ EVALUATION

The evaluation of patients with newly diagnosed FL is directed at risk stratification, including pathologic grade, indentifying the extent of disease burden, and indications for treatment. In general, an excisional biopsy is preferred over core needle biopsies to allow assessment of grade and proliferation index as aforementioned and to exclude areas more consistent with high-grade histology such as DLBCL. A complete history should be taken, including focus on the presence or absence of B symptoms and performance status. A physical exam should be performed, with attention to nodal bearing areas and presence of hepatomegaly or splenomegaly. Laboratory evaluation should include a complete blood count and differential for evaluation of disease related cytopenias, a comprehensive metabolic panel to evaluate for organ involvement, measurement of the LDH, and pregnancy testing in women of child-bearing age from whom therapy is planned. A diagnostic quality CT of the chest, abdomen, and pelvis should be performed to assess stage. A bone marrow biopsy is not required unless needed to document stage I or II disease or to evaluate for disease related cytopenias.

■ LIMITED-STAGE DISEASE

Approximately one-third of patients with FL will present with limited-stage disease defined as disease confined to one side of the diaphragm (10). Pediatric FL and primary intestinal FL are two rare variants that seem to be biologically distinct from other limited-stage FLs. Pediatric FL typically presents as localized cervical adenopathy, lacks BCL-2 protein expression, lacks t(14:18), and has a high proliferation index with a low rate of relapse, even when treated with excision alone (13). Primary intestinal FL frequently presents isolated to the duodenum with BCL-2 protein expression and, similar to pediatric FL, demonstrates an excellent survival, even with excision alone (14). Although radiation therapy is avoided in the pediatric population because of concern for late-treatment effects, patients with primary intestinal FL are frequently candidates for curative radiation therapy.

Definitive Radiation Therapy

For patients with limited-stage FL, many retrospective studies have shown that radiation can be used with curative intent (Table 3). These data are difficult to compare with modern standards, because they contain a wide spectrum of radiation doses, including doses as high as 50 Gy, and use outdated treatment techniques. However, the studies demonstrate a 10 year freedom from relapse of 40% to 50%, with the OS ranging from 58% to 79%. More recently, a prospective trial from the BNLI randomized 289 patients with indolent lymphomas (64% of which were FL) to either 24 Gy or 40 to 45 GY with no difference seen at 5 years in either arm in terms of local recurrence (23% vs. 21%) or in recurrence at any site

TABLE 3 Radiation therapy for limited-stage follicular lymphoma

Center	Number of patients	Stage	Treatment	Survival
Royal Marsden (19)	58	I–II	30–50 GY; 30pts IFRT, 28 extended field	10y PFS 43% 10y OS 79%
Princess Margaret (20)	596	I–II	20–35 Gy	10y FFR 40% 10y OS 58%
BNLI (21)	208	I	35–40 Gy	10y FFR 49% 10y OS 64%
Stanford (22)	177	I–II	35–50 Gy Mix of IFRT, EFRT, TLI	10y FFR 44% 10y OS 64%
Stanford (18)	43	I–II	Observation	10y OS 86%
MDACC (prospective) (15)	85	I–II	30–40 Gy after 3 cycles of COP-Bleo	10y TTTF 76% 10y OS 82%

IFRT = involved field radiotherapy, EFRT = extended field radiotherapy, TLI = total lymphoid irradiation, FFR = Freedom from relapse, TTTF = time to treatment failure, PFS = progression free survival, OS = overall survival, BNLI = British Nation Lymphoma Investigation, MDACC = MD Anderson Cancer center, COP-Bleo = cyclophosphamide, vincristine, prednisone, bleomycin

(51% vs. 55%), suggesting that lower doses may offer similar benefits (Figure 2) (16).

In 2010, Pugh et al. (17) reported the results of a SEER database analysis, investigating the outcomes of 6,568 patients with stage I or II F, grade 1 or 2. They found that upfront radiation therapy resulted in an improved 10 year disease-specific survival (DSS) of 79% in 2,222 patients compared with a DSS of 65% for those not treated with radiation (Figure 3) (17). Combined modality therapy with an anthracycline-based chemotherapy regimen results in a 10 year OS of 82%, suggesting minimal benefit over radiation therapy alone (15). Therefore, definitive radiation therapy should be considered for patients with limited-stage FL, with the intent of long-term disease control. For patients who refuse treatment or are not candidates for radiation therapy, deferred therapy remains a reasonable option. Although DSS is improved with upfront radiation therapy, a retrospective study of 43 patients from Stanford shows a 10 year OS of 86% with observation as the initial therapy (18).

Radiation Techniques

The radiation technique used will vary based on site of disease, but most definitive courses of radiation therapy can be delivered using standard 3-D conformal planning. The gross tumor volume (GTV) will need to be clearly delineated, and alternate imaging modalities or procedures may be required. In the rare instance when PET/CT scan is uses for staging purposes, these images should be used to inform the development of the GTV and clinical target volumes (CTV). For orbital FLs, an orbital MRI or fine-cut orbital CT scan should be obtained to evaluate disease extent (Figure 4A). Diagnostic imaging can then

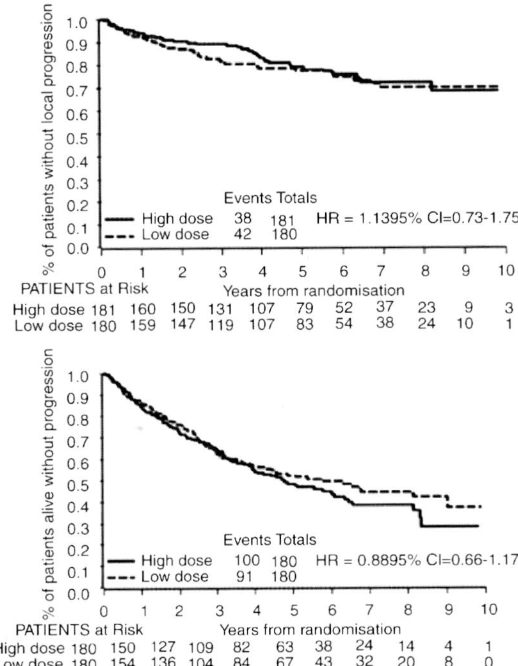

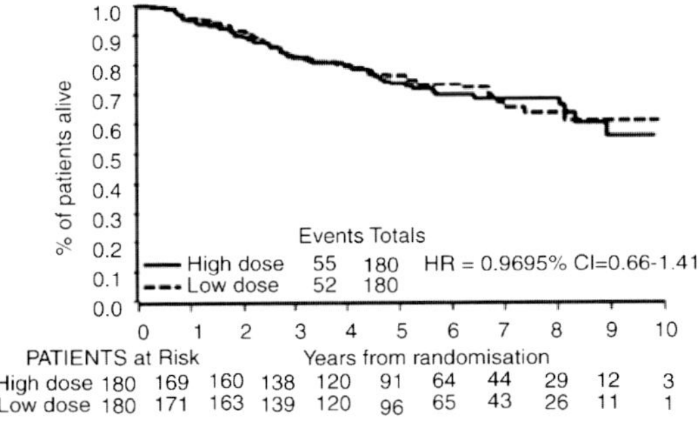

FIGURE 2 Survival curves for patients with indolent lymphoma stratified by treatment with high dose (40 Gy) versus low dose (24 Gy) radiation. (a) Freedom from local progression. (b) Progression-free survival. (c) Overall survival.

Source: From Ref (16). Reprinted with permission from Elsevier.

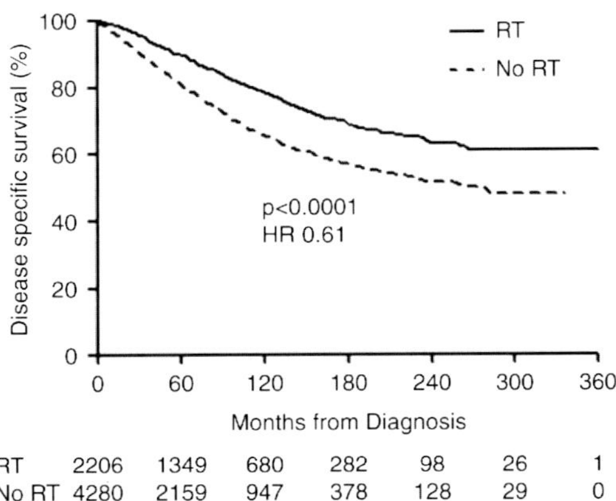

FIGURE 3 Non-Hodgkin lymphoma-specific survival with or without upfront external beam radiation therapy.

Source: From Ref (17). Reprinted with permission from Wiley.

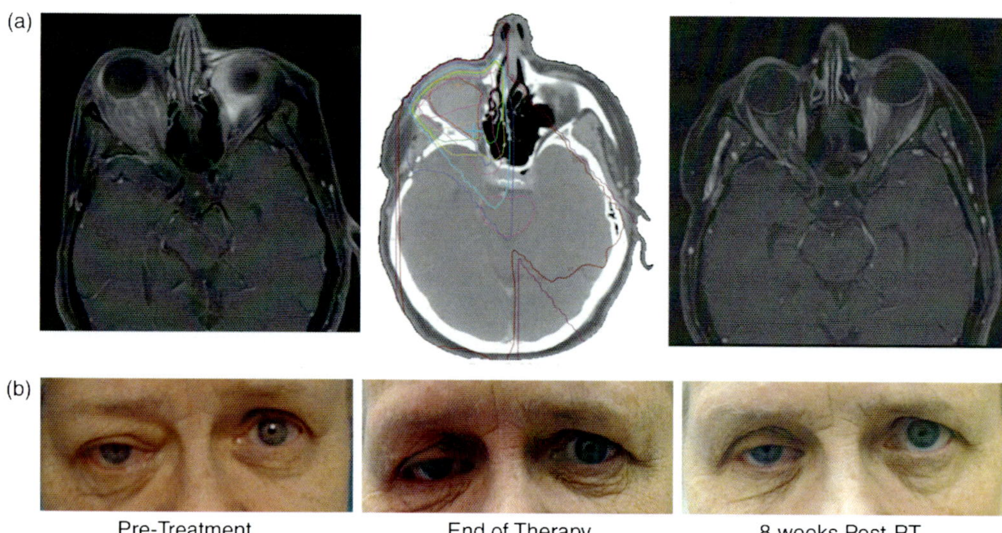

FIGURE 4   Definitive radiation therapy of a retro-orbital follicular lymphoma. (a) Left: T1 postgadolinium (T1-post) orbital MRI showing enhancing soft tissue masses noted within the right orbit along the posterior and inferior margin of the globe, resulting in moderate proptosis. Middle: axial image of planning CT scan showing isodose lines of wedged pair with excellent coverage of the gross tumor volume (100% isodose = green line). Right: repeat T1-post MRI scan, 6 months after completing radiation therapy. (b) Visible changes of orbital and periorbital tissues during the course of therapy; notice proptosis of the right eye before treatment.

be fused with the planning CT scan to delineate the treatment target. In most cases, orbital disease can be adequately treated using a tight wedged-pair, referred to in the past as the "ice-cream cone" technique (Figure 4A). During the course of therapy, patients with orbital FLs can expect to develop periorbital erythema, but frequently see resolution of presenting symptoms during therapy (Figure 4B). Long-term control is monitored with physical exam; comprehensive ophthalmic examination is recommended before and after radiation therapy. If posttreatment imaging is warranted, repeat diagnostic scan can be obtained 4 to 6 months after treatment (Figure 4A).

IMRT can be useful for definitive cases in the head and neck region, because it allows sparing of normal structures, including the oral cavity and salivary glands. This is particularly helpful with older/frailer patients seeking definitive therapy, because they are better able to tolerate treatment. More conformal therapy is appropriate when the tumor involves the nasal cavity or other facial structures. Where available, proton radiation therapy can provide excellent coverage of the CTV while sparing the lens, optic system or other organs at risk (OAR) (Figure 5).

Collaboration with other clinical specialties, such as surgery or gastroenterology, can be vitally important when designing treatment fields. For example, in the case of primary intestinal FL, which can be treated with definitive radiation therapy, the disease extent cannot be fully visualized using radiographic techniques. To ensure all areas of disease are incorporated in the treatment field while sparing uninvolved tissue, a skilled gastroenterologist can place clips within the bowel during endoscopy to define the proximal and distal extent of disease (Figure 6A). This allows a conformal treatment plan to be developed that provides adequate dose to the diseased portion of bowel, whereas sparing uninvolved segments and other OAR (Figure 6B).

■ ADVANCED STAGE DISEASE

Observation

Most patients with FL present with advance stage disease, defined as disease on both sides of the diaphragm

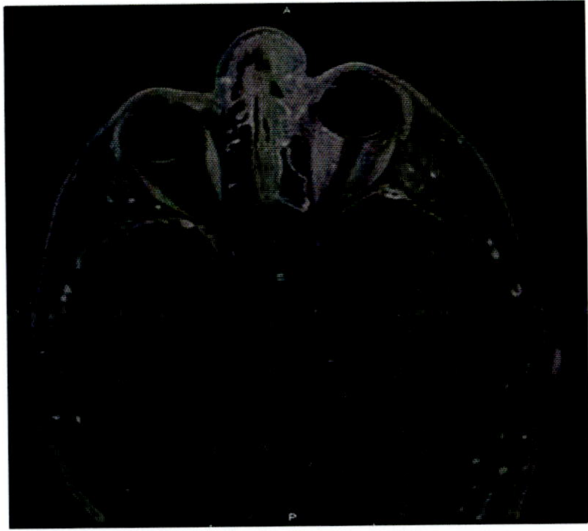
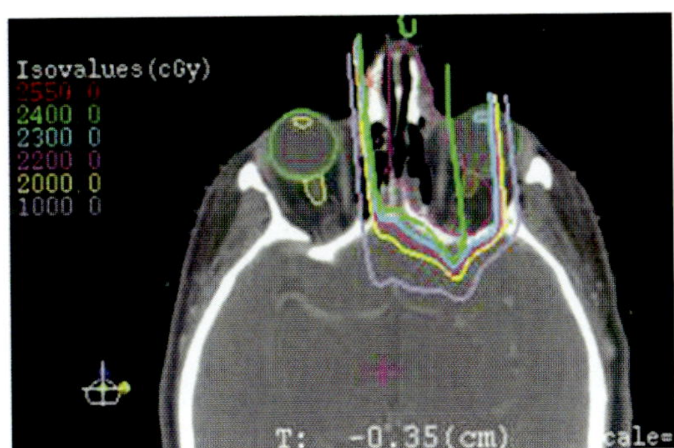

FIGURE 5 Proton radiation therapy for treatment of a follicular lymphoma involving the lacrimal sac. (a) axial T1 Fat Saturated MRI image showing involvement of the left lacrimal sac with extension into ethmoid sinus and retro-orbital space. (b) Proton radiation treatment plan showing high conformality and sparing of organs at risk.

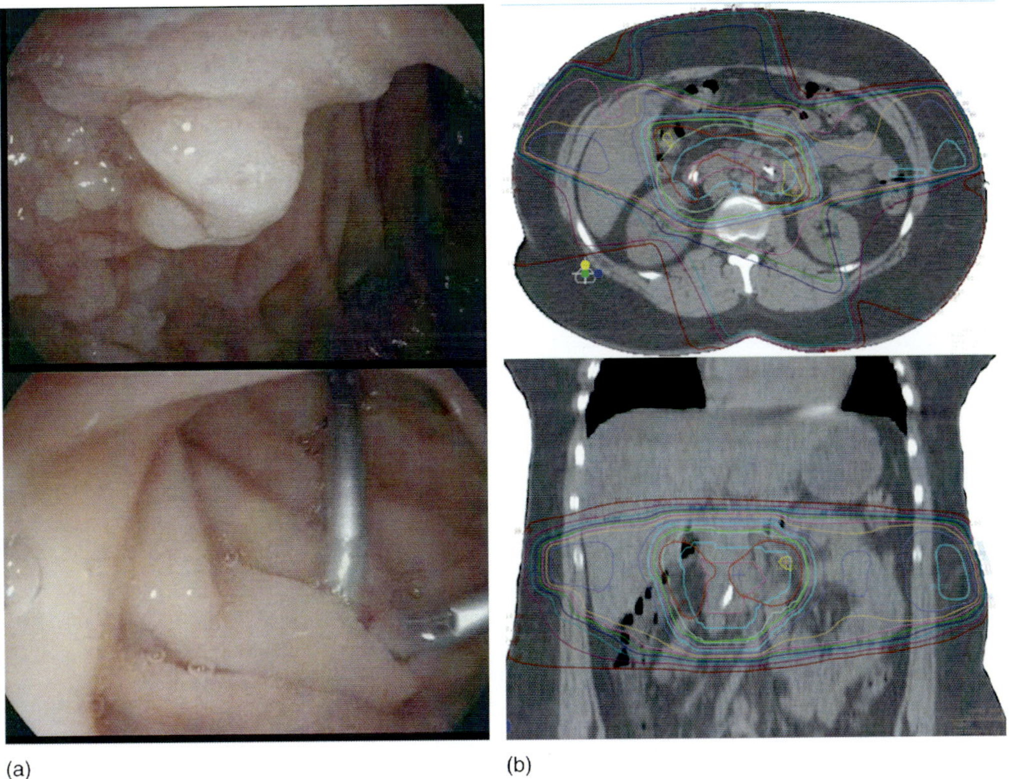

(a) (b)

FIGURE 6 Collaborative approach to the use of radiation therapy to treat primary intestinal follicular lymphoma. (a) Top: Endoscopy reveals firm nodularity involving the fold of the distal duodenum. Bottom: Clip placement proximal to the disease within normal mucosa. (b) Top: Axial image of planning CT scan showing the proximal and distal clips outlining the diseased portion of the duodenum. Isodose lines of 4-field treatment plan show conformality and minimal dose to kidneys. Bottom: Coronal image of planning CT scan with 100% dose (light green) around clinical target volume and dose falloff in surrounding bowel.

Source: Courtesy of Dr. David Forcione.

TABLE 4 Observation as initial therapy for advanced follicular lymphoma

Center	Number of patients	Survival
BNLI (23)	151	10Y OS 35% 10y FFT 20%
GELF (24)	66	5Y OS 78% Median FFT 24 months
Stanford (26)	83	10y OS 73% Median FFT 36 months
Edinburgh (25)	56	Median FFT 33 months

FFT = Freedom from treatment, GELA = Groupe d'Etude des Lymphomes Folliculaires

or with extensive involvement of an extranodal site, mainly the bone marrow. Patients with advanced stage disease are not candidates for curative therapy; this must be kept in mind both when electing to initiate therapy and when determining intensity of therapy. Most patients are candidates for a trial of observation alone as the initial approach (Table 4). The strongest evidence for this approach comes from the BNLI prospective trial of 309 asymptomatic patients randomized to either observation until symptomatic progression or to upfront single agent chlorambucil demonstrating no difference in median survival between the two groups at 16 years (6.7 years vs. 5.9 years) (23). A notable finding in this trial was that approximately 20% of patients at 10 years were still free from therapy in the observation group, suggesting that a substantial number of patients with FL may never require therapy. The equivalent survival with an initial approach of observation alone when compared with upfront treatment has been validated in several additional studies (24–26).

Indications for Treatment

Most patients can be observed at initial presentation as previously detailed. This is especially important, because many patients will have a prolonged period with out progression and a small fraction (up to 6%) may have spontaneous regression of their disease (23,27). Most clinicians use the GELF and BNLI criteria as indications for treatment (23,24), including:

- Cytopenias because of FL
- B symptoms or other symptomatic disease
- Bulky disease
- Compromised organ function because of lymphomatous involvement or compression
- Effusions caused by FL
- Steady or rapid progression.

Palliative Radiation Therapy

Patients with a single site of symptomatic disease may be candidates for radiation therapy and avoid systemic therapy. Low-dose involved field radiation with as little as 4 Gy, 2Gy delivered over 2 days, has shown an overall response rate (ORR) of 92% with 61% of treated patients achieving a complete remission (CR) to therapy (28) These remissions are durable with a median time to local progression of 25 months with those achieving a CR enjoying a longer median time to local progression of 42 months. Patients who progress may be retreated with the same low-dose algorithm and achieve similar excellent response rates (ORR of 98%; 71% CR) with retreatment. The median time to local progression at retreatment is of similar duration to that seen with an initial course of low-dose RT. This approach is especially useful for patients without hard indications for systemic therapy but who might benefit from palliative therapy for disease sites that are uncomfortable (such as bulky axillary nodes), cosmetic benefit (visible neck or facial nodes), or to relieve potentially damaging mass-effect on normal tissues (such as ureteral compression) (see Figure 7).

Choice of Initial Systemic Therapy

Of the many effective systemic agents used to treat FL, none have shown an improved OS benefit that would favor one treatment approach over another, with the exception of rituximab-containing chemotherapy versus chemotherapy alone. Intense chemotherapeutic regimens show improved CR rates and progression-free survival, without improvement in OS. Available treatment strategies currently used in chemotherapy naïve patients include rituximab monotherapy with or without maintenance, rituximab plus bendamustine, R-CVP (cyclophosphamide, vincristine, and prednisone), R-CHOP (cyclophosphamide, doxorubicin, vincristine, and prednisone), fludarabine-based regimens, radioimmunotherapy (RIT), and occasionally single agent oral alkylator therapy. Because no single regimen is superior over another in terms of OS, treatment decisions are made based on tolerability.

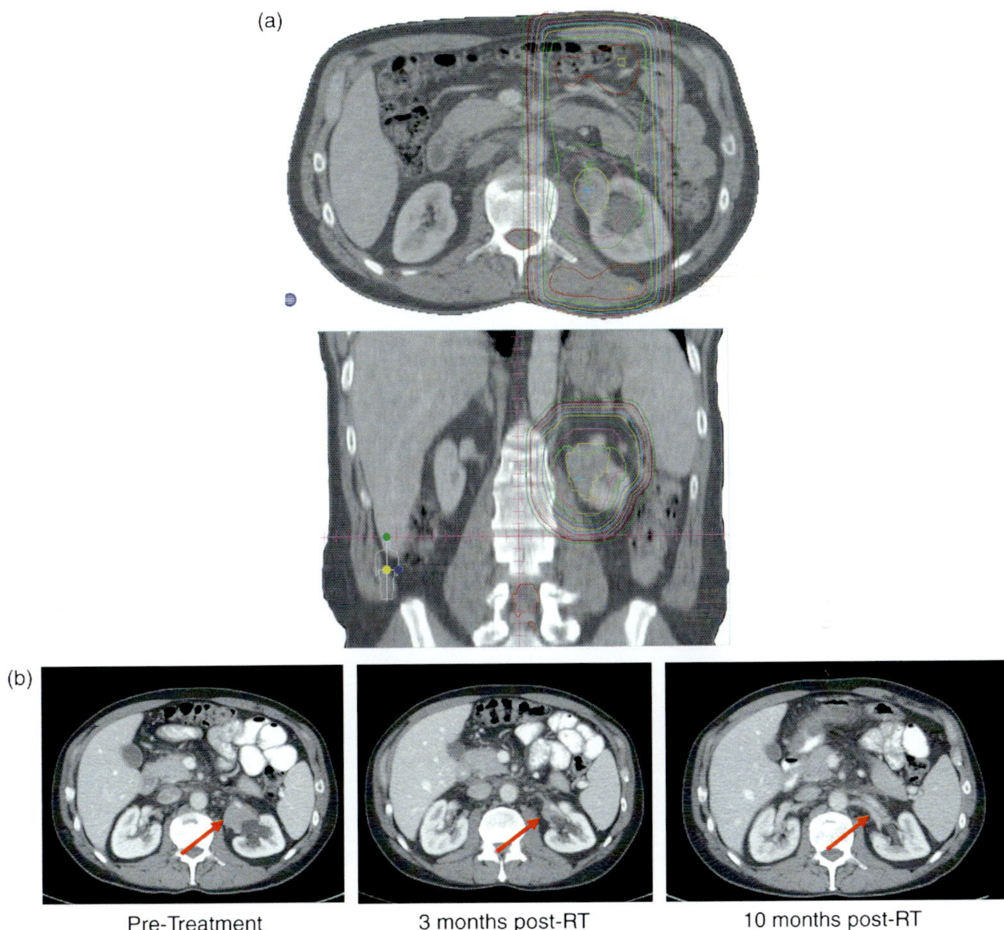

FIGURE 7   Low-dose palliative radiation therapy (2 Gy × 2) relieves ureteral obstruction. (a) Coronal and axial images from planning CT scan showing simple AP/PA beam arrangement. (b) Pretreatment and restaging scans show continued resolution of ureteral mass over time.

Single-Agent Rituximab for Asymptomatic Patients

Rituximab is a genetically engineered, chimeric, murine/human monoclonal antibody directed against the CD20 antigen found on the surface of normal and malignant pre-B and mature B cells. Several mechanisms of action have been proposed in various models including complement-dependent cytotoxicity (CDC), antibody-dependent cell-mediated cytoxicity (ADCC), induction of apoptosis, and a "vaccinal" effect (29). It is likely that rituximab works through a combination of these mechanisms and has been shown to have significant activity in all CD20 positive lymphomas. It has an excellent side effect profile and was therefore studied in two large prospective trials in patient with out indications for treatment.

In a large Intergroup trial, 462 patients with out indications for treatment were randomized to either observation alone, rituximab 375 mg/m² weekly for 4 weeks, or rituximab 375 mg/m² weekly for 4 weeks followed by rituximab maintenance every 2 months for 2 years (30). The freedom from treatment time was similar as to what was seen in previous observational studies with a median of 33 months. The authors report a benefit of improvement of time to new treatment in the rituximab arms but no difference in OS. Similarly, the Eastern Cooperative Oncology Group RESORT (Rituximab Extended Schedule or Re-Treatment) trial evaluated results of asymptomatic patients given rituximab 375 mg/m² weekly for 4 weeks. The 274 patients that responded (70% of patient enrolled) were randomized to either maintenance therapy as a single 375 mg/m² dose every 3 months or observation (31). No significant difference was seen between the groups in terms of time to treatment failure (TTF) suggesting no benefit to maintenance rituximab. Rituximab does have significant single agent activity and is a reasonable approach for older patients who might tolerate chemotherapy poorly. However, in the absence of a survival benefit and with evidence showing treatment free intervals of close to 3 years with observation alone, use of single agent Rituximab for patients without indications for treatment should currently be reserved for clinical trials.

Chemoimmunotherapy

The combination of rituximab with chemotherapy is superior to chemotherapy alone, increasing response rates and survival by approximately 15%. R-CVP administered for 8 cycles has produced comparable findings of an ORR of 81% with CRR of 30% and median TTF 27 months (32). R-CHOP has produced ORR of 96% with CRR of 20% and TTF of 29 months in older patients and not reached in younger patients at limited follow up (33). Recently, the German Study Group Indolent Lymphoma (STiL) NHL1 trial compared RCHOP with bendamustine plus rituximab (BR). This trial of 549 patients 55% of which had FL surprisingly showed that BR was more effective than RCHOP with a median progression free survival (PFS) of 69.5 m compared with 31 m (34). BR was also superior to RCHOP in terms of response rate with CR of 40% compared with 30%. In addition BR was better tolerated with significantly lower rates of neutropenia (11% vs. 47%), stomatitis (6% vs. 19%), and alopecia (15% all grade 1 vs. 62%). This data has been presented but not yet published but suggests that BR may represent an alternative to RCVP and RCHOP with improved efficacy and tolerability.

Maintenance Rituximab after Chemotherapy

Given its excellent side effect profile, several groups have investigated the role of maintenance rituximab after initial therapy. As previously noted, the RESORT trial of maintenance rituximab after initial single agent rituximab failed to show a benefit in delaying future therapy (31). The Intergroup trial also failed to show a benefit in terms of time to next treatment for those who received maintenance rituximab after initial single agent rituximab (30). These trials would suggest that there is not a significant benefit to maintenance rituximab in those receiving rituximab alone. The role of maintenance after chemoimmunotherapy was addressed in the PRIMA trial which took patients with FL with indications for treatment (bulk, >3 nodes, splenomegaly, organ compromise, increased LDH, or B symptoms) and treated them as follows: 885 received RCHOP, 272 received RCVP, and 45 RFCM (fludarabine, cyclophosphamide, mitoxantrone) (35). Patients without progressive disease were then randomized to maintenance rituximab (375 mg/m² every 8 weeks for 2 years) or observation. With a median follow-up of 36 months, there was a benefit for maintenance in terms of PFS (74.9% vs. 57.6%) but OS did not differ significantly between groups (HR 0.87, 95% CI 0.51–1.47). These trials suggest a benefit only in PFS not OS, so the decision to include maintenance rituximab should be made only if PFS is a meaningful goal for an individual patient and must be weighed against the small risks of immunocompromise and hepatitis B reactivation.

Radioimmunotherapy

The radioimmunoconjugates Yttrium-90–Ibritumomab Tiuxetan and Iodine-131-Tositumomab both target CD 20 and have been studied in the upfront treatment of FL. Yttrium-90–Ibritumomab Tiuxetan was studied in a population of FL patients who achieved either a CR or PR to their initial therapy and were then randomized to Yttrium-90–Ibritumomab Tiuxetan (14.8 MBq/kg; maximum of 1,184 MBq) or no further treatment (36). The median PFS favored the treatment group (36.5 vs. 13.3 months) with many patients converting from a PR to a CR. However a majority of the patients in this trial did not receive rituximab as part of there initial therapy. As previously noted, chemoimmunotherapy is more effective than chemotherapy alone and this benefit may have been seen with the naked antibody alone. In addition no OS benefit was reported in this trial. Iodine-131-Tositumomab was also studied in the upfront setting with patients treated with CHOP then randomized to either 6 doses of rituximab or a single therapeutic infusion of I-131-tositumomab labeled with sufficient I-131 (median 85 mCi) to deliver a total body dose of 7.5 Gy (37). Again no significant difference was seen in terms of PFS (76% vs. 80%) or OS (97% vs. 93%) was seen suggesting that their may be little benefit of the radioimmunoconjugate compared with rituximab alone.

Therapy for Relapse

Patients with treated FL have a median PFS survival of 27–70 months and therefore most patients require additional therapy. It is important to note that at the time of relapse if there are not indications for treatment observation remains a reasonable approach. It is also important to remember that for a single site of symptomatic disease, palliative radiation at a dose of 4 Gy remains an option. For patients with indications for systemic therapy, the choice of regimen is made with performance status and prior regimens in mind. Similar themes are seen as in the initial therapy with single agent rituximab having modest activity that is greatly enhanced with the combination with chemotherapy. All the regimens previously detailed have activity in the relapse setting. There are three major differences in the relapsed setting: the role of maintenance rituximab, stem cell transplant, and radioimmunoconjugates.

Maintenance Rituximab in the Relapsed Setting

Unlike in the upfront setting, maintenance rituximab has shown an OS benefit in the relapsed setting but in patients who did not receive rituximab as part of their initial therapy (a population that in general no longer exists). Four hundred and sixty five patients with relapsed FL were randomized to receive CHOP or RCHOP with a second randomization to maintenance rituximab (one dose every three months till progression or two years). RCHOP resulted in a higher CR rate (29.5% vs. 15.6%) and overall response rate (85.1% vs. 72.3%) compared with CHOP alone (38). Three hundred and thirty four responders were then randomized to observation or maintenance rituximab and unlike previous studies maintenance rituximab showed a benefit in both PFS (51.5m vs. 14.9m) and OS at 3 years (85% vs. 77%). However at a longer follow up of 6 years this OS benefit decreased to 74% versus 64% and was no longer statistically significant, perhaps because of the effect of rituximab-containing salvage regimens in the observation arm (39). The benefit of maintenance rituximab in the relapse setting for patients who receive rituximab as part of their initial therapy remains unclear.

Stem Cell Transplant

Autologous stem cell transplant (SCT) for FL can improve the response rate and PFS and unlike other intense chemotherapies can improve OS. In the largest series to date, 140 patients with relapsed FL were treated with four cycles of CHOP and then randomized to receive additional chemotherapy, autologous SCT, or an autologous SCT with the stem cell product purged with an anti CD20 monoclonal antibody (40). With more than 5 years median follow-up, autologous SCT showed an improved PFS (HR 0.30,

p=0.0009) and OS (HR 0.40, p=0.026) compared with further chemotherapy with 4 year OS of 46% for the chemotherapy arm versus 71% for the unpurged and 77% for the purged autologous SCT arms. These results were similar to what was seen in retrospective studies of autologous SCT in relapsed FL with OS of 66%. (41). However, these studies included a patient population that did not receive rituximab as part of their therapy and the role of autologous SCT in the modern patient remains unclear.

Radioimmunotherapy

Both Yttrium-90–Ibritumomab Tiuxetan and Iodine-131-Tositumomab have been studied in relapsed FL. Yttrium-90–Ibritumomab Tiuxetan was compared with single-agent rituximab demonstrating both a higher ORR (80% vs. 56%) and CR rate (30% vs. 16%) but similar duration of response (14.2m vs. 12.1m) and time to progression (11.2m vs. 10.2m) (42). Iodine-131-Tositumomab was studied in patients refractory to rituximab demonstrating ORR of 65% with CR rate of 38% and a median PFS of 10.4 months (43). Despite activity, RIT has been slow to be adopted in the relapsed setting possibly because of the complexity of administration.

Future Directions

FL remains an incurable disease, and although many patients may be observed, a majority require therapy both initial presentation and at relapse. There are several emerging therapeutic strategies under investigation. Targeting the BCL-2 protein with oblimersen, an antisense oligonucleotide drug, in combination with rituximab has resulted in an ORR of 60% with a CR rate of 40% (44). Targeting components of the B cell receptor signaling pathway including inhibitors of the Bruton tyrosine kinase, and SYK are also under development (45,46). Also in development are immunomodulating agents including lenalidomide which in combination with rituximab demonstrated a remarkable CR rate of 87% in untreated FL (47). These strategies with improved efficacy and safety compared with traditional chemotherapy have the potential to change the face of this disease.

■ REFERENCES

1. American Cancer Society. *Cancer Facts and Figures.* 2012; http://www.cancer.org/acs/groups/content/@epidemiologysurveilance/documents/document/acspc-031941.pdf

2. Anderson JR, Armitage JO, Weisenburger DD. Epidemiology of the non-Hodgkin's lymphomas: distributions of the major subtypes differ by geographic locations. *Ann Oncol*. 1998;9(7):717–20.

3. The Non-Hodgkin's Lymphoma Classification Project. A clinical evaluation of the international lymphoma study group classification of non-Hodgkin's lymphoma. *Blood*. 1997;89(11):3909–18.

4. Goldin LR, Björkholm M, Kristinsson SY, Turesson I, Landgren O. Highly increased familial risks for specific lymphoma subtypes. *Br J Haematol*. 2009;146(1):91–4.

5. Swerdlow S, Campo E, Harris NL, Jaffe ES, Pileri S, Stein H, Thiele J, Vardiman JW, eds. who *classification of tumors of haematopoietic and lymphoid tissue*. Lyon,France: IARC; 2008.

6. Wang SA, Wang L, Hochberg EP, Muzikansky A, Harris NL, Hasserjian RP. Low histologic grade follicular lymphoma with high proliferation index: Morphologic and clinical features. *Am J Surg Pathol*. 2005;29(11):1490–6.

7. Wahlin BE, Yri OE, Kimby E, Holte H, Delabie J, Smeland EB, Sundström C, Christensson B, Sander B. Clinical significance of the WHO grades of follicular lymphoma in a population-based cohort of 505 patients with long follow-up times. *Br J Haematol*. 2012; 156(2):225–33.

8. Federico M, Bellei M, Marcheselli L, et al. Follicular lymphoma international prognostic index 2: A new prognostic index for follicular lymphoma developed by the international follicular lymphoma prognostic factor project. *J Clin Oncol*. 2009;27(27):4555–62.

9. Solal-Celigny P, Roy P, Colombat P, et al. Follicular lymphoma international prognostic index. *Blood*. 2004;104(5):1258–65.

10. Friedberg JW, Taylor MD, Cerhan JR, et al. Follicular lymphoma in the United States: first report of the national Lymphocare study. *J Clin Oncol*. 2009;27(8):1202–8.

11. Bastion Y, Sebban C, Berger F, et al. Incidence, predictive factors, and outcome of lymphoma transformation in follicular lymphoma patients. *J Clin Oncol*. 1997;15(4):1587–94.

12. Montoto S, Davies AJ, Matthews J, et al. Risk and clinical implications of transformation of follicular lymphoma to diffuse large B-cell lymphoma. *J Clin Oncol*. 2007;25(17):2426–33.

13. Louissaint A, Ackerman AM, Dias-Santagata D, et al. Pediatric-type nodal follicular lymphoma: An indolent clonal proliferation in children and adults, with high proliferation index and no BCL2 rearrangement. *Blood*. 2012;120(12):2395–404.

14. Misdraji, Joseph Harris, Nancy Lee Hasserjian,Robert P., Lauwers GY, Ferry JA. Primary follicular lymphoma of the gastrointestinal tract. *Am J Surg Pathol*. 2011;35(9):1255–63.

15. Seymour JF, Pro B, Fuller LM, et al. Long-term follow-up of a prospective study of combined modality therapy for stage I-II indolent non-Hodgkin's lymphoma. *J Clin Oncol*. 2003;21(11):2115–22.

16. Lowry L, Smith P, Qian W, Falk S, Benstead K, Illidge T, Linch D, Robinson M, Jack A, Hoskin P. Reduced dose radiotherapy for local control in non-Hodgkin lymphoma: a randomised phase III trial. *Radiother Oncol*. 2011;100(1):86–92.

17. Pugh TJ, Ballonoff A, Newman F, Rabinovitch R. Improved survival in patients with early stage low-grade follicular lymphoma treated with radiation: a surveillance, epidemiology, and end results database analysis. *Cancer*. 2010;116(16):3843–51.

18. Advani R, Rosenberg SA, Horning SJ. Stage I and II follicular non-Hodgkin's lymphoma: Long-term follow-up of no initial therapy. *J Clin Oncol*. 2004;22(8):1454–9.

19. Pendlebury S, el Awadi M, Ashley S, Brada M, Horwich A. Radiotherapy results in early stage low grade nodal non-Hodgkin's lymphoma. *Radiother Oncol*. 1995;36(3):167–71.

20. Gospodarowicz MK, Bush RS, Brown TC, Chua T. Prognostic factors in nodular lymphomas: a multivariate analysis based on the princess Margaret hospital experience. *Int J Radiat Oncol Biol Phys*. 1984;10(4):489–97.

21. Vaughan Hudson B, Vaughan Hudson G, MacLennan KA, Anderson L, Linch DC. Clinical stage 1 non-Hodgkin's lymphoma: Long-term follow-up of patients treated by the British National Lymphoma Investigation with radiotherapy alone as initial therapy. *Br J Cancer*. 1994;69(6):1088–93.

22. Mac Manus MP, Hoppe RT. Is radiotherapy curative for stage I and II low-grade follicular lymphoma? Results of a long-term follow-up study of patients treated at Stanford university. *J Clin Oncol*. 1996;14(4):1282–90.

23. Ardeshna K, Smith P, Norton A, et al. Long-term effect of a watch and wait policy versus immediate systemic treatment for asymptomatic advanced-stage non-Hodgkin lymphoma: A randomised controlled trial. *Lancet*. 2003;362(9383):516–22.

24. Brice P, Bastion Y, Lepage E, et al. Comparison in low-tumor-burden follicular lymphomas between an initial no-treatment policy, prednimustine, or interferon alfa: a randomized study from the Groupe D'etude des Lymphomes Folliculaires. *J Clin Oncol*. 1997;15(3):1110–7.

25. O'Brien ME, Easterbrook P, Powell J, et al. The natural history of low grade non-Hodgkin's lymphoma and the impact of a no initial treatment policy on survival. *Q J Med*. 1991;80(292):651–60.

26. Horning SJ, Rosenberg SA. The natural history of initially untreated low-grade non-Hodgkin's lymphomas. *N Engl J Med*. 1984;311(23):1471–5.

27. Krikorian JG, Portlock CS, Cooney DP, Rosenberg SA. Spontaneous regression of non-Hodgkin's lymphoma: A report of nine cases. *Cancer*. 1980;46(9):2093–9.

28. Haas RLM, Poortmans P, de Jong D, et al. High response rates and lasting remissions after low-dose involved field radiotherapy in indolent lymphomas. *J Clin Oncol*. 2003;21(13):2474–80.

29. Maloney D, Grillo-Lopez A, Bodkin D, et al. IDEC-C2B8: Results of a phase I multiple-dose trial in patients with relapsed non-Hodgkin's lymphoma. *J Clin Oncol.* 1997;15(10):3266–74.

30. Ardeshna KM, Qian W, Smith P, et al. An intergroup randomised trial of rituximab versus a watch and wait strategy in patients with stage II, III, IV, asymptomatic, non-bulky follicular lymphoma (grades 1, 2 and 3a): a preliminary analysis. *Blood.* 2010;116(21):6.

31. Kahl BS, Hong F, Williams ME, et al. Results of eastern cooperative oncology group protocol E4402 (RESORT): a randomized phase III study comparing two different rituximab dosing strategies for low tumor burden follicular lymphoma. *Blood.* 2011;118(21):LBA-6.

32. Marcus R, Imrie K, Belch A, et al. CVP chemotherapy plus rituximab compared with CVP as first-line treatment for advanced follicular lymphoma. *Blood.* 2005;105(4):1417–23.

33. Coiffier B, Lepage E, Briere J, et al. CHOP chemotherapy plus rituximab compared with CHOP alone in elderly patients with diffuse large-B-cell lymphoma. *N Engl J Med.* 2002;346(4):235–42.

34. Rummel MJ, Niederle N, Maschmeyer G, et al. Bendamustine plus rituximab (B-R) versus CHOP plus rituximab (CHOP-R) as first-line treatment in patients with indolent and mantle cell lymphomas (MCL): updated results from the StiL NHL1 study. *ASCO Meeting Abstracts.* 2012;30(18 Suppl):3.

35. Salles G, Seymour JF, Offner F, et al. Rituximab maintenance for 2 years in patients with high tumour burden follicular lymphoma responding to rituximab plus chemotherapy (PRIMA): a phase 3, randomised controlled trial. *Lancet.* 2011;377(9759):42–51.

36. Morschhauser F, Radford J, Van Hoof A, et al. Phase III trial of consolidation therapy with yttrium-90–Ibritumomab tiuxetan compared with no additional therapy after first remission in advanced follicular lymphoma. *J Clin Oncol.* 2008;26(32):5156–64.

37. Press OW, Unger JM, Rimsza LM, et al. A phase III randomized intergroup trial (SWOG S0016) of CHOP chemotherapy plus rituximab vs. CHOP chemotherapy plus iodine-131-tositumomab for the treatment of newly diagnosed follicular non-Hodgkin's lymphoma. *Blood.* 2011;118(21):98.

38. van Oers MHJ, Klasa R, Marcus RE, et al. Rituximab maintenance improves clinical outcome of relapsed/resistant follicular non-Hodgkin lymphoma in patients both with and without rituximab during induction: results of a prospective randomized phase 3 intergroup trial. *Blood.* 2006;108(10):3295–301.

39. van Oers MHJ, Van Glabbeke M, Giurgea L, et al. Rituximab maintenance treatment of Relapsed/Resistant follicular non-Hodgkin's lymphoma: long-term outcome of the EORTC 20981 phase III randomized intergroup study. *J Clin Oncol.* 2010;28(17):2853–8.

40. Schouten HC, Qian W, Kvaloy S, et al. High-dose therapy improves progression-free survival and survival in relapsed follicular non-Hodgkin's lymphoma: results from the randomized European CUP trial. *J Clin Oncol.* 2003;21(21):3918–27.

41. Freedman AS, Neuberg D, Mauch P, et al. Long-term follow-up of autologous bone marrow transplantation in patients with relapsed follicular lymphoma. *Blood.* 1999;94(10):3325–33.

42. Witzig TE, Gordon LI, Cabanillas F, et al. Randomized controlled trial of yttrium-90-labeled ibritumomab tiuxetan radioimmunotherapy versus rituximab immunotherapy for patients with relapsed or refractory low-grade, follicular, or transformed B-cell non-Hodgkin's lymphoma. *J Clin Oncol.* 2002;20(10):2453–63.

43. Horning SJ, Younes A, Jain V, et al. Efficacy and safety of tositumomab and iodine-131 tositumomab (bexxar) in B-cell lymphoma, progressive after rituximab. *J Clin Oncol.* 2005;23(4):712–9.

44. Pro B, Leber B, Smith M, et al. Phase II multicenter study of oblimersen sodium, a bcl-2 antisense oligonucleotide, in combination with rituximab in patients with recurrent B-cell non-Hodgkin lymphoma. *Br J Haematol.* 2008;143(3):355–60.

45. Evans E, Tester R, Aslanian S, et al. Clinical development of AVL-292; A potent, selective covalent btk inhibitor for the treatment of B cell malignancies. *Blood.* 2011;118(21):3485.

46. Pollyea DA, Smith S, Fowler N, et al. A phase I dose escalation study of the btk inhibitor PCI-32765 in relapsed and refractory B cell non-Hodgkin lymphoma and use of a novel fluorescent probe pharmacodynamic assay. *Blood.* 2009;114(22):3713.

47. Fowler N, McLaughlin P, Hagemeister FB, et al. A biologic combination of lenalidomide and rituximab for front-line therapy of indolent B-cell non-Hodgkin's lymphoma. *Blood.* 2009;114(22):1714.

48. Lister, TA, et al, Report of a committee convened to iscuss the evaluation and staging of patients with Hodgkin's disease: Cotswolds meeting. *J Clin Oncol.* 1989;7:1630.

simulation and planning should be used. If available, four-dimensional CT imaging with incorporation of breathing permits more accurate anatomical discrimination of disease, thereby limiting unnecessary dose to uninvolved tissues. It is advisable to perform the simulation and to administer radiation treatments in a fasting state (typically 4–6 hours *nil per os*) to reduce gastric motion. Intensity-modulated radiation therapy (IMRT) provides the ability to administer highly conformal plans, and 3-D conformal techniques are also acceptable. In the setting of more conformal IFRT, image-guided radiotherapy is important, ideally with daily cone beam CT. The target should be treated to 30 Gy in 20 daily fractions and should include the stomach, any pathologically involved lymph nodes, and, electively, perigastric lymph nodes.

Minimizing dose to nearby organs at risk, including the heart, liver, and kidneys is imperative. The dose to one-third of at least one of the kidneys should be less than 20 Gy. At least 50% of the liver should receive less than 20 Gy, with a mean dose of less than 30 Gy. The dose to the heart should be as low as reasonably achievable.

Outcomes after definitive radiotherapy for stage I and II disease are excellent. In an update of the original published series of 17 patients treated for stage I-II MALT lymphoma of the stomach, in which 27 month event-free survival was 100% (60), Yahalom and colleagues reported on 51 patients treated for predominantly stage I and II MALT lymphoma of the stomach with either no prior evidence of *H pylori* infection or persistent disease after antibiotics (62). Patients were treated to 30 Gy to the stomach and adjacent lymph nodes. Ninety-six percent of patients obtained a biopsy proven complete response (CR). Four year freedom from treatment failure was 89% ± 5%, and the cause-specific survival was 100%. At Princess Margaret, between 1989 and 2004, 25 patients were treated with IFRT for stage I and II gastric MALT lymphoma (63). Most patients had no prior evidence of *H.pylori* infection or had persistent/

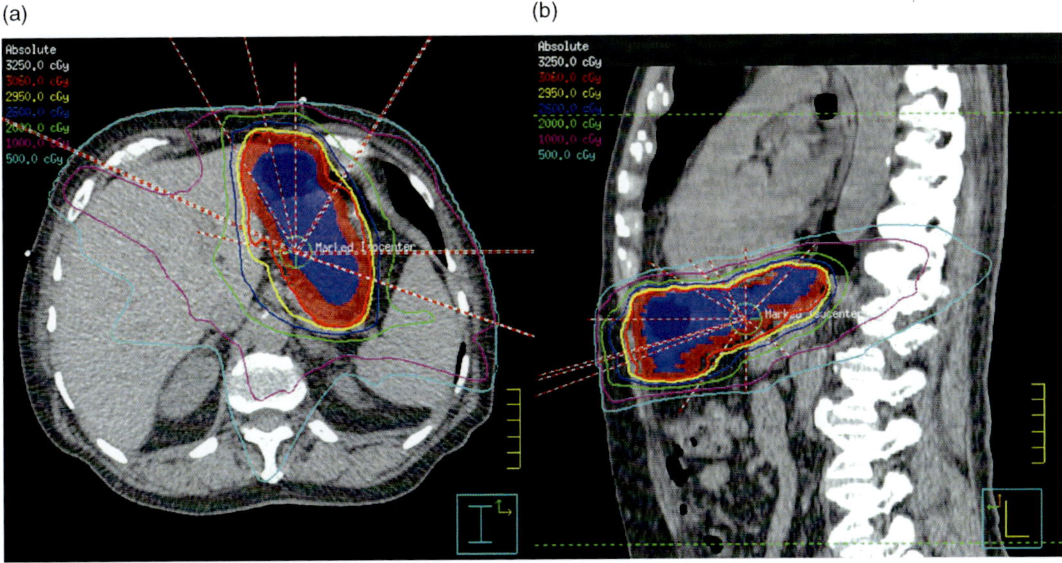

FIGURE 1   Intensity-modulated radiation therapy for gastric mucosa-associated lymphoid tissue (MALT) lymphoma.

Axial (a) and sagittal (b) representative slices of a patient treated for gastric mucosa-associated lymphoid tissue lymphoma of the gastric body and fundus. The patient was simulated on a wing board, with his arms above his head and hands grasping a T-bar. He was *nil per os* 4 hours before the four-dimensional computed tomography–based simulation. An internal target volume that contained the stomach and perigastric lymph nodes (ITV) was created based on 10 phases of the respiratory cycle. The planning target volume was treated to 30 Gy in 20 daily fractions with a 7 field 6 MV photon intensity-modulated radiation therapy–based plan. Daily cone beam computed tomography was used for setup and target verification.

progressive disease after antibiotic therapy. The stomach, perigastric, and celiac lymph nodes were targeted to 30 to 35 Gy. The 10 year recurrence free rate was 92%. Several other retrospective series have reported similar outcomes (64–66). Taken together, these data support the efficacy of IFRT in the treatment of early stage MALT lymphoma of the stomach.

In cases of disseminated stage III and IV disease, typically, the treatment approach parallels that of other indolent lymphomas, such as follicular lymphoma. Observation may be considered, unless the patient is symptomatic (especially GI bleeding), has threatened end organ damage, has bulky or steady progressive disease, is a candidate for a clinical trial, or prefers treatment. In these cases, locoregional radiotherapy can be an excellent treatment modality because of the minimal toxicity. Chemoimmunotherapy can be also considered.

Overall, radiotherapy to the stomach and perigastric lymph nodes to a dose of 30 Gy is well tolerated. The most common acute side effects are nausea, vomiting, and anorexia. These symptoms can be well controlled by antiemetic medications, especially when they are prophylactically administered 1 to 2 hours before radiotherapy. Late side effects are minimal if the dose constraints for organs at risk are respected. Long-term complications because of gastric mucosal damage are not expected at doses of 30 Gy. Some studies suggest a slightly increased risk of secondary malignancy (67–69).

Treatment of Nongastric MALT Lymphoma

Antibiotic therapy for nongastric MALT is more controversial and is currently under investigation. In the case of ocular adnexal MALT lymphoma, an Italian series has reported a prevalence *C. psittaci* infection in 80% of patients, thus providing the rationale for an antimicrobial approach to therapy (6). Other U.S.-based series, however, have not demonstrated an association between *C. psittaci* infection and ocular MALT lymphoma (70,71), suggesting geographical variance in the pathogenesis of this disease. In an Italian-based study, eradication of the bacteria with doxycycline led to complete or partial disease regression in 44% of cases (four of nine patients). The International Extranodal Lymphoma Study Group (IELSG) has an ongoing prospective phase II trial (IELSG 27) to investigate the therapeutic utility of antibiotic therapy for *C. psittaci* eradication in patients with *C. psittaci* positive ocular adnexal MALT lymphoma.

The most common treatment approach for stage I and II nongastric MALT lymphoma is monotherapy-involved field radiation treatment. CT-based planning is essential, especially in cases where limiting normal tissue toxicity is imperative. The most common prescribed dose is 30 Gy in 20 daily fractions. Lower doses (24–25 Gy) may be used for in orbital cases in an effort to spare ocular structures, although a recent retrospective series suggests that doses less than 30.6 Gy result in inferior local control in ocular adnexal MALT lymphoma (72). Several single-institution series have reported excellent outcomes with primary IFRT for the initial management of nongastric MALT lymphoma, with local control and overall survival rates of more than 90% (63,73–77). Surgery can be considered, although undesirable, for some sites (breast, lung, and colon); however, in cases of positive margins, adjuvant radiotherapy is recommended. Therefore, preoperatively, if complete surgical resection is not thought to be feasible, patients should be treated with radiation monotherapy to avoid the morbidity of two treatment modalities. In one multi-institutional series of patients with salivary MALT treated with monotherapy or combined therapy (surgery, radiation or chemotherapy), radiation therapy was the only treatment modality that improved 5 year disease-free survival, with rates of 34.4% when no radiation was used and 66.1% when radiotherapy was administered (77).

The treatment of disseminated disease can vary from a single alkylating agent (cyclophosphamide or chlorambucil) to Fludarabine with a reported CR of 75%. Anthracycline-based chemotherapy has to be reserved for histological transformation, bulky mass, or high LDH. Recently, rituximab has been reported to induce an overall response rate of roughly 75% (78,79).

Follow-Up

After definitive radiotherapy for nongastric MALT lymphoma, patients can be followed clinically every 3 to 6 months for 5 years and then as indicated thereafter. All patients treated for gastric MALT lymphoma should be restaged 3 to 6 months posttreatment with endoscopy and biopsy. Biopsy is important to rule out persistent disease or large cell lymphoma. Subsequently, patients are followed clinically every 3 to 6 months for 5 years and then annually or as clinically indicated. Patients with disease refractory to radiotherapy are typically managed with systemic therapies, similar to those used for patients with follicular lymphoma.

In the population of patients initially treated with antibiotics for *H. pylori* positive disease that ultimately fail anti-microbial treatment and have persistent *H. pylori* infection coupled with persistent biopsy proven lymphoma, radiotherapy or second-line antibiotic treatment are both feasible options. In patients that harbor persistent lymphoma after successful eradication of *H.pylori* however, radiation is indicated, although the timing of treatment is somewhat controversial. It is reasonable to continue to observe these patients for an additional 3 months to await regression of the lymphoma. However, in the case of symptomatic patients with persistent lymphomatous disease, radiotherapy should be administered without an observation period.

■ NODAL MARGINAL ZONE LYMPHOMA

Pathogenesis

Nodal MZL is a rare disease entity, representing less than 2% of all lymphomas (80). It was first described in 1986 as a nodal monocytoid B-cell lymphoma (81). Fifteen years later, it was recognized by the WHO Classification as a category of marginal zone lymphoma (82). The cell origin, as previously mentioned, is thought to be a postgerminal center marginal zone memory B cell. In contrast with other MZLs, nodal MZL cases have not been commonly associated with autoimmune disorders. Some Italian and Spanish series have reported an association with Hepatitis C virus (HCV) (83,84), and there have been a few cases suggesting an association with the Sjögren syndrome (85).

Nodal MZL often poses a diagnostic dilemma, because there are no disease-defining characteristics; it is largely it is a diagnosis of exclusion. To date, no distinctive cytogenetic or immunological abnormalities have been reported for the disease entity as a whole. Cytogenetic analysis is most helpful in identifying hallmark abnormalities of other lymphomas that must be ruled out at the time of diagnosis.

Clinical Presentation and Workup

Affected patients are typically diagnosed in their 50s or early 60s (86,87). Patients may present with peripheral nodal involvement (typically cervical or inguinal) or with abdominal or thoracic lymphadenopathy. Disseminated stage III or IV disease at presentation is typical, with bone marrow involvement in roughly half of the cases and, less commonly, peripheral blood involvement. B symptoms are usually absent. In contrast with other marginal zone lymphomas, these patients also tend to present with poorer performance status (88).

For diagnosis, as is the case for all lymphomas, excisional or incisional nodal biopsy should be performed to provide an adequate diagnostic specimen. The immunophenotype of nodal MZL mirrors extranodal MZL, which can be helpful when trying to exclude other disease entities such as mantle cell lymphoma, follicular lymphoma, lymphoplasmacytic lymphoma, and chronic lymphocytic leukemia. B-cell markers CD 19, CD20 and CD 22 are present. They express surface immunoglobulin (mainly IgM subtype). They are negative for CD 5, CD 10, and CD 23. In many cases, Bcl-2 expression is present. Cytogenetic analysis can be of diagnostic utility in narrowing the differential diagnosis. Despite these efforts, discriminating nodal MZL from other small B lymphomas can be difficult, especially because other lymphomas can have marginal zone differentiation patterns that can masquerade as nodal MZL.

Workup should include CBC with peripheral smear, comprehensive metabolic panel, CT imaging of the neck, chest, abdomen, and pelvis, and a bilateral bone marrow biopsy. It is imperative that extranodal sites of involvement are excluded, because this would suggest a diagnosis of extranodal MZL. For example, in patients that present with cervical nodes, proper evaluation should be performed to exclude ocular, parotid, thyroid and salivary gland involvement.

Treatment

The management of patients with nodal MZL is somewhat controversial but typically parallels treatment for indolent follicular lymphoma. Radiotherapy can be a component of treatment; however, systemic therapy usually predominates, because patients often present with disseminated disease. However, in the case of stage I or II disease, radiation can provide excellent responses, with one series reporting a complete response in 96% of patients treated with single modality radiotherapy for stage I and II disease (88). This is in contrast with patients with early stage disease who were treated with chemotherapy alone who had a CR 67% of the time.

In the setting of advanced stage III and IV disease, the role of radiotherapy is limited to palliation of locally symptomatic disease. It is interesting to note that very low doses of palliative radiation can be effective in local disease control and alleviation of symptoms. The Institut Gustave Roussy pioneered the early studies on low-dose palliative radiotherapy for indolent lymphoma. This concept emerged after an unpublished clinical observation by Ganem and colleagues in 1984 after a patient with a symptomatic bulky abdominal mass had a dramatic clinical response to therapy after 2 Gy of a planned 24 Gy course of radiotherapy (89). Subsequently, the Gustave Russy experience of low-dose radiotherapy in 37 patients was reported in 1994 (4 Gy in two fractions within 3 days, i.e. "boom boom") (90). Since then, several series reporting a mean complete response rate of 55% with a median duration of 15 to 42 months have been published (89).

Prognosis and Follow-Up

Of all the marginal zone lymphomas, some data suggest that nodal MZL tends to have the worse prognosis with 5 year overall survival ranging from 55% to 79% and 5 year freedom from failure survival of 28% (80,86,88,91). A recent retrospective analysis, however, of 275 patients with nodal, extranodal and splenic MZL found that patients with nodal and extranodal MZL have similar outcomes (41). The optimal treatment strategy for these patients has not been established, and as such, treatment on a clinical trial should be considered. Follow-up consists of clinical assessment every 3 to 6 months for up to 5 years with surveillance imaging every 6 months for the first 2 years and not more than annually thereafter.

■ SPLENIC MARGINAL ZONE LYMPHOMA

Pathogenesis

In 1992, the term splenic marginal zone lymphoma was first used to describe a low-grade B-cell lymphoma of the spleen in which a nodular cellular infiltrate occupied the marginal zone (92). It was later recognized that splenic lymphoma with villous lymphocytes (SLVL), a disorder reported several years earlier, was, in fact, an overlapping disease process (93,94). This clinical entity had been characterized by splenomegaly and the presence of lymphoma cells in the peripheral blood and bone marrow that possessed condensed chromatin, round nuclei, and short villi. Splenic marginal zone lymphoma is now recognized as a separate entity within the WHO Classification (95).

The pathogenesis of splenic MZL is not well characterized. It is a rare disease, representing less than 2% of all lymphomatous neoplasms. A recent retrospective study of 330 cases was reported, describing the recurrent chromosomal abnormalities in splenic MZL, which are distinct from other B cell–derived lymphomas. The most common genetic alteration is 7q31 deletion, but this still is only present in less than half of the cases, and a hallmark aberration has not been identified (96). Some postulate that there is a pathologic role for HCV, because splenic MZL has been reported in increased frequency in patients with HCV infection (97).

Clinical Presentation, Workup, and Diagnosis

Most patients present in the sixth decade of life or older with splenomegaly and lymphocytosis without peripheral lymphadenopathy. Cytopenias (typically anemia and thrombocytopenia) related to hypersplenism can happen later in the disease process. B symptoms are typically absent. Bone marrow involvement is the rule, occurring in roughly 85% to 100% of cases, whereas peripheral blood infiltration is less common (25%–65%) (84,91,98–100). A monoclonal M component (typically IgM kappa) has been identified in 13% to 42% of patients (84,91,98–100).

The gold standard for diagnosis is a splenectomy specimen; however, the diagnosis of splenic MZL can be made based on bone marrow involvement in the presence or absence of lymphomatous peripheral blood infiltration in a patient with splenomegaly. There is no specific immuno type in splenic MZL; however, the neoplastic cells do strongly express CD 20. In most cases, Bcl-2 is positive.

Workup should include physical examination, CBC with smear, comprehensive metabolic panel, hepatitis C testing, CT imaging of the chest, abdomen and pelvis, and bilateral bone marrow biopsy. A monoclonal B cell population is identified with flow cytometry of bone marrow or peripheral blood specimen. Serum protein electrophoresis (SPEP) and or quantitative immunoglobulin levels should also be obtained. In cases where rituximab is being considered, Hepatitis B testing should be performed as a result of the risk of reactivation.

Treatment

As the median survival in this disease is 13 years (99) and untreated patients have been reported to have a 5 year survival of 88% (101), long-term observation is feasible, with treatment directed at symptomatic patients. In the absence of splenomegaly or cytopenias, observation is appropriate. In symptomatic patients, HCV status should be determined. Patients with evidence of HCV infection and no contraindications to treatment should be treated by a hepatologist, because complete remission of splenic MZL has been reported after successful antiviral therapy (102).

Because the recognition of splenic MZL is a distinct clinical entity, splenectomy has been the preferred treatment, with 5 year overall survival of 71% to 90%. Splenectomy, however, is not without operative morbidity and mortality, especially in an older patient population. There have only been a few reports of splenic irradiation for the management of splenic MZL. In most reported series, radiotherapy was reserved for patients who were poor surgical candidates or had failed systemic therapy (98,103). Currently, there is no role for radiotherapy in the treatment of patients with splenic MZL.

Rituximab, a chimeric monoclonal antibody to CD-20, has been shown in retrospective series to be extremely effective as an alternative to splenectomy in splenic MZL as monotherapy (104–107). In addition to sparing operative morbidity and mortality in an often elderly patient population, rituximab has the added potential advantage over splenectomy in that disease outside of the spleen (especially the bone marrow) is addressed. In one retrospective study comparing 25 patients who received rituximab monotherapy to 10 patients managed with initial splenectomy, 92% of patients who received rituximab had resolution of splenomegaly (104). Rituximab was superior to splenectomy in normalizing white blood cell, absolute lymphocyte counts and platelet counts. Last, 56% (10 of 18) of patients in the rituximab group had clearance of bone marrow after treatment compared with 0% of the splenectomy patients who had post-splenectomy bone marrow evaluation (nine patients).

Follow-Up

Most patients can be followed clinically for 3 to 6 months from 5 years and then as clinically indicated thereafter. In the setting of disease progression despite first line management or in the case of advanced disease, patients are managed according to guidelines for advanced stage follicular lymphoma. After an average of 3 years postdiagnosis, 13% to 19% of cases can transform to high-grade lymphoma. In these aggressive cases with poor outcome, therapy should mirror that of diffuse large B-cell lymphoma (108,109).

■ CONCLUSION

Extranodal, nodal, and splenic marginal zone lymphomas are a group of heterogenous indolent lymphomas that share a common cell of origin. The prognosis of MZL, in general, is excellent; therefore, a primary goal of treatment is limiting long-term toxicity. Radiotherapy for early stage nodal and extranodal MZL is an excellent primary treatment modality with low morbidity in the setting of treatment delivery advances, dose deescalation, and field size reductions.

■ REFERENCES

1. Swerdlow S.H. CE, Harris N.L. et al. *who classification of tumours of haematopoietic and lymphoid tissues.* Lyon, France: IARC; 2008.

2. A clinical evaluation of the International Lymphoma Study Group classification of non-Hodgkin's lymphoma: the non-Hodgkin's lymphoma classification project. *Blood.* 1997;89:3909–3918.

3. Sagaert X, Sprangers B, De Wolf-Peeters C. The dynamics of the B follicle: understanding the normal counterpart of B-cell-derived malignancies. *Leukemia.* 2007;21:1378–1386.

4. Isaacson PG. Update on MALT lymphomas. *Best Pract Res Clin Haematol.* 2005;18:57–68.

5. Zinzani PL, Magagnoli M, Galieni P, et al. Nongastrointestinal low-grade mucosa-associated lymphoid tissue lymphoma: analysis of 75 patients. *J Clin Oncol.* 1999;17:1254.

6. Ferreri AJ, Guidoboni M, Ponzoni M, et al. Evidence for an association between Chlamydia psittaci and ocular adnexal lymphomas. *J Natl Cancer Inst.* 2004;96:586–594.

7. Royer B, Cazals-Hatem D, Sibilia J, et al. Lymphomas in patients with Sjogren's syndrome are marginal zone B-cell neoplasms, arise in diverse extranodal and nodal sites, and are not associated with viruses. *Blood.* 1997;90:766–775.

8. Derringer GA, Thompson LD, Frommelt RA, et al. Malignant lymphoma of the thyroid gland: a clinicopathologic study of 108 cases. *Am J Surg Pathol.* 2000;24:623–639.

9. Wotherspoon AC, Finn TM, Isaacson PG. Trisomy 3 in low-grade B-cell lymphomas of mucosa-associated lymphoid tissue. *Blood.* 1995;85:2000–2004.

10. Rinaldi A, Mian M, Chigrinova E, et al. Genome-wide DNA profiling of marginal zone lymphomas identifies subtype-specific lesions with an impact on the clinical outcome. *Blood*. 117:1595–1604.

11. Sagaert X, Laurent M, Baens M, et al. MALT1 and BCL10 aberrations in MALT lymphomas and their effect on the expression of BCL10 in the tumour cells. *Mod Pathol*. 2006;19:225–232.

12. Streubel B, Simonitsch-Klupp I, Mullauer L, et al. Variable frequencies of MALT lymphoma-associated genetic aberrations in MALT lymphomas of different sites. *Leukemia*. 2004;18:1722–1726.

13. Dierlamm J, Baens M, Wlodarska I, et al. The apoptosis inhibitor gene API2 and a novel 18q gene, MLT, are recurrently rearranged in the t(11;18)(q21;q21) associated with mucosa-associated lymphoid tissue lymphomas. *Blood*. 1999;93:3601–3609.

14. Zhang Q, Siebert R, Yan M, et al. Inactivating mutations and overexpression of BCL10, a caspase recruitment domain-containing gene, in MALT lymphoma with t(1;14)(p22;q32). *Nat Genet*. 1999;22:63–68.

15. Schreuder MI, Hoeve MA, Hebeda KM, et al. Mutual exclusion of t(11;18)(q21;q21) and numerical chromosomal aberrations in the development of different types of primary gastric lymphomas. *Br J Haematol*. 2003;123:590–599.

16. Alpen B, Neubauer A, Dierlamm J, et al. Translocation t(11;18) absent in early gastric marginal zone B-cell lymphoma of MALT type responding to eradication of Helicobacter pylori infection. *Blood*. 2000;95:4014–4015.

17. Liu H, Ruskon-Fourmestraux A, Lavergne-Slove A, et al. Resistance of t(11;18) positive gastric mucosa-associated lymphoid tissue lymphoma to Helicobacter pylori eradication therapy. *Lancet*. 2001;357:39–40.

18. Ruland J, Duncan GS, Elia A, et al. Bcl10 is a positive regulator of antigen receptor-induced activation of NF-kappaB and neural tube closure. *Cell*. 2001;104:33–42.

19. Ruefli-Brasse AA, French DM, Dixit VM. Regulation of NF-kappaB-dependent lymphocyte activation and development by paracaspase. *Science*. 2003;302:1581–1584.

20. Ruland J, Duncan GS, Wakeham A, et al. Differential requirement for Malt1 in T and B cell antigen receptor signaling. *Immunity*. 2003;19:749–758.

21. Goossens T, Klein U, Kuppers R. Frequent occurrence of deletions and duplications during somatic hypermutation: implications for oncogene translocations and heavy chain disease. *Proc Natl Acad Sci USA*. 1998;95:2463–2468.

22. Wyatt JI, Rathbone BJ. Immune response of the gastric mucosa to Campylobacter pylori. *Scand J Gastroenterol Suppl*. 1988;142:44–49.

23. Stolte M, Eidt S. Lymphoid follicles in antral mucosa: immune response to Campylobacter pylori? *J Clin Pathol*. 1989;42:1269–1271.

24. Genta RM, Hamner HW, Graham DY. Gastric lymphoid follicles in Helicobacter pylori infection: frequency, distribution, and response to triple therapy. *Hum Pathol*. 1993;24:577–583.

25. Wotherspoon AC, Ortiz-Hidalgo C, Falzon MR, et al. Helicobacter pylori-associated gastritis and primary B-cell gastric lymphoma. *Lancet* 1991;338:1175–1176.

26. Eidt S, Stolte M, Fischer R. Helicobacter pylori gastritis and primary gastric non-Hodgkin's lymphomas. *J Clin Pathol* 1994;47:436–439.

27. Nakamura S, Yao T, Aoyagi K, et al. Helicobacter pylori and primary gastric lymphoma. A histopathologic and immunohistochemical analysis of 237 patients. *Cancer*. 1997;79:3–11.

28. Enno A, O'Rourke JL, Howlett CR, et al. MALToma-like lesions in the murine gastric mucosa after long-term infection with Helicobacter felis: a mouse model of Helicobacter pylori-induced gastric lymphoma. *Am J Pathol*. 1995;147:217–222.

29. Hussell T, Isaacson PG, Crabtree JE, et al. The response of cells from low-grade B-cell gastric lymphomas of mucosa-associated lymphoid tissue to Helicobacter pylori. *Lancet*. 1993;342:571–574.

30. Welsh JS, Howard A, Hong HY, et al. Synchronous bilateral breast mucosa-associated lymphoid tissue lymphomas addressed with primary radiation therapy. *Am J Clin Oncol*. 2006;29:634–635.

31. Zucca E, Conconi A, Pedrinis E, et al. Nongastric marginal zone B-cell lymphoma of mucosa-associated lymphoid tissue. *Blood*. 2003;101:2489–2495.

32. Tu PH, Giannini C, Judkins AR, et al. Clinicopathologic and genetic profile of intracranial marginal zone lymphoma: a primary low-grade CNS lymphoma that mimics meningioma. *J Clin Oncol*. 2005;23:5718–5727.

33. George AC, Ozsahin M, Janzer R, et al. Primary intracranial dural lymphoma of mucosa-associated lymphoid tissue (MALT) type: report of one case and review of the literature. *Bull Cancer*. 2005;92:E51–56.

34. Servitje O, Gallardo F, Estrach T, et al. Primary cutaneous marginal zone B-cell lymphoma: a clinical, histopathological, immunophenotypic and molecular genetic study of 22 cases. *Br J Dermatol*. 2002;147:1147–1158.

35. Ferry JA, Fung CY, Zukerberg L, et al. Lymphoma of the ocular adnexa: A study of 353 cases. *Am J Surg Pathol*. 2007;31:170–184.

36. Troch M, Formanek M, Streubel B, et al. Clinicopathological aspects of mucosa-associated lymphoid tissue (MALT) lymphoma of the parotid gland: a retrospective single-center analysis of 28 cases. *Head Neck*. 2011;33:763–767.

37. Borie R, Wislez M, Thabut G, et al. Clinical characteristics and prognostic factors of pulmonary MALT lymphoma. *Eur Respir J*. 2009;34:1408–1416.

38. Anscombe AM, Wright DH. Primary malignant lymphoma of the thyroid—a tumour of mucosa-associated lymphoid tissue: review of seventy-six cases. *Histopathology*. 1985;9:81–97.

39. Koch P, del Valle F, Berdel WE, et al. Primary gastrointestinal non-Hodgkin's lymphoma: I. Anatomic and histologic distribution, clinical features, and survival data of 371 patients registered in the German Multicenter Study GIT NHL 01/92. *J Clin Oncol.* 2001;19:3861–3873.

40. Thieblemont C, Berger F, Dumontet C, et al. Mucosa-associated lymphoid tissue lymphoma is a disseminated disease in one third of 158 patients analyzed. *Blood.* 2000;95:802–806.

41. Mazloom A, Medeiros LJ, McLaughlin PW, et al. Marginal zone lymphomas: factors that affect the final outcome. *Cancer.* 2010;116:4291–4298.

42. Bertoni F, Sanna P, Tinguely M, et al. Association of gastric and Waldeyer's ring lymphoma: a molecular study. *Hematol Oncol.* 2000;18:15–19.

43. Dabaja BS, Ha CS, Wilder RB, et al. Importance of esophagogastroduodenoscopy in the evaluation of nongastrointestinal mucosa-associated lymphoid tissue lymphoma. *Cancer J.* 2003;9:321–324.

44. Mazloom A, Rodriguez A, Ha CS, et al. Incidence of gastric involvement in patients with nongastrointestinal extranodal marginal zone lymphoma. *Cancer.* 2011;117(11):2461–2466.

45. Alinari L, Castellucci P, Elstrom R, et al. 18F-FDG PET in mucosa-associated lymphoid tissue (MALT) lymphoma. *Leuk Lymphoma.* 2006;47:2096–2101.

46. Beal KP, Yeung HW, Yahalom J. FDG-PET scanning for detection and staging of extranodal marginal zone lymphomas of the MALT type: a report of 42 cases. *Ann Oncol.* 2005;16:473–480.

47. Wang G, Auerbach A, Wei M, et al. t(11;18)(q21;q21) in extranodal marginal zone B-cell lymphoma of mucosa-associated lymphoid tissue in stomach: a study of 48 cases. *Mod Pathol.* 2009;22:79–86.

48. Montalban C, Castrillo JM, Abraira V, et al. Gastric B-cell mucosa-associated lymphoid tissue (MALT) lymphoma. Clinicopathological study and evaluation of the prognostic factors in 143 patients. *Ann Oncol.* 1995;6:355–362.

49. Sackmann M, Morgner A, Rudolph B, et al. Regression of gastric MALT lymphoma after eradication of Helicobacter pylori is predicted by endosonographic staging. MALT Lymphoma Study Group. *Gastroenterology.* 1997;113:1087–1090.

50. Ruskone-Fourmestraux A, Lavergne A, Aegerter PH, et al. Predictive factors for regression of gastric MALT lymphoma after anti-Helicobacter pylori treatment. *Gut.* 2001;48:297–303.

51. Rohatiner A, d'Amore F, Coiffier B, et al. Report on a workshop convened to discuss the pathological and staging classifications of gastrointestinal tract lymphoma. *Ann Oncol.* 1994;5:397–400.

52. Ruskone-Fourmestraux A, Dragosics B, Morgner A, et al. Paris staging system for primary gastrointestinal lymphomas. *Gut.* 2003;52:912–913.

53. Radaszkiewicz T, Dragosics B, Bauer P. Gastrointestinal malignant lymphomas of the mucosa-associated lymphoid tissue: factors relevant to prognosis. *Gastroenterology.* 1992;102:1628–1638.

54. Thieblemont C, Bastion Y, Berger F, et al. Mucosa-associated lymphoid tissue gastrointestinal and nongastrointestinal lymphoma behavior: analysis of 108 patients. *J Clin Oncol.* 1997;15:1624–1630.

55. Wundisch T, Thiede C, Morgner A, et al. Long-term follow-up of gastric MALT lymphoma after Helicobacter pylori eradication. *J Clin Oncol.* 2005;23:8018–8024.

56. Bayerdorffer E, Neubauer A, Rudolph B, et al. Regression of primary gastric lymphoma of mucosa-associated lymphoid tissue type after cure of Helicobacter pylori infection. MALT Lymphoma Study Group. *Lancet.* 1995;345:1591–1594.

57. Cohen SM, Petryk M, Varma M, et al. Non-Hodgkin's lymphoma of mucosa-associated lymphoid tissue. *Oncologist.* 2006;11:1100–1117.

58. Chey WD, Wong BC. American College of Gastroenterology guideline on the management of Helicobacter pylori infection. *Am J Gastroenterol.* 2007;102:1808–1825.

59. Koch P, del Valle F, Berdel WE, et al. Primary gastrointestinal non-Hodgkin's lymphoma: II. Combined surgical and conservative or conservative management only in localized gastric lymphoma—results of the prospective German Multicenter Study GIT NHL 01/92. *J Clin Oncol.* 2001;19:3874–3883.

60. Schechter NR, Portlock CS, Yahalom J. Treatment of mucosa-associated lymphoid tissue lymphoma of the stomach with radiation alone. *J Clin Oncol.* 1998;16:1916–1921.

61. Nakamura S, Matsumoto T, Suekane H, et al. Predictive value of endoscopic ultrasonography for regression of gastric low grade and high grade MALT lymphomas after eradication of Helicobacter pylori. *Gut.* 2001;48:454–460.

62. Yahalom J. H. Pylori-Independent MALT Lymphoma of the Stomach: 10-Year Experience with 51 Patients Treated with Radiation Alone. *Cancer J.* 2003;9:495.

63. Goda JS, Gospodarowicz M, Pintilie M, et al. Long-term outcome in localized extranodal mucosa-associated lymphoid tissue lymphomas treated with radiotherapy. *Cancer.* 2010;116:3815–3824.

64. Vrieling C, de Jong D, Boot H, et al. Long-term results of stomach-conserving therapy in gastric MALT lymphoma. *Radiother Oncol.* 2008;87:405–411.

65. Yamashita H, Nakagawa K, Asari T, et al. Radiotherapy for 41 patients with stages I and II MALT lymphoma: a retrospective study. *Radiother Oncol.* 2008;87:412–417.

66. Tomita N, Kodaira T, Tachibana H, et al. Favorable outcomes of radiotherapy for early-stage mucosa-associated lymphoid tissue lymphoma. *Radiother Oncol.* 2009;90:231–235.

67. Raderer M, Streubel B, Wohrer S, et al. Metachronous gastric MALT lymphoma and early gastric cancer. *Ann Oncol.* 2006;17:724.

68. Morgner A, Miehlke S, Stolte M, et al. Development of early gastric cancer 4 and 5 years after complete remission of Helicobacter pylori associated gastric low grade marginal zone B cell lymphoma of MALT type. *World J Gastroenterol*. 2001;7:248–253.

69. Hamaloglu E, Topaloglu S, Ozdemir A, et al. Synchronous and metachronous occurrence of gastric adenocarcinoma and gastric lymphoma: a review of the literature. *World J Gastroenterol*. 2006;12:3564–3574.

70. Rosado MF, Byrne GE, Jr., Ding F, et al. Ocular adnexal lymphoma: a clinicopathologic study of a large cohort of patients with no evidence for an association with Chlamydia psittaci. *Blood*. 2006;107:467–472.

71. Vargas RL, Fallone E, Felgar RE, et al. Is there an association between ocular adnexal lymphoma and infection with Chlamydia psittaci? The University of Rochester experience. *Leuk Res*. 2006;30:547–551.

72. Bayraktar S, Bayraktar UD, Stefanovic A, et al. Primary ocular adnexal mucosa-associated lymphoid tissue lymphoma (MALT): single institution experience in a large cohort of patients. *Br J Haematol*. 2011;152:72–80.

73. Isobe K, Kagami Y, Higuchi K, et al. A multicenter phase II study of local radiation therapy for stage IEA mucosa-associated lymphoid tissue lymphomas: a preliminary report from the Japan Radiation Oncology Group (JAROG). *Int J Radiat Oncol Biol Phys*. 2007;69:1181–1186.

74. Tsang RW, Gospodarowicz MK, Pintilie M, et al. Stage I and II MALT lymphoma: results of treatment with radiotherapy. *Int J Radiat Oncol Biol Phys*. 2001;50:1258–1264.

75. Tsang RW, Gospodarowicz MK, Pintilie M, et al. Localized mucosa-associated lymphoid tissue lymphoma treated with radiation therapy has excellent clinical outcome. *J Clin Oncol*. 2003;21:4157–4164.

76. Son SH, Choi BO, Kim GW, et al. Primary radiation therapy in patients with localized orbital marginal zone B-cell lymphoma of mucosa-associated lymphoid tissue (MALT Lymphoma). *Int J Radiat Oncol Biol Phys*. 2010;77:86–91.

77. Anacak Y, Miller RC, Constantinou N, et al. Primary mucosa-associated lymphoid tissue lymphoma of the salivary glands: a multicenter Rare Cancer Network study. *Int J Radiat Oncol Biol Phys*. 2012;82:315–320.

78. Hammel P, Haioun C, Chaumette MT, et al. Efficacy of single-agent chemotherapy in low-grade B-cell mucosa-associated lymphoid tissue lymphoma with prominent gastric expression. *J Clin Oncol*. 1995;13:2524–2529.

79. Martinelli G, Laszlo D, Ferreri AJ, et al. Clinical activity of rituximab in gastric marginal zone non-Hodgkin's lymphoma resistant to or not eligible for anti-Helicobacter pylori therapy. *J Clin Oncol*. 2005;23:1979–1983.

80. Nathwani BN, Anderson JR, Armitage JO, et al. Marginal zone B-cell lymphoma: a clinical comparison of nodal and mucosa-associated lymphoid tissue types. Non-Hodgkin's Lymphoma Classification Project. *J Clin Oncol*. 1999;17:2486–2492.

81. Sheibani K, Sohn CC, Burke JS, et al. Monocytoid B-cell lymphoma: a novel B-cell neoplasm. *Am J Pathol*. 1986;124:310–318.

82. Ottensmeier C. The classification of lymphomas and leukemias. *Chem Biol Interact*. 2001;135–136:653–664.

83. Luppi M, Longo G, Ferrari MG, et al. Prevalence of HCV infection and second neoplasms in marginal zone lymphomas. *Br J Haematol*. 1997;96:873–874.

84. Arcaini L, Paulli M, Boveri E, et al. Splenic and nodal marginal zone lymphomas are indolent disorders at high hepatitis C virus seroprevalence with distinct presenting features but similar morphologic and phenotypic profiles. *Cancer*. 2004;100:107–115.

85. Mariette X. Lymphomas in patients with Sjogren's syndrome: review of the literature and physiopathologic hypothesis. *Leuk Lymphoma*. 1999;33:93–99.

86. Traverse-Glehen A, Felman P, Callet-Bauchu E, et al. A clinicopathological study of nodal marginal zone B-cell lymphoma. A report on 21 cases. *Histopathology*. 2006;48:162–173.

87. Arcaini L, Lucioni M, Boveri E, et al. Nodal marginal zone lymphoma: current knowledge and future directions of an heterogeneous disease. *Eur J Haematol*. 2009;83:165–174.

88. Oh SY, Ryoo BY, Kim WS, et al. Nongastric marginal zone B-cell lymphoma: analysis of 247 cases. *Am J Hematol*. 2007;82:446–452.

89. Ganem G, Cartron G, Girinsky T, et al. Localized low-dose radiotherapy for follicular lymphoma: history, clinical results, mechanisms of action, and future outlooks. *Int J Radiat Oncol Biol Phys*. 2010;78:975–982.

90. Ganem G, Lambin P, Socie G, et al. Potential role for low dose limited-field radiation therapy (2 × 2 grays) in advanced low-grade non-Hodgkin's lymphomas. *Hematol Oncol*. 1994;12:1–8.

91. Berger F, Felman P, Thieblemont C, et al. Non-MALT marginal zone B-cell lymphomas: a description of clinical presentation and outcome in 124 patients. *Blood*. 2000;95:1950–1956.

92. Schmid C, Kirkham N, Diss T, et al. Splenic marginal zone cell lymphoma. *Am J Surg Pathol*. 1992;16:455–466.

93. Spriano P, Barosi G, Invernizzi R, et al. Splenomegalic immunocytoma with circulating hairy cells: report of eight cases and revision of the literature. *Haematologica*. 1986;71:25–33.

94. Melo JV, Robinson DS, Gregory C, et al. Splenic B cell lymphoma with "villous" lymphocytes in the peripheral blood: a disorder distinct from hairy cell leukemia. *Leukemia*. 1987;1:294–298.

95. Jaffe E.S. HNL, Stein H, Vardiman JW. *Classification of tumours of haematopoietic and lymphoid tissues*. 3rd ed. Lyon, France: International Agency for Research on Cancer; 2001.

96. Salido M, Baro C, Oscier D, et al. Cytogenetic aberrations and their prognostic value in a series of 330 splenic marginal zone B-cell lymphomas: a multicenter

study of the Splenic B-Cell Lymphoma Group. *Blood.* 2010;116:1479–1488.

97. Mele A, Pulsoni A, Bianco E, et al. Hepatitis C virus and B-cell non-Hodgkin lymphomas: an Italian multicenter case-control study. *Blood.* 2003;102:996–999.

98. Chacon JI, Mollejo M, Munoz E, et al. Splenic marginal zone lymphoma: clinical characteristics and prognostic factors in a series of 60 patients. *Blood.* 2002;100:1648–1654.

99. Parry-Jones N, Matutes E, Gruszka-Westwood AM, et al. Prognostic features of splenic lymphoma with villous lymphocytes: a report on 129 patients. *Br J Haematol.* 2003;120:759–764.

100. Thieblemont C, Felman P, Callet-Bauchu E, et al. Splenic marginal-zone lymphoma: a distinct clinical and pathological entity. *Lancet Oncol.* 2003;4:95–103.

101. Troussard X, Valensi F, Duchayne E, et al. Splenic lymphoma with villous lymphocytes: clinical presentation, biology and prognostic factors in a series of 100 patients. Groupe Francais d'Hematologie Cellulaire (GFHC). *Br J Haematol.* 1996;93:731–736.

102. Hermine O, Lefrere F, Bronowicki JP, et al. Regression of splenic lymphoma with villous lymphocytes after treatment of hepatitis C virus infection. *N Engl J Med.* 2002;347:89–94.

103. Mulligan SP, Matutes E, Dearden C, et al. Splenic lymphoma with villous lymphocytes: natural history and response to therapy in 50 cases. *Br J Haematol.* 1991;78:206–209.

104. Tsimberidou AM, Catovsky D, Schlette E, et al. Outcomes in patients with splenic marginal zone lymphoma and marginal zone lymphoma treated with rituximab with or without chemotherapy or chemotherapy alone. *Cancer.* 2006;107:125–135.

105. Bennett M, Sharma K, Yegena S, et al. Rituximab monotherapy for splenic marginal zone lymphoma. *Haematologica.* 2005;90:856–858.

106. Bennett M, Yegena S, Dave HP, et al. Re: Rituximab monotherapy is highly effective in splenic marginal zone lymphoma. *Hematol Oncol.* 2008;26:114.

107. Kalpadakis C, Pangalis GA, Dimopoulou MN, et al. Rituximab monotherapy is highly effective in splenic marginal zone lymphoma. *Hematol Oncol.* 2007;25:127–131.

108. Camacho FI, Mollejo M, Mateo MS, et al. Progression to large B-cell lymphoma in splenic marginal zone lymphoma: a description of a series of 12 cases. *Am J Surg Pathol.* 2001;25:1268–1276.

109. Dungarwalla M, Appiah-Cubi S, Kulkarni S, et al. High-grade transformation in splenic marginal zone lymphoma with circulating villous lymphocytes: the site of transformation influences response to therapy and prognosis. *Br J Haematol.* 2008;143:71–74.

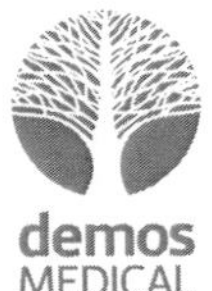 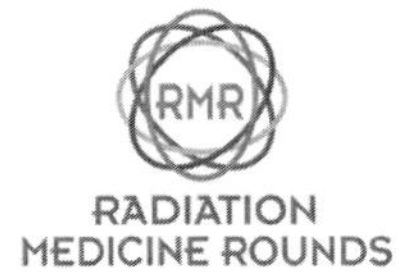

Mycosis Fungoides, Presentation, Diagnosis, and Treatment Strategy

Bouthaina S. Dabaja*

The University of Texas MD Anderson Cancer Center, Houston, TX

■ ABSTRACT

Cutaneous T-cell lymphoma is characterized by the accumulation of malignant T cells in the skin. There are multiple pathologic subtypes that translate into multiple clinical presentations. The diagnosis is often extremely challenging and patients might undergo a long course (years) of being misdiagnosed and mistreated. Therefore, accurate pathologic diagnosis of the subgroup is essential to determine the best therapy. Cutaneous T-cell lymphoma includes many entities; this chapter will address Mycosis Fungoides and its variants. We discuss the different pathologic subtypes, criteria of diagnosis, clinical presentation, treatment options, and outcome.

Keywords: mycosis fungoides, T cell lymphoma, radiation, total skin electron beam

■ INTRODUCTION

The diagnosis of T-cell lymphoma is of paramount importance to distinguish the different subtypes, that can range from a self-limiting disease that have the potential of self-regression like lymphomatoid papillomatosis to aggressive epidermotropic CD8+ CTCL associated with a worse clinical outcome and resistance to current therapy. Using the currently available immunophenotypic, molecular, cytogenetic testing and the histopathologic examination by an experienced pathologist is an unavoidable step before determining therapy. Patients should be staged and stratified according to prognostic factors in an attempt to determine survival/ prognosis; once this step is done, therapy can be tailored accordingly. Treatment has to take into consideration the patient's pathologic diagnosis, stage, comorbidities, and the long-term toxicities of the treatment; the latter should be avoided in patients with early stage disease with an expected long-term survival.

■ PATHOLOGY AND DIAGNOSIS OF MYCOSIS FUNGOIDES

The WHO/European Organization of Research and Treatment of Cancer (EORTC) classification (1) for cutaneous lymphoma divides cutaneous lymphomas according to the cell of origin into B and T cell.

Cutaneous T cell includes mycosis fungoides and its variants, adult T-cell leukemia/lymphoma, primary cutaneous CD30+ lymphoproliferative disorders, subcutaneous panniculitis, Extranodal NK/T-cell lymphoma, nasal type, and primary cutaneous peripheral T-cell lymphoma, unspecified.

* Corresponding author, The University of Texas MD Anderson Cancer Center, 1515 Holcombe Boulevard, Houston, TX

E-mail address: ccpinnix@mdanderson.org

Radiation Medicine Rounds 3:3 (2012) 421–436.

DOI: 10.5003/2151–4208.3.3.421

Mycosis Fungoides and Its Variants

This is an epidermotropic primary cutaneous lymphoma characterized by proliferation of CD4+ small- to medium-sized T lymphocytes with cerebriform nuclei. The disease evolves through different stages clinically (patch, plaque, and tumor) and each stage corresponds to a histopathological features.

Patches is the stage of disease that is commonly misdiagnosed due to non-specific features resembling spongiotic dermatitis (eczema), lichenoid dermatitis, or pigmented purpuric dermatosis. At this stage perinuclear halo, indian filing with lining of the lymphocytes in the basal epidermal layer can be seen, lymphocytes are not atypical, and Pautrier's micro-abscesses are less frequent.

Plaques are the stage that displays a more florid form of epidermal features of patches, more numerous micro-abscesses, collections of neoplastic lymphocytes within a non-spongiotic epidermis, and more appreciated cytologic atypia of lymphocytes.

In the *tumor* stage, the epidermal component of the earlier stages is lost and the disease is now in the full breath of the dermis with large population of lymphocytes, and marked atypia.

The presence of concurrent different stages in the skin is the rule since the tumor d'emblee occurrence is exceedingly rare.

Patients with *erythroderma* show similar features to the patches but with more sparse infiltrate, the sezary syndromes is defined with the presence of sezary cells with cerebriform nuclei in the peripheral blood of >1000/μL with an increased CD4/CD8 T lymphocytes ratio. Sezary cells secrete Th2 cytokines, IL-4 and, IL10–10, causing loss of cellular immunity due to decreased production of Th1 cytokines, interferon gamma, and interleukin2, resulting clinically in erythroderma, staphylococcus colonization, peripheral eosinophilia, increase IgE production, and intractable pruritus

Finally *transformed* mycosis is when cytologically high-grade cells appear and constitute at least 25% of the population.

Immunophenotyping also follow the order of clinical presentation. Lymphocytes at the patch stage are hard to differentiate from eczema they are well-differentiated and express normal complement of T-cell antigens.

Classically CD2, 3, 4, and 5 are positive; while CD45 RO+, CD8, and CD30 are negative.

But as the disease progresses, CD7 is lost and CD30 can be acquired with high grade transformation. Although the dominance of CD4+ is common

in MF, it is also the case of inflammatory dermatosis. There are also cases of abnormal immunophenotyping with CD8+ that are rare.

Polymerase chain reaction helps to identify a T-cell receptor gene and rearrangement can be found in 50% to 80% of cases. The γ region of the T-cell receptor gene is rearranged early on such that it can be readily detectable and expressed at the surface (2).

Chromosomal changes has been identified early in the disease, the extent of gains and losses in chromatin corresponds to the severity of the disease.

Chromosomal aberration included short arm of ch 17, long arm of 13, and was also reported in Ch 6, 7, 10. Loss of chromatin in Ch 6q, 10q, and 13q and gain Ch 7, 8q were associated with lower 5y survival rate (3,4)

Special Variants of MF include:

1. *Folliculotropic*: characterized by the presence of mucin accumulation in hair follicles, although not pathognomonic but the involvement of the hair follicles reflect the deep involvement and might have therapeutic implications (ineffectiveness of skin-directed approaches) (5).
2. *Granulomatous slack skin*: pendulous skin is the whole mark of the disease. Multinucleated giant cells destroy the normal elastic fiber network of the dermis.
3. Pagetoid Reticulosis: a verrucous variant which typically affects acral sites. This disease has a striking epidermotropism that displays variable immunophenotype: CD+/CD8-, CD4-/CD8+, or CD4-/CD8-.
4. *Transformed MF*: characterized by the presence of large atypical lymphocytes that forms more than 25% of the dermal infiltrate, increased mitotic activity, and ki67 proliferation. Immunophenotypically in addition to the classic T-cell associated antigens large cells may express CD30 and CD25. Making the distinction with CD30+ anaplastic large cell lymphoma is essential in this case. Usually the CD30+ epidermotropism along with the small- to medium-cerebrifrom cells in the epidermis is a feature of MF (6).

An algorithm developed by The International Society for Cutaneous Lymphoma facilitates the diagnosis of early mycosis fungoids. The algorithm is based on points and involves a holistic integration of clinical, histopathologic, immunopathologic, and molecular biological characteristics (Table 1) (7).

TABLE 1 Algorithm for diagnosis of early MF*

Criteria	Scoring system
Clinical	
Basic	2 points for basic criteria and two additional criteria
Persistent and/or progressive patches/thin plaques	1 point for basic criteria and two additional criterion
Additional	
1) Non-sun exposed location	
2) Size/shape variation	
3) Poikiloderma	
Histopathologic	
Basic	2 points for basic criteria and two additional criteria
Superficial lymphoid infiltrate	1 point for basic criteria and one additional criterion
Additional	
1) Epidermotropism without spongiosis	
2) Lymphoid atypia +	
Molecular biological	
1) Clonal TCR gene rearrangement	1 point for clonality
Immunopathologic	
1) <50% CD2+, CD3+, and/or CD5+ T cells	1 point for one or more criteria
2) <10% CD7+ T cells	
3) Epidermal/dermal discordance of CD2, CD3, CD5, or CD7+	

MF, Mycosis fungoides; TCR , T -cell receptor.
**A total of 4 points is required for the diagnosis of MF based on any combination of points from the clinical, histopathologic, molecular biological, immunopathologic criteria.*
+Lymphoid atypiais defined as cells with enlarged hyperchromatic nuclei and irregular or cerebriform nuclear contours.
+T-cell antigen deficiency confined to the epidermis.

From Pimpinelli N, Olsen EA, Santucci M, et al. Defining early mycosis fungoides. *J Am Acad Dermatol.* 2005;53:1053–1063. Reproduced with permission of Elsevier Ltd.

■ ETIOLOGY

Infectious agents such as Epstein-Barr virus, cytomegalovirus, HTLV-1, and *Staphylococcus aureus* have been hypothesized as possible triggers. An antigen-driven immune response is suggested by the atypical CD4+ lymphocytes cluster around epidermal Langerhans cells, Pautrier's microabscess (8). Immature dendritic cells (Langerhans cells) in the epidermis are thought to activate T cells through direct contact and provide the stimulus for their clonal expansion by migrating to the dermis (9). It is hypothesized that the loss of activation induced cell death following T-cell proliferation through loss of Fas may lead to accumulation of the T-cells in skin resulting in chronic inflammatory lesions.

Tumor cells expressing Fas ligand may eliminate tumor infiltrating, cytotoxic CD8+ T-cells, allowing disease progression to occur (10). Progression of MF/SS is accompanied by clonal dominance of the malignant cells, and the skin homing CD4+ cells appear in the blood. This appearance can be detected by flow cytometry early on, although the prognostic implications is debatable (11).

■ CLINICAL PRESENTATION

A landmark of MF is the long natural history, and most of the time, presenting with red slightly scaly skin lesions that can wax and wane over years to a decade. Typically, patients are treated with topical steroids, and repeated biopsies are non-diagnostic.

As the disease progresses to plaques, tumors, and/or generalized erythema in some patients, the biopsy will have a higher chance of detecting the disease. The typical patches are slightly scaling and erythematous can be of ring- or crescent-shape involving sun-shaded areas (Figure 1). As they progress to plaques, the lesions are erythematous well defined with palpable edges (Figure 2). The plaques can become hyper- or hypopigmented. As the plaques infiltrate deeply into the dermis and lose their epidermis location, they form tumors with ulceration (Figure 3) and possible superinfection (Figure 3). Pruritus and dryness are a common symptom and complains that eventually lead to a diagnosis. Alopecia can occur early in the disease and is generally associated with follicular mucinosis. Erythroderma (Figure 4) is another generalized skin involvement often accompanied with intense pruritus, burning, tightness, lichenoid skin, and scaling. These patients have the worst quality of life compared to the rest of patients with MF, according to a study done by EORTC (12). The association of lymphadenopathy, peripheral blood cells with same neoplastic features as the skin along with the erythroderma, is the Sezary syndrome.

The disease presentation's median age is 54–60, male/female ratio =1.6–2 with a suggested worse outcome in males (13). There is yet no evidence if ethnicity influences the outcome, and no established etiology. It has been suggested that this may be a source of chronic toxic antigenic exposure, leading eventually to the clonogenic transformation.

In a study by Kim et al, 525 patients were evaluated and the overall survival at 5, 10, and 30 years were 68%, 53%, and 17%, respectively. The disease specific survival was 81%, 74%, and 64%, respectively.

It is worth to note that occasionally, some patients present with a single lesion often around the bathing trunk or chest area, and these can be treated with curative intent since some of them might remain free of disease for a long time (14).

■ CLASSIFICATION AND PROGNOSTIC FACTORS

With the diagnosis being a challenging task, the classification and staging system had to be updated to include the recent advances in areas of molecular, biology, immunohistochemistry, and imaging that proved to have a predictive value of outcome. Therefore, the original Mycosis Fungoides Cooperative Group (MFCG) staging system, which later was modified by the National Cancer Institute and the Veterans Administration and published in 1979 (15), was revised and presented in the updated ISCL/EORTC (International Society for Cutaneous Lymphomas/European Organization of Research and Treatment of Cancer) staging and classification in 2007 (Tables 2–4) (13).

Prognostic Factors

1. *Clinical stage* is the most important predictor of outcome. Patients with early stage IA, IB, and IIA have a median survival of 12 years, while more advanced cases will have a median survival of 5 years and can be as short as 2.5 years with nodal and visceral involvement (13,16).

   a. Patients with limited patches and plaques (low tumor burden) will experience a longer survival compared to expensive patches and plaques; as such the relative risk for death due to disease is reported to be 21.6 times greater for T4 compared to T1a, with erythrodermic patients at diagnosis having the worst prognosis.
   b. Advanced lymph node staging with RR for death of 10 for N2 and N3 compared to 2.8 for N1.
   c. Blood involvement increases the risk of death; although some investigators have questioned T-cell clonality of blood its predictive value (17).

2. *Folliculotropic variant* have an inferior outcome and are resistant to skin-directed therapy. Even when diagnosed at an early stage, they still have a relatively shorter survival estimated to be 41% at 15 years (5).
3. *Large cell transformation* has a poor outcome and it is strongly dependent on stage, the rate of transformation in early disease is low (1.4%, and can be up to 27% in IIB and 56–67% in stage IV (18).
4. *Age at diagnosis* with patients younger than 57 years having better outcome compared to older patients (16).
5. *Elevated LDH and soluble interleukin 2 receptor level*, measurement of serum concentration of soluble alpha-chain receptor for interleukin-2, positively correlates with tumor burden and subsequently with survival (19,20).

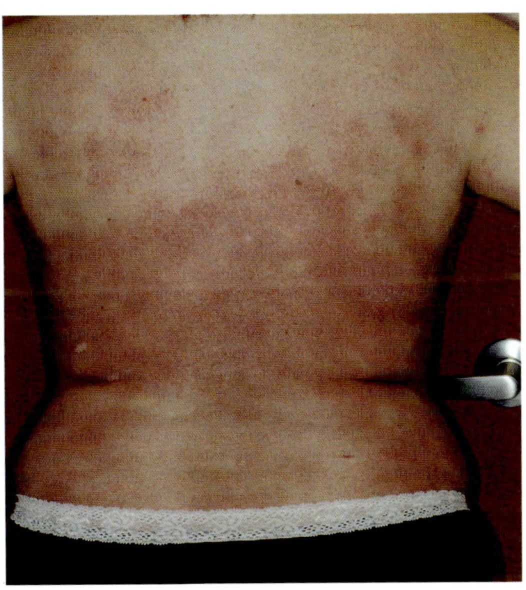

FIGURE 1 Patch stage lesions.

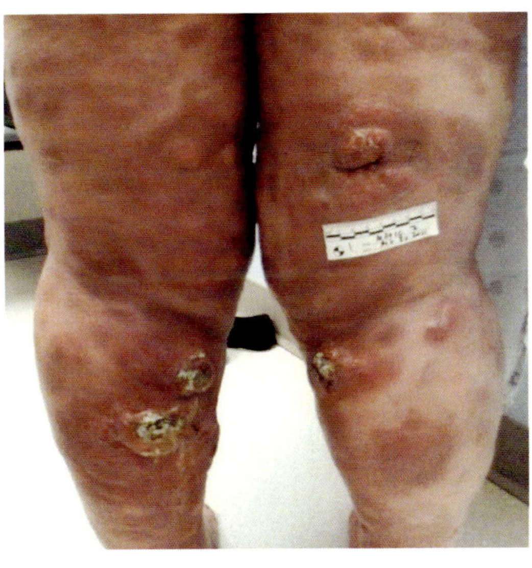

FIGURE 3 Tumors with superimposed infection in some.

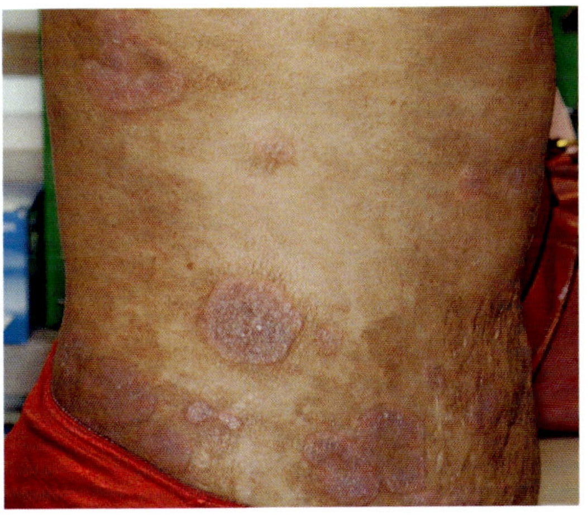

FIGURE 2 Plaque stage lesions.

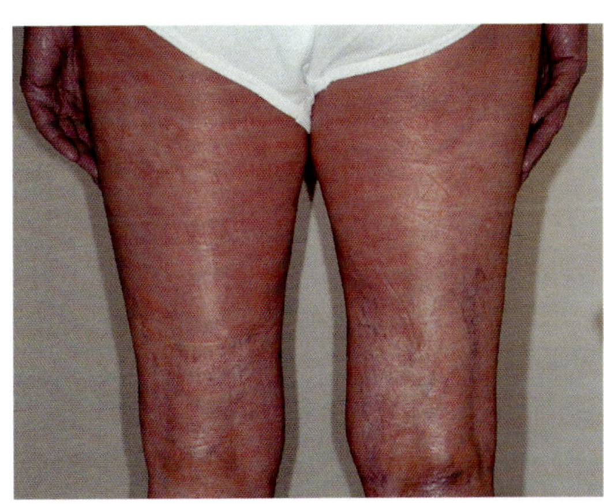

FIGURE 4 Erythrodermic stage.

6. *Low number of CD8+* in the dermis is associated with lower survival, it is suggested that CD8+ T cells can play an important role in the antitumor response (21).
7. *CD30+ dermal expressions* in non-transformed MF are thought to correlate with prognosis (22).

Tumor burden was consistently found to correlate with outcome by different groups. In an effort to validate the revised ISCL/EORTC staging proposal, Agar et al. (13) analyzed 1502 patients. The following factors were found to significantly correlate with the risk of disease progression on

TABLE 2 Original Mycosis Fungoides Cooperative Group TNM Classification of cutaneous T-cell lymphoma (CTCL)

Classification	Description
	T: Skin[a]
T_0	Clinically and/or histopathologically suspicious lesions
T_1	Limited plaques, papules or eczematous patches covering <10% of the skin surface
T_2	Generalized plaque, papules, or erythematous patches covering ≥10% or more of the skin surface
T_3	Tumors, one or more
T_4	Generalized erythroderma
	N: Lymph nodes[b]
N_0	No clinically abnormal peripheral lymph nodes; pathology negative for CTCL
N_1	Clinically abnormal peripheral lymph nodes; pathology negative for CTCL
N_2	No clinically abnormal peripheral lymph nodes; pathology positive for CTCL
N_3	Clinically abnormal peripheral lymph nodes; pathology positive for CTCL
	B: Peripheral blood
B_0	Atypical circulating cells not present (<5%)
B_1	Atypical circulating cells present(>5%); record total white blood count and total lymphocyte counts, and number of atypical cells/ 100 lymphocytes
	M: Visceral organs
M_0	No visceral organ involvement
M_1	Visceral involvement (must have pathology confirmation and organ involved should be specified)

[a]Pathology of T_{1-4} is diagnostic of a CTCL. When more than 1 T exists, both are recorded and the highest is used for staging (e.g., $T_{4(3)}$)

[b]Record number of sites of abnormal nodes (e.g., cervical; left + right), axillary(left + right), inguinal(left + right), epitrochlear, and submandibular/submaxillary.

TABLE 3 Modified ISCL/EORTC revisions to the staging of MF/SS

Stage	T	N	M	B
IA	1	0	0	0, 1
IIB	2	0	0	0, 1
IIA	1–2	1,2, X	0	0, 1
IIIB	3	0–2, X	0	0, 1
IIIIA	4	0–2, X	0	0
IIIIB	4	0–2, X	0	1
IVA$_1$	1–4	0–2, X	0	2
IVA$_2$	1–4	3	0	0–2
IVB	1–4	0–3, X	1	0–2

Abbreviations: ISCL = International Society for Cutaneous Lymphomas; EORTC = European Organization for Research and Treatment of Cancer; MF = mycosis fungoides: SS = Sezary syndrome; X = clinically abnormal lymph nodes without histologic confirmation or inability to fully characterize histologic subcategories.

From Olsen EA, Whittaker S, Kim YH, et al. Clinical end points and response criteria in mycosis fungoides and Sézary syndrome: a consensus statement of the International Society for Cutaneous Lymphomas, the United States Cutaneous Lymphoma Consortium, and the Cutaneous Lymphoma Task Force of the European Organisation for Research and Treatment of Cancer. *J Clin Oncol.* 2011;20;29(18):2598–2607. Reproduced with permission of the American Society of Clinical Oncology.

TABLE 4 ISCL/EORTC revision to the classification of mycosis fungoides and Sezary syndrome

TNMB stages

Skin

T_1		Limited patches,[a] papules, and/or plaques[b] covering <10% of the skin surface. May further stratify into T_{1a} (patch only) versus T_{1b} (plague ± patch)
T_2		Patches, papules or plagues covering ≥10% of the skin surface. May further stratify into T_{2a} (patch only) versus T_{2b} (plague ± patch)
T_3		One or more tumors[c] (≥1 cm diameter)
T_4		Confluence of erythema covering ≥ 80% body surface area

Node

N_0		No clinically abnormal peripheral lymph nodes[d] biopsy not required
N_1		Clinically abnormal peripheral lymph nodes; histopathology Dutch grade 1 or $NCILN_{0-2}$
	N_{1a}	Clone negative[g]
	N_{1b}	Clone positive[g]
N_2		Clinically abnormal peripheral lymph nodes; histopathology Dutch grade 2 or $NCILN_3$
	N_{2a}	Clone negative[g]
	N_{2b}	Clone positive[g]
N_3		Clinically abnormal peripheral lymph nodes; histopathology Dutch grades 3 to 4 or $NCILN_4$:clone positive or negative
N_x		Clinically abnormal peripheral lymph nodes;no histologic confirmation

Visceral

M_0		No visceral organ involvement
M_1		Visceral involvement (must have pathology confirmation[e] and organ involved should be specified

Blood

B0		Absence of significant blood involvement: ≤5% of peripheral blood lymphocytes are atypical(Sezary) cells
	B_{0a}	Clone negative[g]
	B_{0b}	Clone positive[g]
B1		Low blood tumor burden:>5% of peripheral blood lymphocytes are a typical(Sézary) cells but does not meet the criteria of B_2
	B_{1a}	Clone negative[g]
	B_{1b}	Clone positive[g]
B2		High blood tumor burden: ≥1000/μL Sézary cells[f] with positive clone[g]

[a]For skin, patch indicates any size skin lesion without significant elevation or induration. Presence/absence of hypo- or hyperpigmentation, scale, crusting, and/or poikiloderma should be noted.

[b]For skin, plaque indicates any size skin lesion that is elevated or indurated. Presence or absence of scale, crusting and/or poikiloderma features such as folliculotropism or large-cell transformation (>25% large cells), CD30[+] or CD30[-], and clinical features such as ulceration are important to document.

[c]For skin, tumor indicates at least one 11-cm diameter solid or nodular lesion with evidence of depth and/or vertical growth. Note total number of lesions, total volume of lesions, largest size lesion, and region of body involved. Also note if histologic evidence of large-cell transformation has occurred. Phenotyping for CD30 is encouraged.

[d]For node, abnormal peripheral lymph node(s) indicates any palpable peripheral node that on physical examination is firm, irregular, clustered, fixed or 1.5 cm or larger in diameter. Node groups examined on physical examination include cervical, supraclavicular, epitrochlear, axillary, and inguinal. Central nodes, which are not generally amenable to pathologic assessment, are not currently considered in the nodal classification unless used to establish N_3 histopathologically.

[e]For viscera, spleen and liver may be diagnosed by imaging criteria.

[f]For blood, Sezary cells are defined as lymphocytes with hyperconvoluted cerebriform nuclei. If Sezary cells are not able to be used to determine tumor burden for B_2, then one of the following modified ISCL criteria along with a positive clonal rearrangement of the TCR may be used instead:(a) expanded CD4[+] or CD3[+] cells with CD4/CD8 ratio of 10 or more, (b) expanded CD4[+] cells with abnormal immunophenotype including loss of CD7 or CD26.

[g]A T-cell clone is defined by PCR or Southern blot analysis of the T-cell receptor gene.

From Olsen EA, Whittaker S, Kim YH, et al. Clinical end points and response criteria in mycosis fungoides and Sézary syndrome: a consensus statement of the International Society for Cutaneous Lymphomas, the United States Cutaneous Lymphoma Consortium, and the Cutaneous Lymphoma Task Force of the European Organisation for Research and Treatment of Cancer. *J Clin Oncol.* 2011;20;29(18):2598–2607. Reproduced with permission of the American Society of Clinical Oncology.

multivariate analysis: T classification, blood clonality, high LDH, tumor distribution (generalized versus solitary), the presence of folliculotropic MF, and large cell transformation. On the other hand node status, blood classification and age did not affect the risk of disease progression.

TREATMENT STRATEGY

With the long-term survival and no advantage for early cytotoxic therapeutic application (23), the risk of therapy related side effects has to be carefully considered in each patient. Another essential reality to keep in mind is that this is not a curable disease and treating with several consecutive therapeutic approaches even in advanced disease failed in several publications to show a benefit or the ability to prevent relapse (24–29) although others showed a benefits. Since most patients are symptomatic, symptom control is an essential part of the approach, thus, supportive measures with aggressive moisturization, topical steroids, and antipruritic medicines are frequently used. Options used to control pruritus includes: antihistamines, gabapentin, mirtazapine (which helps with sleeping) (30,31), naloxone, and Aprepitant (neurokinin-1-receptor) (32). Also, since superinfection is common, clinicians should be able to differentiate disease flare from an infection that can be easily managed with antibiotics and local care (33).

The stage of the disease should determine the type of therapy. When the disease is limited to patches and plaques with no extra-cutaneous involvement, skin-directed therapy is the rule keeping in mind that none of the options are curative. Therapy choice depends on stage of disease, age, presence of comorbidities, and socioeconomic situations. When the stage is advanced specifically in the case of SS, the following has to be taken into consideration: burden of disease, degree of skin infiltration, presence of tumors, extent of lymphadenopathy, burden of circulating malignant T cells, and the level of LDH. Subsequently and when choosing therapy, preservation of the immune system is essential to decrease the risk of infection that can be fatal, therefore, skin-directed therapy and immune modulatory therapy is advised as first option followed by more intense multi-agents chemotherapy/transplant when disease progress or with sign of transformation.

OPTIONS FOR EARLY STAGE DISEASE

Topical steroids: can be used for many years alone or in combination with other skin-directed therapy. Class I potent topical corticosteroids, such as betamethasone dipropionate 0.05% or mometasone furoate 0.1%, are indicated. Intralesional corticosteroids can be also effective for thicker plaques. The CR achieved with steroids in T1 lesions can be as high as 65%.

Topical chemotherapy: Mechlorethamine (topical nitrogen mustard) mixed with an ointment or in an aqueous solution at 10–20 mg/100cc is applied to affected skin or to the whole skin. The application is on daily basis until clearance of the disease, which might take several months. Concentration might be modified according to response, and maintenance therapy can be useful in some patients. Since half of the patients will relapse after discontinuation, repeated courses are the usual, the chance of attaining a response in early stage is 70% to 80%, but only 20% to 25% will have a durable response (34). Nitrogen mustard can produce skin hypersensitivity but has no systemic side effects since it is not absorbed unlike BCNU (carmustine), which has the potential of myelo-suppression.

Phototherapy: readily available in dermatology practices and it is in the form of UVB shortwave or UVA longwave which has more skin penetration. Phototherapy can be used alone or with psoralen as a photosensitizing agent. Patients are treated two to three times a week during the clearing phase. Then they move to a maintenance phase. The benefit of this treatment varies from 50% to 90% depending of the extent of disease. The primary toxicity includes nausea, skin dryness, blistering, and on the long-term cataract (35,36).

Topical and oral retinoids: a novel synthetic retinoid binding selectively with retinoid X receptor, Targretin (bexarotene), a 1% gel is indicated for limited disease and can be combined with PUVA or PUVB, used twice daily with a limited durable response rate. It can cause skin irritation lasting for few weeks making it hard to differentiate disease from reaction. Systemic oral therapy has been FDA approved since 1999 and reported a response rate of 44% with 9% complete response, and median response duration of 8 months (37). Initial dose is 300 mg/m^2, side effects include: photosensitivity, xerosis, myalgia, arthralgia, headaches and impaired night vision; in addition hepatotoxicity, hyperlipidism and hypothyroidism

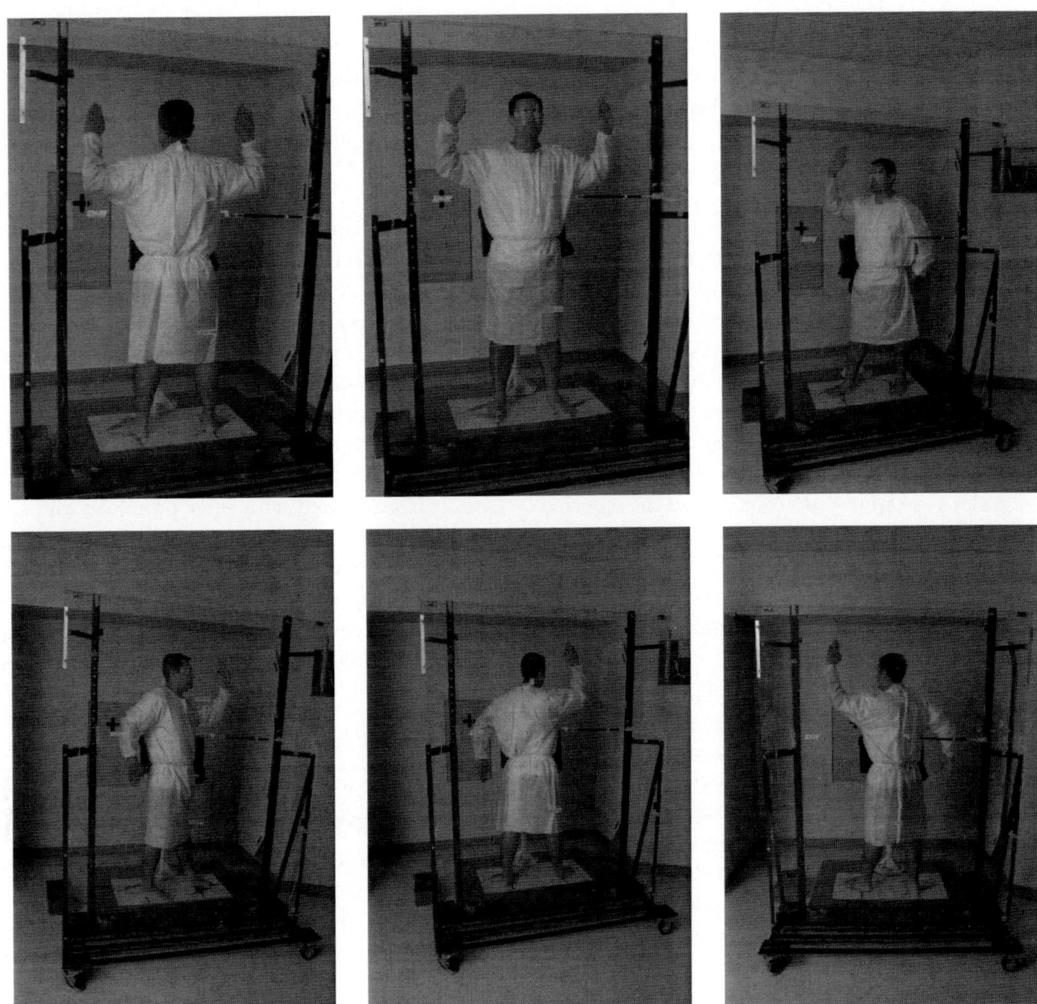

FIGURE 6   Total skin electron beam, patient's six different positions.

irradiated normal and neoplastic lymphocytes while enhancing differentiation of monocytes towards immature dendritic cells the overall response rate estimated to be 60% and can be combined with other immunomodulated agents like interferon or retinoids or TSEB. To date the mechanism of action is not fully understood. Generally it is used every 4 weeks although in some cases can be every 2 weeks followed by maintenance after the clearance phase of the disease.

Photophoresis is considered an effective treatment of erythrodermic MF and Sezary syndrome compared to other therapies with little side effects. Recently it has been looked at in early stage disease with a reported response duration of 6 months (49).

Vorinostat: Epigenetic regulation of gene transcription by small molecule inhibitors of histone deacetylases (HDAC) is the first FDA-approved HDAC-inhibitor for the treatment of patients with cutaneous T-cell lymphoma. At an oral dose of 400mg/day the reported overall response rate is 24%–30% (51) in refractory advanced patients to systemic chemotherapy. It is generally indicated for extra-cutaneous disease, response is usually short. Many combinations have been used including CHOP, CAVE (adding etoposide), or COMP (adding methotrexate). Common side effects include fatigue, nausea, vomiting, thrombocytopenia, and elevated creatinine.

Romidepsin is a potent pan HDAC inhibitor, with phase II studies completed with a reported ORR of 34%, with up to 43% of patients improved pruritus (52,53). Reported side effects include nausea, anorexia, fatigue, transient thrombocytopenia and granulocytopenia, and T wave flattening.

Alemtuzumab (MabCampath): humanized monoclonal antibody targeted against CD52. This is FDA approved for the treatment of CLL and it induces a complement and antibodies dependent cellular toxicity. Doses used varied from 10–30 mg three times a week for 4 to 12 weeks and the reported outcome was as high as an ORR of 86%–100% with 21% CR. Side effects including fever/chills during infusion and CMV reactivation has been reported (54,55) other common toxicities includes immune suppression and infection.

Chemotherapy typically including anthracyclines, purine analogs, alkylating agents, and etoposide. Typically responses are not durable. If used as single agents such as gemcitabine or liposomal doxorubicin they are better tolerated; multiple combinations can be considered including cyclophosphamide, MTX, etoposide dexamethasone, or doxorubicin bleomycin and vinblastine, or cyclophosphamide and fludarabine, or cyclophosphamide, vincristine, Adriamycin, and prednisone.

Allogeneic transplant: The failure of autologous transplant (56) to achieve a long-term remission suggests that the graft versus lymphoma effect in allogeneic SCT is an important factor for durable responses in MF. Allogeneic SCT reported by the European Bone Marrow Transplant registry (57) on 46 patients had a non relapse mortality of 20% for myeloablative regimens versus reduced intensity (9%), and only 17% had a complete remission. At 2 years after transplantation the cumulative incidence of disease relapse was 33% and post transplantation progression-free survival was 46%.

Reduced intensity allogeneic bone marrow transplant was developed to reduce the known associated risks of morbidity and mortality of this approach. In a study from MD Anderson Cancer Center (59), 19 patients with transformed disease or sezary syndromes were treated with reduced intensity myeloablative regimens; patients were conditioned with 32 Gy TSEB, postulated to reduce skin antigen presenting cell, and

Fludarabine-Melphalan. HLA compatible donors selected with no more than one antigen mismatch. Two patients died with disease, four died in complete remission, and eight relapsed. Eleven of the remaining 13 patients remained in remission. The current belief is that the outcome of advanced cases is superior with allogeneic transplant compared to conventional therapy. Efforts are concentrating at managing infections and GVHD that remains that leading cause of nondisease-related death.

Transformed disease is defined as large cells in more than 25% of the infiltrate or if these cells formed microscopic nodules. Whenever suspected with a rapid formation of aggressive tumor a biopsy should be performed. It is reported to occur in up to 27% in stage IIB, and up to 67% in stage IV disease. It is associated with poor prognosis and short overall survival of median of 2 years (60,61). In these cases chemotherapy should be initiated early and allogeneic transplantation is a consideration coupled with radiation therapy mostly as total skin electron therapy.

■ CONCLUSIONS

Diagnosing MF remains a challenge requiring multiple biopsies. Once diagnosis is obtained, a thorough classification has to be conducted to determine the prognostic grouping that will help determine the optimal therapy to be used. Therapy is not only governed by the stage but also by an effort to minimize long-term side effects in this patient population where living for many years is possible and obtaining a cure is challenging to say the least.

■ REFERENCES

1. Willemze R, Jaffe ES, Burg G, et al. WHO–EORTC classification for cutaneous lymphomas. *Blood. [Review].* 2005;105(10):3768–3785.

2. Kohler S, Jones CD, Warnke RA, Zehnder JL. PCR-heteroduplex analysis of T-cell receptor gamma gene rearrangement in paraffin-embedded skin biopsies. *Am J Dermatopathol.* [Research Support, Non-U.S. Gov't Research Support, U.S. Gov't, P.H.S.]. 2000;22(4):321–327.

3. Karenko L, Kahkonen M, Hyytinen ER, et al. Notable losses at specific regions of chromosomes 10q and 13q in the Sezary syndrome detected by comparative genomic hybridization. *J Invest Dermatol.* [Comparative

Study Letter Research Support, Non-U.S. Gov't]. 1999;112(3):392–395.

4. Mao X, Lillington D, Scarisbrick JJ, et al. Molecular cytogenetic analysis of cutaneous T-cell lymphomas: identification of common genetic alterations in Sezary syndrome and mycosis fungoides. *Br J Dermatol*. [Research Support, Non-U.S. Gov't]. 2002;147(3):464–475.

5. Gerami P, Rosen S, Kuzel T, et al. Folliculotropic mycosis fungoides: an aggressive variant of cutaneous T-cell lymphoma. *Arch Dermatol*. [Comparative Study]. 2008;144(6):738–746.

6. Herrmann JL, Hughey LC. Recognizing large-cell transformation of mycosis fungoides. *J Am Acad Dermatol*. 2012;67:665–672.

7. Pimpinelli N, Olsen EA, Santucci M, et al. Defining early mycosis fungoides. *J Am Acad Dermatol*. [Research Support, N.I.H., Extramural Research Support, U.S. Gov't, Non-P.H.S.Review]. 2005;53(6):1053–1063.

8. Girardi M, Heald PW, Wilson LD. The pathogenesis of mycosis fungoides. *N Engl J Med*. [Review]. 2004;350(19):1978–1988.

9. Berger CL, Hanlon D, Kanada D, et al. The growth of cutaneous T-cell lymphoma is stimulated by immature dendritic cells. *Blood*. [Research Support, Non-U.S. Gov't Research Support, U.S. Gov't, P.H.S.]. 2002;99(8):2929–2939.

10. Ni X, Zhang C, Talpur R, Duvic M. Resistance to activation-induced cell death and bystander cytotoxicity via the Fas/Fas ligand pathway are implicated in the pathogenesis of cutaneous T cell lymphomas. *J Invest Dermatol*. [Research Support, Non-U.S. Gov't Research Support, U.S. Gov't, P.H.S.]. 2005;124(4):741–750.

11. Vega F, Luthra R, Medeiros LJ, et al. Clonal heterogeneity in mycosis fungoides and its relationship to clinical course. *Blood*. [Comparative Study Research Support, U.S. Gov't, P.H.S.]. 2002;100(9):3369–3373.

12. Sampogna F, Frontani M, Baliva G, et al. Quality of life and psychological distress in patients with cutaneous lymphoma. *Br J Dermatol*. [Research Support, Non-U.S. Gov't]. 2009;160(4):815–822.

13. Agar NS, Wedgeworth E, Crichton S, et al. Survival outcomes and prognostic factors in mycosis fungoides/Sezary syndrome: validation of the revised International Society for Cutaneous Lymphomas/European Organisation for Research and Treatment of Cancer staging proposal. *J Clin Oncol*. [Research Support, Non-U.S. Gov't Validation Studies]. 2010;28(31):4730–4739.

14. Wilson LD, Kacinski BM, Jones GW. Local superficial radiotherapy in the management of minimal stage IA cutaneous T-cell lymphoma (Mycosis Fungoides). *Int J Radiat Oncol Biol Phys*. 1998;40(1):109–115.

15. Bunn PA, Jr., Lamberg SI. Report of the committee on staging and classification of cutaneous T-cell lymphomas. *Cancer Treatment Reports*. 1979;63(4):725–728.

16. Kim YH, Liu HL, Mraz-Gernhard S, et al. Long-term outcome of 525 patients with mycosis fungoides and Sezary syndrome: clinical prognostic factors and risk for disease progression. *Arch Dermatol*. [Research Support, Non-U.S. Gov't]. 2003;139(7):857–866.

17. Delfau-Larue MH, Laroche L, Wechsler J, Lepage E, et al. Diagnostic value of dominant T-cell clones in peripheral blood in 363 patients presenting consecutively with a clinical suspicion of cutaneous lymphoma. *Blood*. 2000;96(9):2987–2992.

18. Benner MF, Jansen PM, Vermeer MH, et al. Prognostic factors in transformed mycosis fungoides: a retrospective analysis of 100 cases. *Blood*. 2012;119(7):1643–1649.

19. Wasik MA, Vonderheid EC, Bigler RD, et al. Increased serum concentration of the soluble interleukin-2 receptor in cutaneous T-cell lymphoma. Clinical and prognostic implications. *Arch Dermatol*. [Research Support, Non-U.S. Gov't Research Support, U.S. Gov't, Non-P.H.S.Research Support, U.S. Gov't, P.H.S.]. 1996;132(1):42–47.

20. Abeni D, Frontani M, Sampogna F, et al. Circulating CD8+ lymphocytes, white blood cells, and survival in patients with mycosis fungoides. *Br J Dermatol*. [Research Support, Non-U.S. Gov't]. 2005;153(2):324–330.

21. Vermeer MH, van Doorn R, Dukers D, et al. CD8+ T cells in cutaneous T-cell lymphoma: expression of cytotoxic proteins, Fas Ligand, and killing inhibitory receptors and their relationship with clinical behavior. *J Clin Oncol*. 2001;19(23):4322–4329.

22. Edinger JT, Clark BZ, Pucevich BE, et al. CD30 expression and proliferative fraction in nontransformed mycosis fungoides. *Am J Surg Pathol*. [Research Support, N.I.H., Extramural]. 2009;33(12):1860–1868.

23. Kaye FJ, Bunn PA, Jr., Steinberg SM, et al. A randomized trial comparing combination electron-beam radiation and chemotherapy with topical therapy in the initial treatment of mycosis fungoides. *N Engl J Med*. [Clinical Trial Comparative Study Randomized Controlled Trial]. 1989;321(26):1784–1790.

24. Duvic M, Apisarnthanarax N, Cohen DS, et al. Analysis of long-term outcomes of combined modality therapy for cutaneous T-cell lymphoma. *J Am Acad Dermatol*. [Research Support, Non-U.S. Gov't Research Support, U.S. Gov't, P.H.S.]. 2003;49(1):35–49.

25. Hallahan DE, Griem ML, Griem SF, et al. Combined modality therapy for tumor stage mycosis fungoides: results of a 10-year follow-up. *J Clin Oncology*. 1988;6(7):1177–1183.

26. Braverman IM, Yager NB, Chen M, et al. Combined total body electron beam irradiation and chemotherapy for mycosis fungoides. *J Am Acad Dermatol*. [Comparative Study Research Support, U.S. Gov't, P.H.S.]. 1987;16:45–60.

27. Wilson LD, Licata AL, Braverman IM, et al. Systemic chemotherapy and extracorporeal photochemotherapy for T3 and T4 cutaneous T-cell lymphoma patients who have achieved a complete response to total skin electron beam therapy. *Int J Radiat Oncol Biol Phys*. 1995;32(4):987–995.

28. Griem ML, Tokars RP, Petras V, et al. Combined therapy for patients with mycosis fungoides. *Cancer Treatment Reports.* [Research Support, U.S. Gov't, P.H.S.]. 1979;63(4):655–657.

29. Bunn PA, Jr., Fischmann AB, Schechter GP, et al. Combined modality therapy with electron-beam irradiation and systemic chemotherapy for cutaneous T-cell lymphomas. *Cancer Treatment Reports.* 1979;63(4):713–717.

30. Davis MP, Frandsen JL, Walsh D, et al. Mirtazapine for pruritus. *J Pain Symptom Manag.* [Case Reports]. 2003;25(3):288–291.

31. Rose MA, Kam PC. Gabapentin: pharmacology and its use in pain management. *Anaesthesia.* [Review]. 2002;57(5):451–462.

32. Duval A, Dubertret L. Aprepitant as an antipruritic agent? *N Engl J Med.* [Case Reports Letter]. 2009;361(14):1415–1416.

33. Talpur R, Bassett R, Duvic M. Prevalence and treatment of Staphylococcus aureus colonization in patients with mycosis fungoides and Sezary syndrome. *Br J Dermatol.* [Research Support, N.I.H., Extramural Research Support, Non-U.S. Gov't]. 2008;159(1):105–112.

34. Vonderheid EC, Tan ET, Kantor AF, et al. Long-term efficacy, curative potential, and carcinogenicity of topical mechlorethamine chemotherapy in cutaneous T cell lymphoma. *J Am Acad Dermatol.* [Research Support, Non-U.S. Gov't]. 1989;20(3):416–428.

35. Berthelot C, Rivera A, Duvic M. Skin directed therapy for mycosis fungoides: a review. *J Drugs Dermatol.* [Research Support, N.I.H., Extramural Research Support, Non-U.S. Gov't Review]. 2008;7(7):655–666.

36. Geskin L. ECP versus PUVA for the treatment of cutaneous T-cell lymphoma. *Skin Therapy Lett.* [Review]. 2007;12(5):1–4.

37. Abbott RA, Whittaker SJ, Morris SL, et al. Bexarotene therapy for mycosis fungoides and Sezary syndrome. *Br J Dermatol.* 2009;160(6):1299–1307.

38. Zackheim HS, Kashani-Sabet M, McMillan A. Low-dose methotrexate to treat mycosis fungoides: a retrospective study in 69 patients. *J Am Acad Dermatol.* [Research Support, Non-U.S. Gov't]. 2003;49(5):873–878.

39. Papa G, Tura S, Mandelli F, Vegna ML, et al. Is interferon alpha in cutaneous T-cell lymphoma a treatment of choice? *Br J Haematol.* 1991;79 Suppl 1:48–51.

40. Olsen E, Duvic M, Frankel A, et al. Pivotal phase III trial of two dose levels of denileukin diftitox for the treatment of cutaneous T-cell lymphoma. *J Clin Oncol.* [Clinical Trial Clinical Trial, Phase III Multicenter Study Randomized Controlled Trial]. 2001;19(2):376–388.

41. Hoppe RT. Total skin electron beam therapy in the management of mycosis fungoides. *Front Radiat Ther Oncol.* [Research Support, U.S. Gov't, P.H.S.]. 1991;25:80–89; discussion 132–123.

42. Jones GW, Tadros A, Hodson DI, et al. Prognosis with newly diagnosed mycosis fungoides after total skin electron radiation of 30 or 35 GY. *Int J Radiat Oncol Biol Phys.* 1994;28(4):839–845.

43. Chinn DM, Chow S, Kim YH, et al. Total skin electron beam therapy with or without adjuvant topical nitrogen mustard or nitrogen mustard alone as initial treatment of T2 and T3 mycosis fungoides. *Int J Radiat Oncol Biol Phys.* 1999;43(5):951–958.

44. Navi D, Riaz N, Levin YS, et al. The Stanford University experience with conventional-dose, total skin electron-beam therapy in the treatment of generalized patch or plaque (T2) and tumor (T3) mycosis fungoides. *Archives Dermatol.* [Research Support, Non-U.S. Gov't]. 2011;147(5):561–567.

45. Hoppe RT. Mycosis fungoides: radiation therapy. *Dermatol Ther.* [Review]. 2003;16(4):347–354.

46. Jones G, Wilson LD, Fox-Goguen L. Total skin electron beam radiotherapy for patients who have mycosis fungoides. *Hematol Oncol Clin North Am.* [Research Support, Non-U.S. Gov't Review]. 2003;17(6):1421–1434.

47. Jones GW, Kacinski BM, Wilson LD, et al. Total skin electron radiation in the management of mycosis fungoides: Consensus of the European Organization for Research and Treatment of Cancer (EORTC) Cutaneous Lymphoma Project Group. *J Am Acad Dermatol.* 2002;47(3):364–370.

48. Harrison C, Young J, Navi D, et al. Revisiting low-dose total skin electron beam therapy in mycosis fungoides. *Int J Radiat Oncol Biol Phys.* 2011;81(4):e651–7.

49. Talpur R, Demierre MF, Geskin L, et al. Multicenter photopheresis intervention trial in early-stage mycosis fungoides. *Clin Lymphoma Myeloma Leuk.* [Clinical Trial Multicenter Study Research Support, Non-U.S. Gov't]. 2011;11(2):219–227.

50. Zic JA. Photopheresis in the treatment of cutaneous T-cell lymphoma: current status. *Curr Opin Oncol.* [Research Support, Non-U.S. Gov't Review]. 2012;24:S1–S10.

51. Duvic M, Talpur R, Ni X, et al. Phase 2 trial of oral vorinostat (suberoylanilide hydroxamic acid, SAHA) for refractory cutaneous T-cell lymphoma (CTCL). *Blood.* [Clinical Trial, Phase II Comparative Study Research Support, N.I.H., Extramural Research Support, Non-U.S. Gov't]. 2007;109(1):31–39.

52. Piekarz RL, Frye R, Turner M, et al. Phase II multi-institutional trial of the histone deacetylase inhibitor romidepsin as monotherapy for patients with cutaneous T-cell lymphoma. *J Clin Oncol.* [Clinical Trial, Phase II Multicenter Study Research Support, N.I.H., Extramural Research Support, N.I.H., Intramural Research Support, Non-U.S. Gov't]. 2009; 27(32):5410–5417.

53. Whittaker SJ, Demierre MF, Kim EJ, et al. Final results from a multicenter, international, pivotal study of romidepsin in refractory cutaneous T-cell lymphoma. *J Clin Oncol.* [Clinical Trial, Phase II Multicenter Study Research Support, Non-U.S. Gov't]. 2010;28(29):4485–4491.

54. Lenihan DJ, Alencar AJ, Yang D, et al. Cardiac toxicity of alemtuzumab in patients with mycosis fungoides/Sezary syndrome. *Blood.* [Case Reports Review]. 2004;104(3):655–658.

55. Zinzani PL, Alinari L, Tani M, et al. Preliminary observations of a phase II study of reduced-dose alemtuzumab treatment in patients with pretreated T-cell lymphoma. Haematologica. [Clinical Trial, Phase II Letter]. 2005;90(5):702–703.

56. Ingen-Housz-Oro S, Bachelez H, Verola O, et al. High-dose therapy and autologous stem cell transplantation in relapsing cutaneous lymphoma. *Bone Marrow Transplant*. 2004;33(6):629–634.

57. Duarte RF, Schmitz N, Servitje O, et al. Haematopoietic stem cell transplantation for patients with primary cutaneous T-cell lymphoma. *Bone Marrow Transplant*. [Review]. 2008;41(7):597–604.

58. Giralt S, Khouri I, Champlin R. Non myeloablative "mini transplants." *Cancer Treat Res*. [Review]. 1999;101:97–108.

59. Duvic M, Donato M, Dabaja B, et al. Total skin electron beam and non-myeloablative allogeneic hematopoietic stem-cell transplantation in advanced mycosis fungoides and Sezary syndrome. *J Clin Oncol*. [Clinical Trial Research Support, Non-U.S. Gov't]. 2010;28(14):2365–2372.

60. Arulogun SO, Prince HM, Ng J, et al. Long-term outcomes of patients with advanced-stage cutaneous T-cell lymphoma and large cell transformation. *Blood*. [Research Support, Non-U.S. Gov't]. 2008; 112(8):3082–3087.

61. Diamandidou E, Colome-Grimmer M, Fayad L, et al. Transformation of mycosis fungoides/Sezary syndrome: clinical characteristics and prognosis. *Blood*. 1998;92(4):1150–1159.

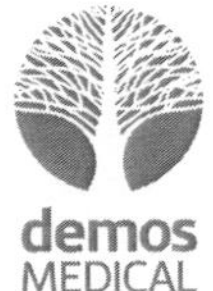

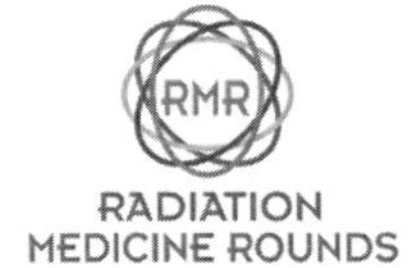

Natural Killer Cell Lymphomas

Timur Mitin and Karen M. Winkfield*

Department of Radiation Oncology, Massachusetts General Hospital Cancer Center, Boston, MA

■ ABSTRACT

Natural killer (NK) cell lymphomas are rare malignancies. They are almost exclusively Epstein-Barr virus (EBV) driven and disproportionally affect Asian and South American populations. The World Health Organization classification divides NK cell lymphomas into two subtypes: the extranodal NK/T-cell lymphoma, nasal type, and the aggressive NK cell leukemia. From the standpoint of prognosis and treatment algorithm, NK cell lymphomas can be divided into three categories: nasal, non-nasal, and aggressive NK leukemia. This review focuses on pathobiology, diagnosis, and staging and prognosis of NK cell lymphomas and then analyzes the evidence behind current treatment modalities for nasal NK cell lymphoma. Radiation therapy techniques, doses, and concurrent systemic agents are discussed in depth. Finally, salvage strategies are also reviewed for patients who fail the initial course of aggressive multi-modality therapy.

Keywords: natural killer cell lymphoma, Epstein-Barr virus, radiation therapy, chemotherapy, salvage

■ INTRODUCTION

Natural killer (NK) cells are cytotoxic cells that protect the host by lysing cells infected with viruses and bacteria, as well as recognizing and eliminating tumor cells (1). A bipotential T/NK cell progenitor has the ability to develop into an NK cell or a T cell. Because of a common ontogeny, some antigens are shared by both lineages, including CD2, CD7, and CD8. T cells express surface CD3, whereas NK cells express cytoplasmic CD3 epsilon. More specific markers of NK cells include CD16, CD56, and CD57. Although CD56 is commonly viewed as the most specific marker of NK lineage, some T cells, neural and neuroendocrine tissues, and occasionally skeletal muscles have also been shown to express CD56 (2).

NK cell lymphomas (NKCL) are a recently recognized lymphoma subtype within WHO classification (3). These rare malignancies were previously known as lethal midline granuloma, midline malignant reticulosis, or progressive lethal granulomatous ulceration. They are almost exclusively Epstein-Barr virus (EBV) driven (2,4) and disproportionally affect Asian and South American populations (5–7). Due to the angiocentricity and angiodestruction in these destructive midline facial lesions, NKCL were categorized as angiocentric T-cell lymphomas in the Revised European American Lymphoma (REAL) classification (8). With the development of clinically

*Corresponding author, Department of Radiation Oncology, Massachusetts General Hospital Cancer Center, 100 Blossom Street, Cox 3, Boston, MA

E-mail address: kwinkfield@partners.org

Radiation Medicine Rounds 3:3 (2012) 437–450.

DOI: 10.5003/2151–4208.3.3.437

useful anti-CD56 antibodies, most angiocentric T-cell lymphomas of the nose and upper aerodigestive tract were found to express CD56 (9).

The 2008 WHO classification divides NKCLs into two subtypes: aggressive NK cell leukemia and extranodal NK/T-cell lymphoma, nasal type (10). Although "NK/T cell" refers to the very rare subset of true surface CD3+ and CD56+ cytotoxic T-cell lymphomas, these are clinically indistinguishable from NKCL. It is unclear whether the malignancy originates from an NK cell or if it represents a T cell with abnormal cell markers. Due to this ambiguity, investigators often use the term NK/T-cell lymphoma when classifying NKCLs.

■ PATHOBIOLOGY

EBV belongs to the herpes family and is one of the most common viruses in humans. EBV was originally isolated from tissue samples of patients with endemic Burkitt's lymphoma (11), and subsequently an association with EBV for other B-cell neoplasms was described. The EBV oncogene, *LMP1*, is essential for EBV transformation of lymphocytes. The encoded viral protein LMP1 interacts with signal transducer proteins belonging to the tumor necrosis factor (TNF) family of receptors (TRAFs) (12). LMP1 acts as a constitutively activated TRAF molecule, inducing nuclear factor kappa-B (NF-kB) activation (13). LMP1 induces expression of several important cellular genes, such as BCL2, A20, activation markers, adhesion molecules and proteins involved in invasion and metastasis, such as matrix metalloproteinase (MMP) 9 and vascular epidermal growth factor.

Molecular mechanisms of malignant transformation of NK cells remain poorly defined. The strong association with EBV, irrespective of the ethnic origin of the patients, suggests a probable pathogenic role of the virus (7,14–17). NK and T cells are infected with EBV (always of subtype A), which is present in a clonal episomal form, with type II latency pattern (EBNA1+, EBNA2-, LMP1+) and with a common 30-bp deletion in the *LMP1* gene (18).

■ EPIDEMIOLOGY

NKCL is uncommon in the US, accounting for 0.4% to 2.2% of all extranodal lymphomas, but is more prevalent in Asian countries, such as China, Korea, and Japan, and South American countries, including Peru, Mexico, and Guatemala. Based on strong association with race/ethnicity, it has been postulated that a genetic-based impaired immune response against EBV may contribute to disease development (19). NKCL may be preceded by systemic diseases related to EBV infection. Chronic active EBV infection (CAEBV) is an infectious mononucleosis-like syndrome persisting for at least 6 months and associated with high titers of antibodies to EBV-capsid antigen and early antigen. (20) Whereas in mononucleosis B-cells are infected with EBV, in CAEBV the targets are T and NK cells. It has been described predominantly in children and young adults of Japanese, Korean, and Chinese decent (20). This disease is progressive, culminating in either NK or T-cell lymphoma or leukemia. Another condition which might precede the development of NKCL is a dermatological disease termed mosquito bite hypersensitivity. Patients present with severe blistering reactions to insect bites, occasionally accompanied by fever or hepatosplenomegaly. The condition is indolent and most lesions heal with scarring, however, occasionally the lesions can deteriorate and develop into a cutaneous lymphoma or either T cell (most commonly) or NK cell lineages.

■ CLINICAL PRESENTATION

Although the 2008 WHO classification divides NKCLs into two subtypes, the clinical presentation and prognosis of these malignancies differ based on anatomic location and degree of organ involvement (Table 1). Although nasal and non-nasal NKCLs represent the same spectrum of disease, they are managed differently due to differences in pattern of spread and prognosis. Aggressive lymphoma/leukemia can be difficult to distinguish from the terminal leukemic form of a nasal/non-nasal NKCLs and is uniformly fatal.

Nasal NK Cell Lymphoma

Nasal NKCL typically peaks in the fifth decade of life and has a male predominance (male:female = 3). They often present as destructive lesions involving the nasal cavity, nasopharynx, paranasal sinuses, tonsils, hypopharynx, and larynx. This group of malignancies may also involve Waldeyer's ring. Patients with nasal involvement tend to present with symptoms of nasal obstruction, or epistaxis, or with extensive midfacial destructive lesions. Neoplastic cells can disseminate to other sites, including skin, gastrointestinal tract,

TABLE 1 Clinical features of NK cell lymphomas

	Nasal NKCL	Non-nasal NKCL	Aggressive NKCL/leukemia
Age at presentation	50 to 60 years	50 to 60 years	30 to 40 years
Sex (Male: Female)	3:1	3:1	1:1
Involved organs	Upper aerodigestive tract (nasal cavity, nasopharynx, oral cavity, oropharynx, hypopharynx) and Waldeyer ring	Skin, GI tract, bone marrow, lung, extremities, orbit, adrenal gland, testis, CNS	Disseminated disease. Blood, bone marrow, liver, spleen, lymph nodes
Clinical presentation	Based on location of lesion	Based on location of lesion	Fever, jaundice, hepatosplenomegaly, lymphadenopathy
Prognosis	Stage I/II: good Stage III/IV: poor 73% to 85% of patients present with early stage (22,44)	Stage I/II: good Stage III/IV: poor 32% to 41% of patients present with early stage (22,44)	Fatal within several weeks

testis, or cervical lymph nodes, however distant organ involvement occurs in only about 10% of patients at presentation. Fewer than 10% of cases show bone marrow involvement (21). Nodal involvement at the time of presentation ranges between 17% and 46% (22–26), however 80% of patients with Waldeyer ring involvement were found to have nodal disease at presentation (27,28). A hemophagocytic syndrome occurs in 2% to 8% of patients and can alter the clinical scenario (22,29). Peripheral blood cytopenias are predominantly due to active hemophagocytosis in the marrow. The hemophagocytic cells represent activated reticuloendothelial cells and on their own do not indicate marrow infiltration. Establishment of the lymphomatous infiltration requires EBV-encoded RNA-1 in-situ hybridization (EBER ISH).

Non-Nasal NK Cell Lymphoma

Age of presentation and male predominance are similar to nasal NKCLs. Any anatomic site can be involved, with the common primary sites being skin, gastrointestinal tract, salivary glands, spleen and testis. It should be noted that primary sites of non-nasal NKCL are the same sites that can be involved by disseminated nasal NKCL. Therefore, patients with evidence of non-nasal NKCL should undergo imaging studies and nasal endoscopy to exclude an occult nasal primary. Some authors argue that with modern imaging techniques, most apparently non-nasal cases can be found to have nasal involvement, implying

that they are in fact disseminated nasal NKCLs (30). Non-nasal NKCLs are associated with significantly higher proportions of advanced stage disease, two or more extranodal sites, elevated LDH levels, B symptoms, and poor performance status (22).

Aggressive NK Cell Leukemia/Lymphoma

Men and women are equally affected with this catastrophic disorder. They present with high fever, weight loss, jaundice, skin infiltration, lymphadenopathy, and hepatosplenomegaly. Marrow hemophagocytosis is often present, which can lead to severe anemia and thrombocytopenia. Disseminated intravascular coagulopathy is progressive and patients usually succumb within weeks of diagnosis. Clinically, aggressive NK cell leukemia is similar to the rare terminal leukemic form of nasal or non-nasal NKCL. The diagnostic clues are more aggressive course, younger age of presentation, and the absence of previous history consistent with NKCLs.

■ WORKUP AND STAGING

Careful history and physical exam are critical for timely and accurate diagnosis. Special attention must be paid to the racial/ethnic background of a patient presenting with a sinonasal tumor. NKCL is a much more likely diagnosis in Asian and South American patients, whereas in Caucasian patients, Wegener's granulomatosis, sarcoidosis, carcinomas, and conventional sinonasal diffuse large B cell lymphomas are higher on the differential (31). Involved organ should be biopsied, with special care of submitting a large specimen, since zonal necrosis is common and can preclude timely diagnosis. The biopsies should be sent fresh unfixed to the pathology laboratory for cryostat sectioning and flow cytometry to distinguish between T-cell and NK-cell lymphoma based on the surface CD3 positivity. If fresh tumor biopsies are unavailable, TCR gene rearrangement studies may be used to distinguish between the two lineages, since TCR genes are clonally rearranged only in T-cell lymphomas (2,4). Diagnosis requires a biopsy showing a diffuse, nonadhesive proliferation of medium-size lymphoid cells, surface CD3-, cytoplasmic CD3ε+, CD56+, CD20- phenotype and a cytotoxic profile (TIA-1, perforin or granzyme B positivity). Demonstration of EBV in the biopsy either by EBV-encoded small nuclear RNA (with in-situ hybridization) or LMP1 (by immunohistochemistry) is mandatory.

A careful ENT exam and a baseline ophthalmologic evaluation are critical, both for nasal and non-nasal NKCLs. CNS involvement is uncommon in early stage disease and routine lumbar puncture is not recommended. Laboratory tests should include full blood count and differential, renal and hepatic panels, LDH, beta2 microglobulin, albumin, serum calcium, uric acid and markers of hemophagocytic syndrome (serum ferritin, triglyceride and fibrinogen). Bone marrow biopsy should be examined for EBV-encoded RNA-1 in-situ hybridization.

Imaging

Radiologic imaging is critical for initial evaluation and staging of NKCLs. CT scan is preferred for detection of bony involvement and MRI is superior for evaluation of soft tissue infiltration. PET scan is useful for staging, as NKCLs are invariably 18-FDG avid with standardized uptake value maximum reported between 5 and 25 (32,33) and usually lower than that of aggressive B-cell lymphomas (34). The largest published series concluded that PET/CT successfully detected active disease in the nasopharynx in all five cases of involvement, with a mean SUVmax of 16. PET/CT detected extranasal disease in three of five cases in lymph nodes, bones, and skin, missing disease diffusely involving the bone marrow and liver. The mean SUVmax in PET-positive extranasal lesions was 10.9. There were no false-positive PET/

CT readings (33). High tumor FDG uptake has been shown to be associated with local tumor invasion and worse treatment outcomes (35).

Quantification of Circulating Plasma EBV DNA

EBV DNA quantification can be performed in plasma or whole blood, however peripheral blood mononuclear cells are not a suitable source, since circulating lymphoma cells are absent. Most patients will have circulating EBV DNA in the peripheral blood that is derived from the malignant cells, however EBV DNA is not specific for NKCL. Therefore, serum EBV DNA detection does not replace tissue biopsy and negativity does not eliminate the diagnosis. EBV DNA levels at diagnosis range from 10^5 to 10^{10} copies/mL, correlate with disease stage and LDH levels (36). EBV quantification can assist with assessment of tumor load and prognosis at diagnosis and also for monitoring response and relapse (36,37). In a retrospective series from Hong Kong, high levels of EBV DNA on presentation (>7.3 × 10^7 copies/mL) were associated with worse disease-free survival (0.5 vs. 8.7 months, SS) and overall survival (2 vs. 36 months, SS) (36).

■ PROGNOSIS

Several studies have shown that the Ann Arbor staging is not an effective prognostic tool for NKCL. No difference in overall survival could be found between patients with early stage and advanced stage NKCL (38) or Stage I and Stage II disease (39,40) when classified per the Ann Arbor staging system. The International Prognostic Index (IPI) is a clinical tool that provides as a predictive model to estimate prognosis of patients with aggressive NHL (Table 2). The IPI was developed from the results of a retrospective analysis of 1385 patients who were treated with doxorubicin-based chemotherapy between 1982 and 1987 (41), and is still widely used in practice. Although the IPI failed to predict survival in patients with NKCL in several studies (40,42), a low IPI score is consistently associated with better overall survival. More applicable prognostic models have been designed based on retrospective analysis of patients with NKCL. The Korean Prognostic Index (KPI), depicted in Table 3, is based on multicenter retrospective analysis of 262 patients (26). A more recent prognostic model has been proposed by a Japanese group (Table 4), based on a retrospective analysis of 172 patients with NKCL (43). Many additional parameters have been reported to correlate with prognosis, including high plasma EBV DNA levels, low expression of CD94 transcripts, absence of granzyme B inhibitor PI9, levels of KI-67 expression, absolute lymphocyte counts, local tumor invasiveness, high tumor 18F-fluorodeoxyglucose uptake (2,36,39,44–46), however these factors require further validation by other research groups.

■ MANAGEMENT OF NK CELL LYMPHOMAS

The optimal treatment strategy depends on the stage and location of the disease. Localized nasal NKCL is best managed by a combination of chemotherapy and radiation therapy (RT). Radiation does not appear to benefit patients with disseminated disease, or with non-nasal variant. Within the past 20 years, the application of more appropriate chemotherapy regimens and the refinement of RT techniques have improved both local control and overall survival in patients with NKCL.

Treatment of Localized Nasal NKCL

Initial response to RT is generally rapid (Figure 1), which established RT as the cornerstone of management of localized nasal NKCL. However, 20% to 30% of patients treated with RT alone develop systemic failure, highlighting the importance of chemotherapy in the management of NKCL. Moreover, concurrent chemo-RT appears to improve both local and decrease distant metastases, arguing for

TABLE 2 International Prognostic Index

Risk Factors	No. of Risk Factors	Risk Groups	5-year RFS	5-year OS
Age >60	0 to 1	Low	70%	73%
Serum LDH >1X normal	2	Low intermediate	50%	51%
PS 2–4	3	High intermediate	49%	43%
Stage III/IV	4 to 5	High	40%	26%
Extranodal involvement >1 site				

TABLE 3 Korean Prognostic Index

Risk Factors	No. of Factors	Risk Groups	5-year OS	RR of Death
B symptoms	0	Group 1	80.9%	1.0
Serum LDH >1X normal	1	Group 2	64.2%	1.8
Regional lymph node involvement	2	Group 3	34.4%	4.1
Ann Arbor Stage III/IV	3–4	Group 4	6.6%	13.6

TABLE 4 Japanese Prognostic Index

Risk Factors	No. of Factors	Risk Groups	4-year OS
Non-nasal type	0	Group 1	55%
Stage	1	Group 2	33%
Performance status	2	Group 3	15%
No extranodal involvement	3–4	Group 4	6%

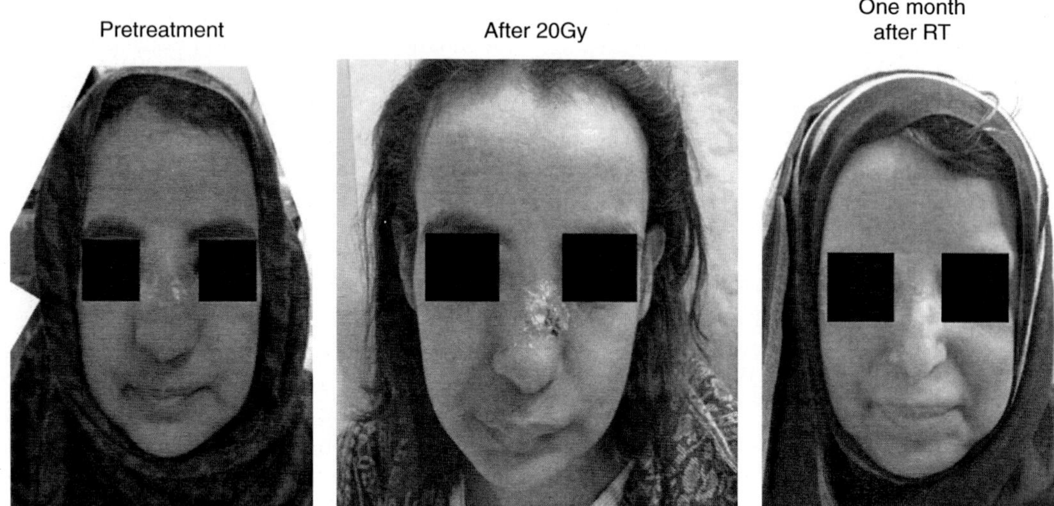

FIGURE 1   Facial NK cell lymphoma demonstrating tumor response to radiation therapy.

synergistic effect of two modalities. While there are no randomized trials comparing the effectiveness of RT alone versus combined modality therapy, retrospective studies have shown improved outcomes with the combination of chemotherapy and RT (Table 5). The majority of these studies have used doxorubicin-based chemotherapy regimens, with CHOP being the most common multi-drug therapy.

Radiation Therapy in Localized NKCL

Effective Radiation Dose

Several retrospective studies have established the association of RT dose and treatment outcome. Koom et al. (47) analyzed the outcome in 102 patients with Stage I/II NKCL treated with RT alone to a median dose of 45 Gy, with a range between 20 and 70 Gy in early 1980s and 1990s. The dose–response curve (Figure 2) was sigmoid in shape within the range of 20–54 Gy, which followed the plateau at doses in excess of 54 Gy. Isobe et al. (48) reported an analysis of 35 patients treated with RT or chemo-RT with a median tumor dose of 50 Gy, with a range between 22 and 60 Gy. The 5-year local control for patients who received ≥50 Gy vs patients received <50 Gy was 69.2% vs 53.3% (P = .13). In the study by Wu et al. (49), patients who received >50 Gy of RT had a better local control and a greater median survival than those who received <50 Gy of RT (P < .05). Huang et al. (50) reported improvement of OS and DFS in patients receiving ≥54 Gy of RT as compared with <54 Gy (5-year OS 75.5% vs 46.1%, P = .019; 5-year DFS 60.3% vs 33.4%, P = .004).

Target Volumes and Tumor Coverage

While there is general agreement around the minimal dose is required for treatment of nasal NKCL, there is greater uncertainty regarding the appropriate target volumes. Many original articles contain terms such as "adequate margin" around gross tumor volume and "elective nodal coverage." In one study evaluating outcomes of 214 patients who received RT for NKCL, regional lymph node failure was only observed in 4 (1.9%), 3 of whom had received nodal irradiation (51). One of 23 (4.3%) stage I patients and 2 of 32 (6.3%) stage II patients who received neck RT had a nodal relapse (51). One patient (0.6%) of 159 who had not received elective nodal RT developed subsequent regional lymph node failure. Koom et al. observed no regional nodal failures among 36 node-negative patients who received elective neck RT, and 1 of 46 (2.2%) node-negative patients had cervical nodal failure in the absence of elective nodal RT (47). Conversely, 2 of the 20 node-positive patients (10%) subsequently experienced a nodal recurrence within the RT field. (47) Results of these studies suggest that patients with stage II disease have a higher rate of nodal failure even with the use of local therapy (Table 6).

In the study noted above, Li et al. achieved excellent 5-yrs OS and PFS rates for patients with stage I and II disease of (77.6% and 72.3%, respectively)

TABLE 5 Retrospective studies comparing the outcome of RT alone versus chemo-RT in the management of localized NK cell lymphoma

				Treatment		RT Dose (Gy)			Overall Survival		PFS		Failure Rate (%)	
Study	Year of publication	No of patients	Study Period	Type	No of patients	Median	Range	CR Rate (%)	Type	Rate (%)	Type	Rate (%)	Local	Systemic
Li et al. (73)	2006	105	1983–2003	RT alone	31	50	40–65	83	5 years	66	5 years	61	29	81
				CT + RT				81	5 years	76	5 years	61		
Cheung et al. (29)	2002	79	1977–2001	RT alone	18	50	30–60	77.8	5 years	29.8	5 years	30.5	46.7	75.6
				CT + RT	61			65.6	5 years	40.3	5 years	35.8		
Li et al. (51)	2011	182	1987–2009	RT alone	96	53	50–56	89.7	5 years	69.8	5 years	59.5	12	25.5
				CT + RT	118				5 years	74.4	5 years	68.2		
Ma et al. (74)	2010	64	1993–2005	RT alone	23	54	45.2–60.4	69.6	5 years	57.9	5 years	52.3		
				CT + RT	41			87.8	5 years	61.5	5 years	52.2		
Kim et al. (52)	2001	143	1976–1995	RT alone	104	50.4	40–54	69%	5 years	38	5 years	32	48	24
				RT + CT	39			67%	5 years	35	5 years	27	41	33

TABLE 6   Neck failure in patients with stage IE with and without elective RT and in patients with Stage IIE with neck RT

Study	Failure rate among IE with no neck RT	Failure rate among IE with neck RT	Failure rate among IIE with neck RT
Li et al. (51)	0.6% (1/159)	4.3% (1/23)	6.3% (2/32)
Koom et al. (47)	2.2% (1/46)	0 (0/36)	10% (2/20)

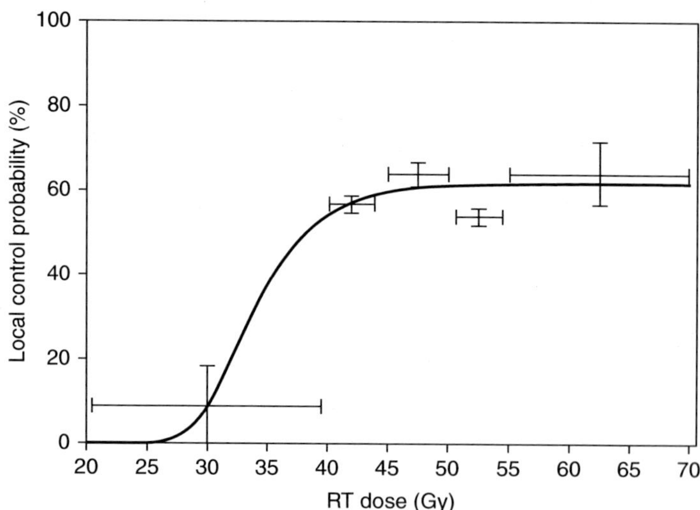

FIGURE 2 Dose-response curve for NK cell lymphoma. Local control probability as function of radiation dose in patients treated with radiotherapy alone. Horizontal lines indicate range of RT doses delivered; vertical lines represent 95% CI of local control probability.

Source: Adapted from Ref (17). Reproduced with permission by Elsevier.

(51). Based on their experience, the Department of Radiation Oncology from Beijing issued the following guidelines for radiation planning. GTV is determined by the analysis of all available imaging modalities (CT scan, PET/CT, MRI) as well as clinical examination. Clinical target volume (CTV) for patients with Stage IE disease limited to the nasal cavity, includes the nasal cavity, bilateral frontal ethmoid sinuses, and ipsilateral maxillary sinus. For patients with extensive or limited stage IE diseases close to the choanae, CTV is extended to encompass involved paranasal tissues, nasopharynx, and other adjacent organs. For patients with involvement of Waldeyer's ring, CTV includes the entire lymphoid ring (nasopharynx, tonsil, base of tongue, and oropharynx) and any localized disease extension. Based on the failure rates with and without elective nodal RT, prophylactic cervical node irradiation should not be given to patients with stage IE nasal NKCL, unless Waldeyer's ring is involved.

Timing of Chemotherapy

Due to the excellent response of NKCL to RT, it is frequently used as first-line therapy, as opposed to initiating systemic therapy and consolidating with RT. The complete remission (CR) rate with doxorubicin-based chemotherapy alone is poor. Kim et al. report a 5% CR rate with chemotherapy alone in patients treated for NKCL, as compared with 69% in those treated with up-front RT (52). The CR rate improved to 67% if consolidative RT was employed after systemic therapy (52). Huang et al. show improved survival for Stage I patients who receive up-front RT when compared with patients treated with chemotherapy followed by RT (5-year OS 90.0% versus 48.9%, $P = .012$; DFS 78.7% vs 39.9%, $P = .021$) (50). Similar results were shown by You et al. who reported 5-year OS of 83% versus 29%, following up-front versus consolidative RT (53).

RT Technique

Most institutions use intensity modulated radiation therapy (IMRT) in the treatment of NKCL to improve dose distribution and decrease treatment toxicity. Wang et al. (54) reported on their use of IMRT in patients with localized NKCL treated to a median dose of 50 Gy and showed excellent 2-year

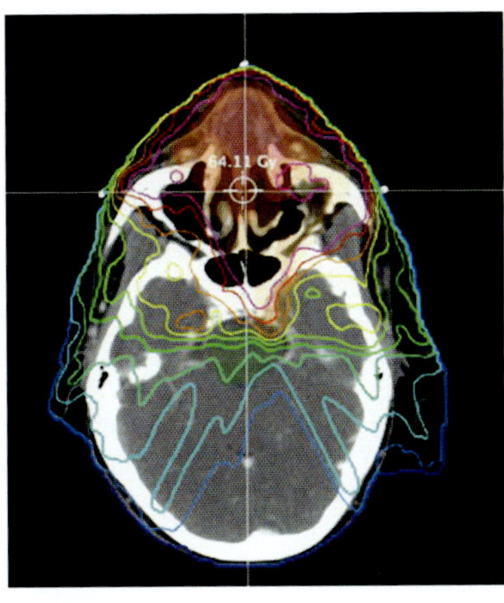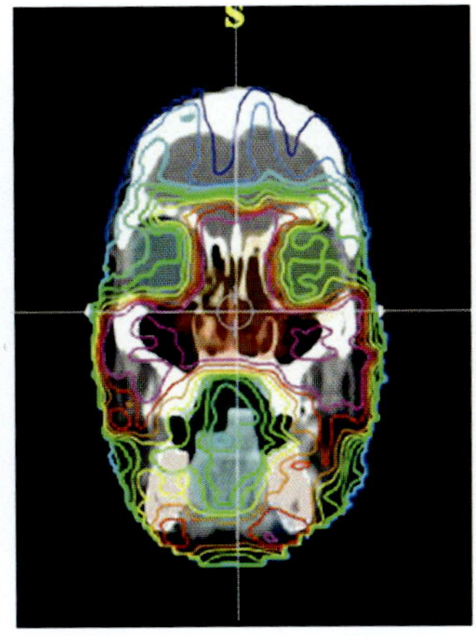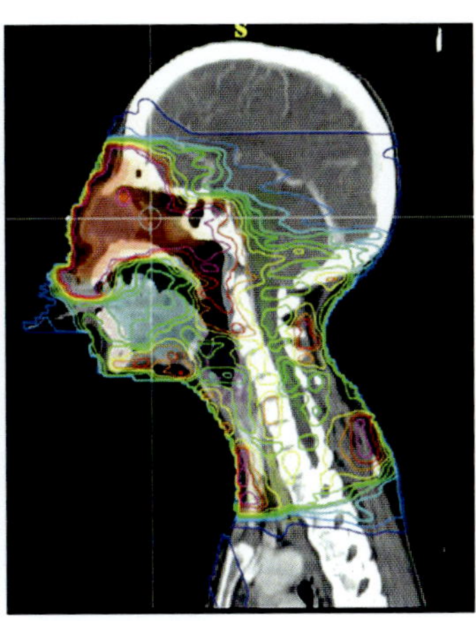

FIGURE 3 Treatment plan for stage II disease with nodal involvement. Axial, coronal, and sagittal view of treatment plan. Tumor visualized within the nasal cavity in both the axial and sagittal planes.

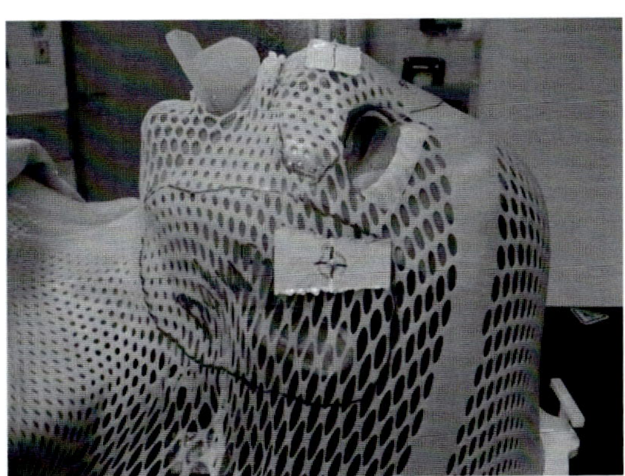

FIGURE 4 Immobilization for radiation therapy. The patient is immobilized using a custom Aquaplast mask. The head is placed with chin slightly extended; a bite block is used to separate tongue from hard palate. Custom bolus is applied to areas outlined; need for bolus is determined during the course of planning.

outcomes with mild toxicity. The authors were able to deliver less than 20 Gy to parotid glands in all their patients, with the mean parotid dose of 15 Gy. Tomita et al. (55) compared radiation treatment plans generated with IMRT or 3D-CRT for nasal cell lymphoma patients treated at their institution. IMRT achieved a better PTV coverage (with more than 99% of the PTV receiving 90% and 95% of the prescribed dose with IMRT, vs 89.1% and 84.5% of the PTV receiving 90% and 95% of the prescribed

dose with 3D-CRT.) The homogeneity index was 0.29 for IMRT and 0.046 for 3D-CRT ($P < .0001$).

The use of IMRT is particularly advantageous when nodal volumes need to be included in the treatment field (Figure 3), or if an additional dose is prescribed to the GTV for particularly large or destructive lesions. When IMRT is employed, patients should be immobilized in an Aquaplast mask to ensure reproducibility of position. Appropriate use of bite blocks and bolus are essential (Figure 4). The clinician will ensure quality assurance by evaluating portal imaging; air gaps around the tumor volume should be avoided to ensure the accurate delivery of the planned dose distribution (Figure 5).

Concurrent Chemo-RT for Localized NK Cell Lymphoma

Conventional CHOP or CHOP-like regimens give poor outcome, with CR achieved in <20% of patients (4). This in part may be due to the expression of the multi-drug resistance 1 (MDR-1) gene, leading to high levels of P-glycoprotein and therefore active export of many chemotherapeutic drugs, such as anthracyclines. The two most recent prospective trials, summarized in Table 7 have achieved substantial improvements in both CR and OS by combining upfront RT with non-anthracycline multiagent chemotherapy regimens.

The longer follow-up is necessary to determine whether this combination can be termed curable, and dose-escalation studies in the setting of these systemic agents will determine whether RT dose of at

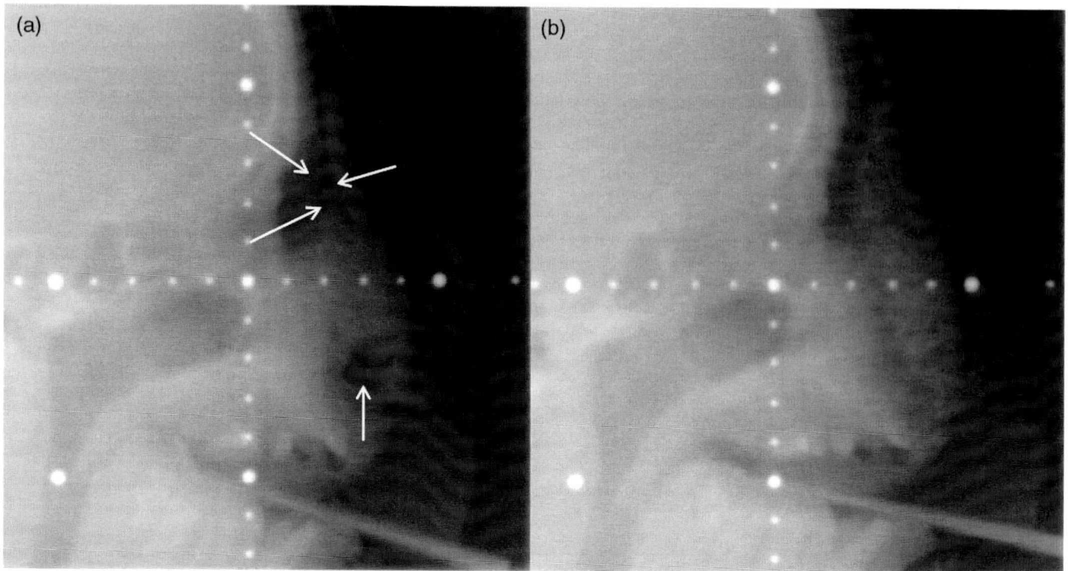

FIGURE 5 Treatment quality assurance. Portal imaging (a) demonstrating air gaps as designated by the white arrows; (b) with bolus materials adequately filling in air gaps.

Portal imaging is typically obtained on a weekly basis. Some institutions are moving toward the use of cone-beamed CT to ensure accurate set-up of patients getting radiation therapy for head and neck tumors.

TABLE 7 Prospective trials of concurrent chemo-RT for stage I/IIE Nasal NK Cell Lymphoma

Study	Treatment	N	Stage IE	Stage IIE	CR (%)	OR (%)	Local/systemic relapse	Main toxicity	OS
Yamaguchi et al. (64)	RT: 50 Gy for Stage IE, 50.4 Gy for Stage IIE CT: 3 courses of DeVIC	27	18	9	77	81	4%/33%	Mucositis	78% at 2 years
Kim et al. (75)	RT median 40 Gy CT: weekly cisplatin 30 mg/m^2 with RT, then 3 courses of VIPD	30	15	15	80	83	7%/7%	Leucopenia	86% at 3 years

DeVIC: Dexamethasone 40 mg D1–3, etoposide 67 mg/m^2 D1–3, ifosfamide 1 g/m^2 D1–3, carboplatin 200 mg/m^2 D1 (q3 weeks)

VIPD: Etoposide 100 mg/m^2 D1–3, ifosfamide 1.2 g/m^2 D1–3, cisplatin 33 mg/m^2 D1–3, dexamethasone 40 mg D1–4 (q3 weeks)

least 54 Gy is still beneficial in the presence of these radiosensitizer, and whether toxicity is tolerable. Until such data is available, these combinations of chemo-RT, with clinical decision on the appropriate RT dose with a careful clinical monitoring during the therapy for toxicity, should be considered the standard of care for patients with localized nasal NKCL.

CNS Prophylaxis

Secondary CNS involvement is a devastating complication that leads to death in most patients. Several studies report a variable incidence of CNS involvement in NKCL, from 0% to 6% (24,51,56,57). Kim et al. (58) analyzed 208 patients for incidence of CNS invasion. Overall 12 patients (5.76%) experienced

CNS disease during treatment or follow-up, with a median time from diagnosis to CNS involvement of 11.6 months. The clinical variables associated with CNS disease were Ann Arbor stage III/IV (15.87%), regional lymph node involvement (10.41%), group III/IV on NK/T-cell lymphoma prognostic index (NKPI; 10.2%) and extra-upper aerodigestive primary sites (9.75%). In multivariate analysis, NKPI retained the strongest statistical power to predict CNS disease (RR 9.29) in NKCL. Therefore it is not a standard practice to offer CNS prophylaxis to patients with localized NKCL. Prophylaxis could be considered in patients with advanced-stage disease.

Response Evaluation and Patient Follow-up

With new non-anthracycline based chemo-RT the cure rate could be as high as 70%. As NKCLs are FDG-avid, PET/CT scan is a useful modality for response evaluation, and quantification of circulating EBV DNA is another way of measuring tumor load. Au et al. analyzed EBV DNA in patients with NKCL and observed an association between EBV DNA levels and treatment response. In 7 patients who achieved CR, EBV DNA became undetectable, however in 14 refractory or relapsing cases, EBV DNA remained high (range: 6.7×10^7–2.4×10^{11}, median: 2.8×10^8 copies/mL) with persistent disease and until death (36). However, a small study of a novel agent in refractory and/or relapsing NKCL detected EBV serum DNA in only 68% of patients (13 out of 19), and did not find a difference in survival between positive and negative patients ($P = .6$) or between patients with low and high EBV serum DNA ($P = .46$) (37). The use of PET/CT and EBV DNA quantification in documenting clinical and molecular remission will have to be validated prospectively. Very late relapses of early-stage nasal NKCL as local or systemic recrudescence have been described as late as 10 to 30 years after initial treatments (59,60). Therefore, life-long follow up is recommended even for patients who are in prolonged remission.

Treatment of Elderly Patients with Early Stage NKCL

NKCL is rare in elderly patients. Wang et al. (61) reported their experience with 24 elderly patients (age >60 years) with early stage disease, treated with RT, chemotherapy or chemo-RT. Five-year overall, cancer-specific and progression-free survival rates were 54.3%, 42% and 40.2%, respectively. Eight out of 24 patients had disease relapse, with only one out of 8 local relapse. Of concern, four patients died of treatment-related mortality. It is important to realize that elderly patients have an unfavorable prognosis and they should be managed with a greater care to avoid toxicity and treatment-related mortality.

The Role of Surgery in Localized Disease

Surgery is rarely used in the management of lymphomas. The experience of surgical management of NKCL is extremely limited and is summarized in Table 8. It appears that surgery may be an important component of the local management, and its use with RT or instead of RT should be further studied.

Management of Advanced-Stage Nasal and Non-Nasal NK Cell Lymphoma.

For patients initially advanced nasal cell lymphoma, as well as non-nasal NKCL, chemotherapy is the mainstay of treatment; historically, the prognosis was dismal. An anthracycline-based regimen by itself achieves a very low CR due to the frequent expression of MDR1 protein. Non-anthracycline regimen (combination of ifosfamide, methotrexate, etoposide and prednisolone) achieved CR rate of 13% and a median overall survival of 2.7 months (62). A novel regimen SMILE

TABLE 8 Summary of results of surgical management of NK cell lymphoma

Study	Number of patients	Number of patients who underwent surgery	Outcome
Pagano et al. (38)	26	2 (chemo after surgery) and 1 (surgery only)	All 3 patients with surgery were the only long-term survivors
Lee et al. (76)	262	2 (surgery only)	Information is not available
Chim et al. (77)	67	1 (surgery only)	Scrotal relapse 10 years later, died of systemic relapse
Nair et al. (78)	1	1 (failed chemo, RT and immunotherapy; surgery followed by HD chemo and autologous hematopoietic stem cell rescue	In CR 4 years after surgery

(dexamethasone 40 mg, D2–4, methotrexate 2 g/m², D1, ifosfamide 1.5 g/m² D2–4, etoposide 100 mg/m² D2–4, l-asparaginase 6,000 U/m², D8, 10, 12, 14, 16, 18, 20; q28 days) has been shown in phase I (63) and phase II (64) studies to be promising. This regimen is based on the use of drugs which are not transported by MDR1 gene product P-glycoprotein, together with l-asparaginase, which has been used in relapsed NKCLs as a single agent (37,65), and has also been shown to have anti-tumor activity in vitro (66). In patients with relapsed or refractory NKCL, SMILE regimen resulted in an overall response rate of 74% and CR of 35%–50% (63,64). Despite promising early outcomes, long-term results need to be awaited. Nevertheless, this combination appears to be the most effective systemic therapy for the advanced disease at the present time. Novel drugs, such as NK-kB inhibitors and proteasome inhibitors are studied in vitro (67) and clinically (68), and with time might form the backbone of systemic management of this aggressive disease.

Salvage Therapies for Relapsed Disease

Salvage treatment significantly prolongs overall survival compared with the best supportive care alone (5-years OS 38% vs 0%, *P* < .0001). However, salvage RT is more effective in improving survival in relapsed stage III/IV patients, than anthracycline-based chemotherapy in relapsed patients with early stage disease (69). In retrospective studies, l-asparaginase-based regimen was demonstrated to have an overall response rate of 82% with a 5-year overall survival of 67% (65), whereas the Phase II trial of SMILE regimen results in the overall response rate of 74% (64). Different preparations of l-asparaginase, including *E. coli* derived, Erwinia derived and pegylated forms, appear to have similar treatment results (37,65). The main side effects of l-asparaginase include hyperbilirubinemia, liver dysfunction, leucopenia, infections, hyperglycemia, and hypersensitivity reactions.

Hematopoietic Stem Cell Transplantation

HSCT has been explored as consolidation or salvage therapy, however, prospective trials have not been performed. In a large retrospective multi-institutional analysis, NKCL patients who received autologous HSCT were matched to patients treated with chemotherapy or RT and analyzed. Although patients undergoing HSCT appeared to have a slightly lower relapse rate, HSCT was associated with a 8.5% treatment-related mortality, and the overall survival between the two groups was similar (70). In a review of cases treated with allogeneic HSCT and reported in the literature, half of the patients were alive after HSCT, but 25% died from transplantation-related complications, with the remaining dying from progressive disease (71). In the largest retrospective series, the 2-year OS after allogeneic HSCT was 40% (72). Given the high rate of complications and poor short-term results, further trials need to elucidate which patient population might derive the most benefit from HSCT.

■ REFERENCES

1. Spits H, Lanier LL, Phillips JH. Development of human T and natural killer cells. *Blood*. 1995;85(10):2654–2670.

2. Oshimi K. Progress in understanding and managing natural killer-cell malignancies. *Br J Haematol*. 2007:139(4):532–544.

3. Harris NL, et al. World Health Organization classification of neoplastic diseases of the hematopoietic and lymphoid tissues: report of the Clinical Advisory Committee meeting-Airlie House, Virginia, November 1997. *J Clin Oncol*. 1999;17(12):3835–3849.

4. Kwong YL. Natural killer-cell malignancies: diagnosis and treatment. *Leukemia*. 2005;19(12):2186–2194.

5. Li CC, et al. Treatment outcome and pattern of failure in 77 patients with sinonasal natural killer/T-cell or T-cell lymphoma. *Cancer*. 2004;100(2):366–375.

6. Jaffe ES, et al. Report of the workshop on nasal and related extranodal angiocentric T/natural killer cell lymphomas. Definitions, differential diagnosis, and epidemiology. *Am J Surg Pathol*. 1996;20(1):103–111.

7. Arber DA, et al. Nasal lymphomas in Peru. High incidence of T-cell immunophenotype and Epstein-Barr virus infection. *Am J Surg Pathol*. 1993;17(4):392–399.

8. Harris NL, et al. A revised European-American classification of lymphoid neoplasms: a proposal from the International Lymphoma Study Group. *Blood*. 1994;84(5):1361–1392.

9. Wong KF, et al. CD56 (NKH1)-positive hematolymphoid malignancies: an aggressive neoplasm featuring frequent cutaneous/mucosal involvement, cytoplasmic azurophilic granules, and angiocentricity. *Hum Pathol*. 1992;23(7):798–804.

10. Campo E, et al. The 2008 WHO classification of lymphoid neoplasms and beyond: evolving concepts and practical applications. *Blood*. 117(19):5019–5032.

11. Pagano JS, et al. Infectious agents and cancer: criteria for a causal relation. *Semin Cancer Biol*. 2004;14(6):453–471.

12. Mosialos G, et al. The Epstein-Barr virus transforming protein LMP1 engages signaling proteins for the tumor necrosis factor receptor family. *Cell*. 1995;80(3):389–399.

13. Miller WE, Cheshire JL, Raab-Traub N. Interaction of tumor necrosis factor receptor-associated factor signaling proteins with the latent membrane protein 1 PXQXT motif is essential for induction of

epidermal growth factor receptor expression. *Mol Cell Biol.* 1998;18(5):2835–2844.

14. Chan JK, et al. Nonnasal lymphoma expressing the natural killer cell marker CD56: a clinicopathologic study of 49 cases of an uncommon aggressive neoplasm. *Blood.* 1997;89(12):4501–4513.

15. Chan JK, et al. Detection of Epstein-Barr viral RNA in malignant lymphomas of the upper aerodigestive tract. *Am J Surg Pathol.* 1994;18(9):938–946.

16. Elenitoba-Johnson KS, et al. Cytotoxic granular protein expression, Epstein-Barr virus strain type, and latent membrane protein-1 oncogene deletions in nasal T-lymphocyte/natural killer cell lymphomas from Mexico. *Mod Pathol.* 1998;11(8):754–761.

17. van Gorp J, et al. Epstein-Barr virus in nasal T-cell lymphomas (polymorphic reticulosis/midline malignant reticulosis) in western China. *J Pathol.* 1994;173(2):81–87.

18. Chiang AK, et al. Comparative analysis of Epstein-Barr virus gene polymorphisms in nasal T/NK-cell lymphomas and normal nasal tissues: implications on virus strain selection in malignancy. *Int J Cancer.* 1999;80(3):356–364.

19. Tabanelli V, et al. Systemic Epstein-Barr-virus-positive T cell lymphoproliferative childhood disease in a 22-year-old Caucasian man: A case report and review of the literature. *J Med Case Reports.* 2011;5:218.

20. Cohen JI, et al. Epstein-Barr virus-associated lymphoproliferative disease in non-immunocompromised hosts: a status report and summary of an international meeting, 8–9 September 2008. *Ann Oncol.* 2009;20(9):1472–1482.

21. Wong KF, et al. Bone marrow involvement by nasal NK cell lymphoma at diagnosis is uncommon. *Am J Clin Pathol.* 2001;115(2):266–270.

22. Kim TM, et al. Clinical heterogeneity of extranodal NK/T-cell lymphoma, nasal type: a national survey of the Korean Cancer Study Group. *Ann Oncol.* 2008;19(8):1477–1484.

23. Liang R, et al. Treatment outcome and prognostic factors for primary nasal lymphoma. *J Clin Oncol.* 1995;13(3):666–670.

24. Cheung MM, et al. Primary non-Hodgkin's lymphoma of the nose and nasopharynx: clinical features, tumor immunophenotype, and treatment outcome in 113 patients. *J Clin Oncol.* 1998;16(1):70–77.

25. Kim GE, et al. Angiocentric lymphoma of the head and neck: patterns of systemic failure after radiation treatment. *J Clin Oncol.* 2000;18(1):54–63.

26. Lee J, et al. Extranodal natural killer T-cell lymphoma, nasal-type: a prognostic model from a retrospective multicenter study. *J Clin Oncol.* 2006;24(4):612–618.

27. Li YX, et al. Clinical features and treatment outcome of nasal-type NK/T-cell lymphoma of Waldeyer ring. *Blood.* 2008;112(8):3057–3064.

28. Li YX, et al. Variable clinical presentations of nasal and Waldeyer ring natural killer/T-cell lymphoma. *Clin Cancer Res.* 2009;15(8):2905–2912.

29. Cheung MM, et al. Early stage nasal NK/T-cell lymphoma: clinical outcome, prognostic factors, and the effect of treatment modality. *Int J Radiat Oncol Biol Phys.* 2002;54(1):182–190.

30. Yok-Lam K, The diagnosis and management of extranodal NK/T-cell lymphoma, nasal-type and aggressive NK-cell leukemia. *J Clin Exp Hematop.* 51(1):21–28.

31. Batsakis JG, Luna MA. Midfacial necrotizing lesions. *Semin Diagn Pathol.* 1987;4(2):90–116.

32. Khong PL, et al. Fluorine-18 fluorodeoxyglucose positron emission tomography in mature T-cell and natural killer cell malignancies. *Ann Hematol.* 2008;87(8):613–621.

33. Karantanis D, et al. The value of [(18)F] fluorodeoxyglucose positron emission tomography/computed tomography in extranodal natural killer/T-cell lymphoma. *Clin Lymphoma Myeloma,* 2008;8(2):94–99.

34. Chan WK, et al. Metabolic activity measured by F-18 FDG PET in natural killer-cell lymphoma compared to aggressive B- and T-cell lymphomas. *Clin Nucl Med.* 2010;35(8):571–575.

35. Suh C, et al. Prognostic value of tumor 18F-FDG uptake in patients with untreated extranodal natural killer/T-cell lymphomas of the head and neck. *J Nucl Med.* 2008;49(11):1783–1789.

36. Au WY, et al. Quantification of circulating Epstein-Barr virus (EBV) DNA in the diagnosis and monitoring of natural killer cell and EBV-positive lymphomas in immunocompetent patients. *Blood.* 2004;104(1):243–249.

37. Jaccard A, et al. Efficacy of l-asparaginase with methotrexate and dexamethasone (AspaMetDex regimen) in patients with refractory or relapsing extranodal NK/T-cell lymphoma, a phase 2 study. *Blood.* 2011;117(6):1834–1839.

38. Pagano L, et al. NK/T-cell lymphomas 'nasal type': an Italian multicentric retrospective survey. *Ann Oncol.* 2006;17(5):794–800.

39. Kim TM, et al. Local tumor invasiveness is more predictive of survival than International Prognostic Index in stage I(E)/II(E) extranodal NK/T-cell lymphoma, nasal type. *Blood.* 2005;106(12):3785–790.

40. Kim SJ, et al. Ki-67 expression is predictive of prognosis in patients with stage I/II extranodal NK/T-cell lymphoma, nasal type. *Ann Oncol.* 2007;18(8):1382–1387.

41. No Authors. A predictive model for aggressive non-Hodgkin's lymphoma. The International Non-Hodgkin's Lymphoma Prognostic Factors Project. *N Engl J Med.* 1993;329(14):987–994.

42. Aviles A, et al. Angiocentric nasal T/natural killer cell lymphoma: a single centre study of prognostic factors in 108 patients. *Clin Lab Haematol.* 2000;22(4):215–220.

43. Suzuki R et al. Prognostic factors for mature natural killer (NK) cell neoplasms: aggressive NK cell leukemia and extranodal NK cell lymphoma, nasal type. *Ann Oncol.* 2010;21(5):1032–1040.

44. Au WY, et al. Clinical differences between nasal and extranasal natural killer/T-cell lymphoma: a study of 136 cases from the International Peripheral T-Cell Lymphoma Project. *Blood.* 2009;113(17):3931–3937.

45. Huang JJ, et al. Absolute lymphocyte count is a novel prognostic indicator in extranodal natural killer/T-cell lymphoma, nasal type. *Ann Oncol.* 2011;22(1):149–155.

46. Lin CW, et al. CD94 transcripts imply a better prognosis in nasal-type extranodal NK/T-cell lymphoma. *Blood.* 2003;102(7):2623–2631.

47. Koom WS, et al. Angiocentric T-cell and NK/T-cell lymphomas: radiotherapeutic viewpoints. *Int J Radiat Oncol Biol Phys.* 2004;59(4):1127–1137.

48. Isobe K, et al. Extranodal natural killer/T-cell lymphoma, nasal type: the significance of radiotherapeutic parameters. *Cancer.* 2006;106(3):609–615.

49. Wu X, et al. A clinical study of 115 patients with extranodal natural killer/T-cell lymphoma, nasal type. *Clin Oncol (R Coll Radiol).* 2008;20(8):619–625.

50. Huang MJ, et al. Early or up-front radiotherapy improved survival of localized extranodal NK/T-cell lymphoma, nasal-type in the upper aerodigestive tract. *Int J Radiat Oncol Biol Phys.* 2008;70(1):166–174.

51. Li YX, et al. Failure patterns and clinical implications in early stage nasal natural killer/T-cell lymphoma treated with primary radiotherapy. *Cancer.* 2011;117(22):5203–5211.

52. Kim GE, et al. Combined chemotherapy and radiation versus radiation alone in the management of localized angiocentric lymphoma of the head and neck. *Radiother Oncol.* 2001;61(3):261–269.

53. You JY, et al. Radiation therapy versus chemotherapy as initial treatment for localized nasal natural killer (NK)/T-cell lymphoma: a single institute survey in Taiwan. *Ann Oncol.* 2004;15(4):618–625.

54. Wang H, et al. Mild toxicity and favorable prognosis of high-dose and extended involved-field intensity-modulated radiotherapy for patients with early-stage nasal NK/T-cell lymphoma. *Int J Radiat Oncol Biol Phys.* 2012;82(3):1115–1121.

55. Tomita N, et al. A comparison of radiation treatment plans using IMRT with helical tomotherapy and 3D conformal radiotherapy for nasal natural killer/T-cell lymphoma. *Br J Radiol.* 2009;82(981):756–763.

56. Cuadra-Garcia I, et al. Sinonasal lymphoma: a clinicopathologic analysis of 58 cases from the Massachusetts General Hospital. *Am J Surg Pathol.* 1999;23(11):1356–1369.

57. Kim GE, et al. Clinical relevance of three subtypes of primary sinonasal lymphoma characterized by immunophenotypic analysis. *Head Neck,* 2004;26(7):584–593.

58. Kim SJ, et al. When do we need central nervous system prophylaxis in patients with extranodal NK/T-cell lymphoma, nasal type? *Ann Oncol.* 2010;21(5):1058–1063.

59. Ishida F, et al. Late relapse of extranodal natural killer/T cell lymphoma, nasal type, after more than ten years. *Leuk Lymphoma.* 2010;51(1):171–173.

60. Au WY, et al. Clinicopathological features and outcome of late relapses of natural killer cell lymphomas 10–29 years after initial remission. *Am J Hematol.* 2010;85(5):362–363.

61. Wang ZY, et al. Unfavorable prognosis of elderly patients with early-stage extranodal nasal-type NK/T-cell lymphoma. *Ann Oncol.* 2011;22(2):390–396.

62. Lee KW, et al. First-line ifosfamide, methotrexate, etoposide and prednisolone chemotherapy +/- radiotherapy is active in stage I/II extranodal NK/T-cell lymphoma. *Leuk Lymphoma.* 2006;47(7):1274–1282.

63. Yamaguchi M, et al. Phase I study of dexamethasone, methotrexate, ifosfamide, l-asparaginase, and etoposide (SMILE) chemotherapy for advanced-stage, relapsed or refractory extranodal natural killer (NK)/T-cell lymphoma and leukemia. *Cancer Sci.* 2008;99(5):1016–1020.

64. Yamaguchi M, et al. Phase I/II study of concurrent chemoradiotherapy for localized nasal natural killer/T-cell lymphoma: Japan Clinical Oncology Group Study JCOG0211. *J Clin Oncol.* 2009;27(33):5594–5600.

65. Yong W, et al. l-asparaginase in the treatment of refractory and relapsed extranodal NK/T-cell lymphoma, nasal type. *Ann Hematol.* 2009;88(7):647–652.

66. Ando M, et al. Selective apoptosis of natural killer-cell tumours by l-asparaginase. *Br J Haematol.* 2005;130(6):860–868.

67. Kim K, et al. Effects of nuclear factor-kappaB inhibitors and its implication on natural killer T-cell lymphoma cells. *Br J Haematol.* 2005;131(1):59–66.

68. Shen L, et al. Proteasome inhibitor bortezomib-induced apoptosis in natural killer (NK)-cell leukemia and lymphoma: an in vitro and in vivo preclinical evaluation. *Blood.* 2007;110(1):469–470.

69. Zhang XX, et al. Salvage treatment improved survival of patients with relapsed extranodal natural killer/t-cell lymphoma, nasal type. *Int J Radiat Oncol Biol Phys.* 2009;74(3):747–752.

70. Lee J, et al. Autologous hematopoietic stem cell transplantation in extranodal natural killer/T cell lymphoma: a multinational, multicenter, matched controlled study. *Biol Blood Marrow Transplant.* 2008;14(12):1356–1364.

71. Kwong YL. High-dose chemotherapy and hematopoietic SCT in the management of natural killer-cell malignancies. *Bone Marrow Transplant.* 2009;44(11):709–714.

72. Murashige N, et al. Allogeneic haematopoietic stem cell transplantation as a promising treatment for natural killer-cell neoplasms. *Br J Haematol.* 2005;130(4):561–567.

73. Li YX, et al. Radiotherapy as primary treatment for stage IE and IIE nasal natural killer/T-cell lymphoma. *J Clin Oncol.* 2006;24(1):181–189.

74. Ma, HH, et al. Treatment outcome of radiotherapy alone versus radiochemotherapy in early stage nasal natural killer/T-cell lymphoma. *Med Oncol.* 2010;27(3):798–806.

75. Kim SJ, et al. Phase II trial of concurrent radiation and weekly cisplatin followed by VIPD chemotherapy in newly diagnosed, stage IE to IIE, nasal, extranodal NK/T-Cell Lymphoma: Consortium for Improving Survival of Lymphoma study. *J Clin Oncol.* 2009;27(35):6027–6032.

76. Moser EC, et al. Risk of second cancer after treatment of aggressive non-Hodgkin's lymphoma; an EORTC cohort study. *Haematologica.* 2006;91(11):1481–1488.

77. Chim CS, et al. Primary nasal natural killer cell lymphoma: long-term treatment outcome and relationship with the International Prognostic Index. *Blood.* 2004;103(1):216–221.

78. Nair RR, et al. Surgery for nasal NK/T-cell lymphoma. *Leuk Lymphoma.* 2008;49(11):2206–2208.

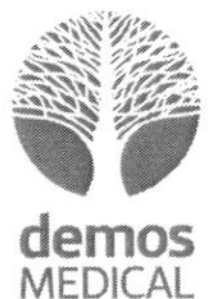

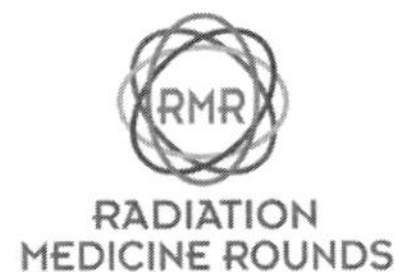

Mantle Cell and Other Aggressive B-Cell Non-Hodgkin Lymphoma Subtypes

Shripal Bhavsar[1] and Michael B. Tomblyn[2*]

[1]*Department of Radiation Oncology, SUNY-Upstate Medical University, Syracuse, NY*

[2]*Department of Radiation Oncology, H. Lee Moffitt Cancer Center and Research Institute, Tampa, FL*

■ ABSTRACT

In addition to diffuse large B-cell lymphoma, there are a number of additional aggressive B-cell subtypes seen in clinical practice, each with its unique pathologic and molecular profile. Histologies include mantle cell lymphoma, Burkitt lymphoma, plasmablastic lymphoma, and lymphomatoid granulomatosis. We review each of these aggressive B-cell malignancies, including epidemiology, pathology, staging and prognosis, and therapy.

Keywords: mantle cell lymphoma, Burkitt lymphoma, Lymphomatoid granulomatosis

■ MANTLE CELL LYMPHOMA

Mantle cell lymphoma (MCL) has only recently been officially recognized as an independent non-Hodgkin lymphoma (NHL) subtype, originally described as a group of centrocytic lymphomas in the Kiel classification (1). Today, MCL is a distinct NHL histology and is generally considered to represent a nonindolent lymphoma (2). MCL represents approximately 4% of all lymphomas in the U.S. and about 8% in Europe (3). The median age at diagnosis is in the seventh decade of life, with a strong male predominance (4). Patients generally present with stage III or IV disease, with frequent involvement of the bone marrow (5).

In contrast with other NHL histologies, MCL frequently involves the gastrointestinal (GI) tract (6).

Diagnosis and Pathology

The diagnosis of MCL is made upon pathologic review of a sample from a lymph node, bone marrow, or tissue biopsy, with the malignant cells typically exhibiting a lymphoid morphology with irregular nuclear contours. The typical immunophenotype of the MCL cell is CD20+, CD5+, CD10-, Bcl6-, and cyclin D1+ (2). Most MCL cases are significant for a hallmark chromosomal translocation, t(11;14), leading to the aberrant expression of cyclin D1 (7). Overexpression of transcription factor SOX11 is commonly seen in MCL, and its absence in the disease predicts for a more indolent course (8). Other molecular predictors for aggressive MCL include p53 mutations, p16 deletions, and a high Ki-67 index (9).

*Corresponding author, Department of Radiation Oncology, H. Lee Moffitt Cancer Center and Research Institute, 12902 Magnolia Drive, MCC-RAD ONC, Tampa, FL

E-mail address: michael.tomblyn@moffitt.org

Radiation Medicine Rounds 3:3 (2012) 451–458.

DOI: 10.5003/2151-4208.3.3.451

Staging and Prognosis

Staging for MCL includes the typical history and physical, complete blood counts, chemistry panel including lactate dehydrogenase (LDH), a bone marrow biopsy, and computed tomography (CT) of the chest, abdomen and pelvis. The use of PET/CT for MCL is not fully characterized, but the lesions typically have low to intermediate uptake (10). Upper and lower endoscopy is usually encouraged, given the frequent GI involvement, particularly lymphomatous polyposis of the intestine (11). A number of poor prognostic factors have been found in univariate analysis for MCL, including age greater than 60 years, poor performance status, presence of B symptoms, advanced stage, extranodal involvement, and elevated LDH (12). More recently, a well-validated mantle cell international prognostic index (MIPI) has been developed with good discrimination between MIPI risk groups (13).

Systemic Therapy

MCL is generally responsive to a number of frontline therapies, with overall response rates from 70% to 90% with anthracyclines (14–16). Rituximab as a single agent offers very modest response rates (17). Nevertheless, complete response rates are generally around 50%, and the median duration of remission only 2 to 3 years (18). For this reason, asymptomatic or elderly patients are often merely observed, with therapy to begin only for symptomatic disease (19). For the young, symptomatic patient, most oncologists pursue an aggressive therapeutic approach. Historically, the choice of induction therapy had been cyclophosphamide, doxorubicin, oncovin and prednisone (CHOP), now given with rituximab (20). More recently, improvement in survival has been seen with a more intensive induction regimen: hyperfractionated cyclophosphamide, vincristine, doxorubicin, and dexamethasone alternating with high-dose cytarabine and methotrexate (HyperCVAD) plus rituximab (21). Perhaps, the most controversial question in the management of newly diagnosed MCL is the role for autologous transplantation in first remission. A retrospective analysis of 167 patients with MCL receiving either R-CHOP of R-HyperCVAD followed by autologous transplant in the first remission showed a superior progression-free survival to chemoimmunotherapy alone (22). Ongoing prospective trials aim at answering this question.

Radiation Therapy

Because of the relative rarity of MCL, there are no randomized data on radiation therapy for this entity. Because the vast majority of patients present with advanced stage disease, radiotherapy is not commonly used in the up-front management of MCL. However, there are data on the role for radiation in patients presenting with stage IA or IIA MCL. An early prospective trial of extended field irradiation versus total central lymphatic irradiation in patients diagnosed based on the old Kiel classification revealed good control for patients with stage I disease but poor control for others (23). A retrospective series of 26 patients with stage IA or IIA MCL showed a superior progression-free survival and a trend toward improved overall survival with the use of involved-field radiotherapy over systemic therapy alone (24). Of the 15 patients with early stage MCL treated with radiotherapy alone, 11 obtained a complete response, with four patients enjoying durable remissions (25). The National Comprehensive Cancer Network (NCCN) guidelines advise the inclusion of involved-field radiotherapy for early stage MCL (26). Given the radiosensitivity of MCL (27), doses in the range of 30 to 36 Gy are generally used.

■ BURKITT LYMPHOMA

Burkitt lymphoma (BL), originally described in Africa, is a high-grade lymphoma of germinal center origin. It is uniquely characterized by a translocation deregulating c-MYC expression. Endemic, sporadic, and immunodeficient forms exist, and we will not discuss the endemic variety, because it is quite rare in North America. Sporadic BL does not have the typical associations of Epstein Barr Virus (EBV) or holoendemic malaria that characterize 'African' BL. It accounts for 1% of adult NHL in the Western world and approximately 30% of pediatric lymphomas (28).

Diagnosis and Pathology

Morphologically, BL is a tumor of B-cell origin with very high growth fraction (Ki-67 >95%), with uniform, medium-sized cells, with basophilic cytoplasmic inclusions, round open nuclei, multiple basophilic nucleoli, and lipid vacuoles. It has a 'starry-sky' appearance because of active macrophages interrupting the diffuse, monotonous lymphoma cells.

The typical histological features of higher grade are apparent. Immunophenotype staining will reveal CD19, CD20, CD22, CD79a, CD10, BCL-6, CD43, surface IgM, and Ig-kappa light chain positivity. CD5 and BCL-2 are not expressed, as well as CD21, because sporadic BL is usually EBV negative (29). Characteristic genetic abnormalities include a translocation of the c-MYC oncogene at 8q24 and can include t(8;14), t(2;8), and t(8;22) (30). The mechanism of how BL acquires c-MYC rearrangements is unclear; however, the upregulation of c-MYC gene expression in a constitutive fashion produces more MYC protein transcription factor which promotes cell-cycle progression (31,32).

Clinical Presentation

Sporadic BL presents most commonly in the abdomen, often as bleeding or a bowel obstruction. The jaw can be involved in 10% to 25% of cases, less than half as commonly as in endemic BL (33). Mesenteric sites can involve visceral organs or localized lymphadenopathy, and the upper aerodigestive tract can be a presenting site (34). There is a modest chance of bone marrow and CNS involvement at presentation; 30% and 15%, respectively. A leukemic form also exists. There is a male preponderance of cases, >3:1 ratio, and the greatest incidence in pre-adolescent children. The average age of BL in adults is 30, because there is a wide distribution of sporadic BL in adults. There are actually more cases of BL in adults than in children, given that the span of adulthood is temporally greater than childhood. Nodal involvement and bulky disease (>10cm) are both more common in adults (35).

Staging

The basic staging procedures for BL are the same as those for other NHLs: history and physical, labs, bone marrow biopsy, and imaging. Strong consideration should be given to a lumbar puncture to evaluate for involvement of the central nervous system (CNS). The role for PET/CT is unclear at the present. Over the decades, a number of staging systems have been used. The first, described by Ziegler and Magrath, was based on surgical resection and extent of involvement (36). Today, BL staging is typically performed with the Ann Arbor classification for adults and the St. Jude staging system for children and adolescents (37).

Systemic Therapy

The treatment of BL has evolved considerably over the past several decades (38). Prompt supportive care and risks to minimize tumor lysis syndrome are important features of therapy. Treatment should not be withheld to complete staging. Initial treatment regimens were modified B-cell acute lymphoblastic leukemia (ALL) protocols. Outcomes were poor until CHOP-like regimens were introduced and radiotherapy was used for bulky disease. Numerous reports showed a benefit to accelerating intense therapy instead of prolonged therapy which is used in B-cell ALL (39,40).

The routine use of radiotherapy fell out of favor following CALGB 9251 which showed high rates of neurotoxicity with 12 cycles of intrathecal (IT) chemotherapy and craniospinal irradiation (CSI). The initial experience called for 2400 cGy in 12 fractions to the craniospinal axis and 12 cycles of IT chemotherapy in all patients but excessive neurologic toxicity including three instances of transverse myelitis and an instance of blindness prompted revision of the protocol to reduce the intensity of CNS-directed therapy. CSI was then used in very high-risk patients with bone marrow involvement and the number of IT cycles was reduced to 6. There were no significant differences in EFS, DFS, or OS for patients with reduced intensity CNS therapy (41). The above therapeutic regimens have CR rates above 80% and overall survival of approximately 70% at 2 to 3 years. More recent evolutions in treatment regimens have shown 90% 3 year survival rates in BL.

The Magrath regimen, CODOX-M/IVAC (cyclophosphamide, vincristine, doxorubicin, high-dose methotrexate with ifosfamide, cytarabine, etoposide, and intrathecal methotrexate) is the most commonly used regimen presently. The initial report and subsequent follow-up yielded promising results (42–44). However, the regimen has significant hematologic toxicity and a treatment mortality rate of 8%.

An MD Anderson study looking at HyperCVAD, another regimen derived from B-cell ALL, showed EFS and OS rates of 52% and 53%, with an older cohort of patients (45). The addition of rituximab to this regimen did not change the CR rates (86%) but improved EFS to 80% and OS to 89%. This is a regimen that shows promise and lends evidence that immunotherapy should be further investigated, particularly for older patients. Trials with rituximab have not shown a difference in outcomes for different age groups, which is compelling, because age is a significant prognostic factor for aggressive lymphomas.

Another promising regimen is DA-EPOCH (dose-adjusted etoposide, prednisone, vincristine, cyclophosphamide, and doxorubicin) which has been used with modest success in immunodeficiency-associated BL. The addition of rituximab to this regimen demonstrated a 55% CR rate (46). Immunodeficiency related BL has poor response to treatment, higher association with EBV, and has not shown reduced incidence since the advent of HAART like in other AIDS-related lymphomas (38). The addition of HAART has improved performance status and immune function in these patients such that they can tolerate the intensive, accelerated regimens discussed above.

Radiation Therapy

As mentioned above, radiotherapy has largely fallen out of favor in the treatment of BL. When used, standard fractionation has typically led to poor tumor response (47), likely a function of the high proliferative index of the lymphoma. Hyperfractionation may offer superior responses to radiotherapy (48). In general, radiation is limited to palliative intent for BL in the modern era (26).

■ PLASMABLASTIC LYMPHOMA

Plasmablastic lymphoma (PBL) is a recently recognized and distinct subtype of diffuse large B-cell lymphoma, typically arising in the immunosuppressed, particularly in patients positive for the human immunodeficiency virus (HIV). Originally described in the oral cavity (49,50), PBL is found in a variety of extranodal sites with a strong predominance of the GI tract. Rarely seen in the immunocompetent, PBL represents only about 2% to 3% of HIV-associated NHL (51).Patients with PBL tend to be significantly younger than those with other NHL histologies, although immunodeficiency of old age has also been associated with the diagnosis.

Diagnosis and Pathology

The etiology of PBL is incompletely elucidated, although it does not seem that HIV is a direct cause. PBL cells are typically EBV positive and are always negative for human herpes virus type 8 (HHV8), distinguishing the lymphoma from Kaposi sarcoma. Pathology reveals a diffuse proliferation of plasma blastoid cells with a prominent central nucleolus (52). Specific cytogenetic abnormalities have been isolated in PBL including c-MYC and t(8:14), but PBL does not fit the 'double-hit' paradigm evident in other aggressive lymphomas such as Burkitt (53). The World Health Organization 2008 classification identifies PBL as a diffuse immunoblastic lymphoma (54). The immunophenotype is characteristic of plasma cells, with expression of CD138, CD38, VS38c, and IRF4/MUM1, and do not express mature B-cell markers such as CD-20, CD-45, or PAX-5. Morphologically, PBL may seem as a spectrum from immature immunoblasts to differentiated plasma cells and must be differentiated from extramedullary plasmablastic myeloma due significant differences in treatment (55). EBV-encoded RNA (EBER) is a viral transcript that is expressed almost universally in latent EBV infection. Patients with HIV have almost double the rate of expression as those without HIV, and it may prove useful in differentiating from plasmablastic myeloma (56).

Staging and Prognosis

PBL is staged as any other NHL, and the Ann Arbor system is used. Because most patients present with advanced disease and have elevated IPI scores, the prognosis is generally quite poor. In HIV+ patients, the prognosis is better if they have earlier stage disease, and improves if they have a complete response to multi-agent induction chemotherapy (57). EBER has been shown to correlate to disease levels during treatment and may be a marker which can be followed to track remission or non-response to therapy.

Systemic Therapy

Given the relative rarity of the disease, there is no defined standard of care for PBL. Most patients are treated with multi-agent chemotherapy or involved-field radiation. CHOP is considered inadequate therapy for PBL, and the NCCN guidelines recommend CODOX-M/IVAC, DA-EPOCH, or HyperCVAD (26). The role of rituximab and anti-CD20 radioimmunotherapy in PBL is undefined but could be beneficial for the small percentage of patients whose lymphoma expresses CD20. Liu et al. outline a promising strategy of aggressive induction followed by autologous transplant in which 7 of 9 HIV negative patients were alive at 2 years follow-up (58). Of note, the use of highly active antiretroviral therapy (HAART) has improved survival in most AIDS-related lymphomas but does not seem to improve CR rates in PBL (57,59). Given the many similarities to plasma cell myeloma, bortezomib is being investigated as a treatment option (60,61).

Radiation Therapy

There have been no reported prospective studies of radiotherapy for PBL. One case report of an elderly Japanese HIV negative man with stage IIA PBL involving the left paranasal sinuses described only a partial response to 50 Gy involved field radiation (62). In contrast, an HIV negative man with PBL of the ano-rectal junction was treated with three cycles of CHOP followed by involved field radiation, achieved a complete response, and remained disease free at five years (63). A 38-year-old woman presented with a maxillary alveolar ridge PBL and was subsequent discovered to be HIV positive. Treatment consisted of HAART therapy and external beam radiotherapy to 23.4 Gy with a complete and durable response (64).Tsachouridou et al. reported two cases of HIV positive patients with oral PBL (65). One treated with chemoradiation enjoyed a durable complete remission, and the other treated with chemotherapy alone relapsed after six months and died of the disease. Rao et al. reported on two HIV negative patients with oral PBL lesions treated with chemoradiation, both of whom obtained complete responses (66). Sarode et al. provide a recent excellent review of the published cases of PBL of the oral cavity (67). Radiotherapy seems to play an important role in the treatment of localized PBL, either alone or in combination with systemic therapy.

■ LYMPHOMATOID GRANULOMATOSIS

Lymphomatoid granulomatosis (LYG) is a rare B-cell entity, originally considered to represent a gray zone between aggressive lymphoma and vasculitic conditions such as Wegener granulomatosis (68). The tumor cells are highly infiltrative, particularly for vascular invasion causing necrosis (69). LYG most frequently is found in the lungs, although it is not uncommon to also see involvement of the liver, kidneys, or CNS (70).There is a male predominance, with the disease typically arising in patients in their 50s.

Diagnosis and Pathology

LYG is now recognized as a distinct subtype of T-cell-rich DLBCL. In nearly all cases, it is associated with EBV, which has been confirmed with *in situ* hybridization techniques in LYG pathologic series (71–73). On pathologic examination, the infiltrates exhibit significant necrosis, a diffuse background of T lymphocytes, and varying numbers of atypical large B cells. The WHO recognizes three grades for LYG, with increasing numbers of EBV positive large B cells per high-power field (74).

Staging and Prognosis

LYG patients typically present with B symptoms and often respiratory complaints. Imaging with CT generally reveals multifocal nodular lung lesions with necrosis. LYG can initially be confused with sarcoidosis, vasculitis, or hypersensitivity pneumonitis based on radiographic appearance (75).Transbronchial or CT-guided biopsy is often attempted but can provide insufficient tissue to make the diagnosis. An open lung biopsy may be necessary. Grades 1 and 2 LYG can be observed in the asymptomatic patient and can even spontaneously regress. Grade 3 LYG is treated as a DLBCL and carries a very poor prognosis.

Therapy

Corticosteroid therapy has shown some activity against low-grade LYG (76). Interferon-alpha 2b has also been used with some efficacy (77). Grade 3 LYG is typically treated more aggressively, using rituximab plus CHOP or other systemic cytotoxic regimens, and autologous transplantation has been attempted (78–80).Given the typically multifocal nature of LYG, the role of radiotherapy is unclear. A few case reports document efficacy of radiation in cases of cutaneous or intracranial involvement (81–84), and the responses described suggest good radiosensitivity of LYG. Given the CD20-expression, radioimmunotherapy may be an effective option for more diffuse disease. We (MT) recently treated a male with highly refractory LYG with ^{90}Y ibritumomab tiuxetan, obtaining a near complete response, durable for at least 1 year (unpublished).

■ CONCLUSIONS

MCL, BL, plasmablastic lymphoma, and LYG all represent aggressive B-cell NHL subtypes seen in clinical practice. With the exception of MCL, all are associated with EBV infection, often in the immunocompromised. Each histology exhibits unique clinicopathologic and molecular features distinguishing them from other entities included in the differential diagnosis. With the exception of BL, these lymphomas seem to respond well to conventionally fractionated radiotherapy; however, systemic therapy remains the treatment of choice in the front-line setting.

■ REFERENCES

1. Gerard-Marchant R, Hamlin I, Lennert K, et al. Classification of non-Hodgkin's lymphomas. *Lancet.* 1974;2:405–408.

2. Swerdlow SH, Campo E, Harris N, et al. *WHO classification of tumors of the hematopietic and lymphoid tissues.* Lyon, France: IARC, 2008.

3. Non-Hodgkin's Lymphoma Classification Project. A clinical evaluation of the International Lymphoma Study Group. *Blood.* 1997;89:3909–3918.

4. Velders GA, Kluin-Nelemans JC, DeBoer CJ, et al. Mantle-cell lymphoma: a population-based clinical study. *J Clin Oncol.* 1996;14:1269–1274.

5. Tiemann M, Schrader C, Klapper W, et al. Histopathology, cell proliferation indices and clinical outcome in 304 patients with mantle cell lymphoma (MCL): A clinico-pathological study from the European MCL Network. *Br J Hematol.* 1005;131:29–38.

6. Romaguera JE, Medeiros LJ, Hagemeister FB, et al. Frequency of gastrointestinal involvement and its clinical significance in mantle cell lymphoma. *Cancer.* 2003;97:586–591.

7. Bertoni F, Rinaldi A, Zucca E, et al. Update on the molecular biology of mantle cell lymphoma. *Hematol Oncol.* 2006;24:22–27.

8. Fernandez V, Salamero O, Espinet B, et al. Genomic and gene expression profiling defines indolent forms of mantle cell lymphoma. *Cancer Res.* 2010;70:1408–1418.

9. Bernard M, Gressin R, Lefrere F, et al. Blastic variant of mantle cell lymphoma: A rare but highly aggressive subtype. *Leukemia.* 2001;15:1785–1791.

10. Gill S, Wolf M, Prince HM, et al. [18F] fluorodeoxyglucose positron emission tomography scanning for staging, response assessment, and disease surveillance in patients with mantle cell lymphoma. *Clin Lymphoma Myeloma.* 2008;8:159–165.

11. Kadayifci A, Benekli M, Savas MC, et al. Multiple lymphomatous polyposis. *J Surg Oncol.* 1997;64:336–340.

12. Hiddemann W, Brittinger G, Tiemann M, et al. Presentation features and clinical course of mantle cell lymphomas–results of a European survey. *Ann Oncol.* 1996;7:22.

13. Hoster E, Dreyling M, Klapper W, et al. A new prognostic index (MIPI) for patients with advanced mantle cell lymphoma. *Blood.* 2008;111:558–565.

14. Meusers P, Engelhard M, Bartels H, et al. Multicentre randomized therapeutic trial for advanced centrocytic lymphoma: anthracycline does not improve the prognosis. *Hematol Oncol.* 1989;7:365–380.

15. Unterhalt M, Hermann R, Tiemann M, et al. Prednimustine, mitoxantrone (PmM) vs cyclophosphamide, vincristine, prednisone (COP) for the treatment of advanced low-grade non-Hodgkin's lymphoma. German Low-Grade Lymphoma Study Group. *Leukemia.* 1996;10:836–843.

16. Zinzani PL, Magagnoli M, Moretti L, et al. Randomized trial of fludarabine versus fludarabine and idarubicin as frontline treatment in patients with indolent or mantle-cell lymphoma. *J Clin Oncol.* 2000;18:773–779.

17. Foran JM, Rohatiner AZ, Cunningham D, et al. European phase II study of rituximab (chimeric anti-CD20 monoclonal antibody) for patients with newly diagnosed mantle-cell lymphoma and previously treated mantle-cell lymphoma, immunocytoma, and small B-cell lymphocytic lymphoma. *J Clin Oncol.* 2000;18:317–324.

18. Vose JM. Mantle cell lymphoma: 2012 update on diagnosis, risk-stratification, and clinical management. *Am J Hematol.* 2012;87:605–609.

19. Martin P, Chadburn A, Christos P, et al. Outcome of deferred initial therapy in mantle-cell lymphoma. *J Clin Oncol.* 2009;27:1209–1213.

20. Weisenburger DD, Vose JM, Greiner TC, et al. Mantle cell lymphoma: a clinicopathologic study of 68 cases from the Nebraska Lymphoma Study Group. *Am J Hematol.* 2000;64:190–196.

21. Romaguera JE, Fayad L, Rodriguez MA, et al. High rate of durable remission after treatment of newly diagnosed aggressive mantle-cell lymphoma with rituximab plus HyperCVAD alternating with rituximab plus high-dose methotrexate and cytarabine. *J Clin Oncol.* 2005;23:7013–7023.

22. LeCase AS, Vandergrift JL, Rodriguez MA, et al. Comparative outcome of initial therapy for younger patients with mantle cell lymphoma: An analysis from the NCCN NHL database. *Blood.* 2012;119:2093–2099.

23. Stuschke M, Hoederath A, Sack H, et al. Extended field and total central lymphatic radiotherapy in the treatment of early stage lymph node centroblastic-centrocytic lymphomas: results of a prospective multicenter study. Study Group NHL-früheStadien. *Cancer.* 1997;80:2273–2284.

24. Leitch HA, Gascoyne RD, Chhanabhai M, et al. Limited-stage mantle-cell lymphoma. *Ann Oncol.* 2003;14:1555–1561.

25. Vandenberghe E, De Wolf-Peeters C, Vaughan Hudson G, et al. The clinical outcome of 65 cases of mantle cell

lymphoma initially treated with non-intensive therapy by the British National Lymphoma Investigation Group. *Br J Haematol.* 1997;99:842–847.

26. National Comprehensive Cancer Network. Non-Hodgkin's Lymphomas. Version 3.2012. Accessed August 13, 2012. http://www.nccn.org/professionals/physician_gls/pdf/nhl.pdf

27. Schaffner C, Idler I, Stilgenbauer S, et al. Mantle cell lymphoma is characterized by inactivation of the ATM gene. *Proc Natl Acad Sci USA.* 2000;97:2773–2778.

28. Morton LM, Wang SS, Devesa SS, et al. Lymphoma incidence patterns by WHO subtype in the United States, 1992–2001. *Blood.* 2006;107:265–276.

29. Harris NL, Jaffe ES, Diebold J, et al. World Health Organization classification of neoplastic diseases of the hematopoietic and lymphoid tissues: report of the Clinical Advisory Committee Meeting, Airlie House, Virginia, November 1997. *J Clin Oncol.* 1997; 17:3835–3849.

30. Dalla-Favera R, Bregni M, Erikson J, et al. Human c-mycconc gene is located on the region of chromosome 8 that is translocated in Burkitt lymphoma cells. *Proc Natl Acad Sci USA.* 1982;79:7824–7827.

31. Eilers M, Eisenman RN. Myc's broad reach. *Genes Dev.* 2008;22:2755–2766.

32. Walker W, Zhou ZQ, Ota S, et al. Mnt-Max to Myc-Max complex switching regulates cell cycle entry. *J Cell Biol.* 2005;169:405–413.

33. Sariban E, Donahue A, Magrath IT. Jaw involvement in American Burkitt's lymphoma. *Cancer.* 1984;53:141–146.

34. Magrath IT, Sariban E. Clinical features of Burkitt's lymphoma in the USA. *IARC Sci Publ.* 1985;60:119–127.

35. Boerma EG, van Imhoff GW, Appel IM, et al. Gender and age-related differences in Burkitt lymphoma—epidemiological and clinical data from The Netherlands. *Eur J Cancer.* 2004;40:2781–2787.

36. Ziegler JL, Magrath IT. Burkitt's lymphoma. *Pathobiol Annual* 1974;4:129–142.

37. Sandlund JT. Burkitt lymphoma: staging and response evaluation. *Br J Haematol.* 2012;156:761–765.

38. Linch DC. Burkitt lymphoma in adults. *Br J Haematol.* 2012;156:693–703.

39. Lopez TM, Hagemeister FB, McLaughlin P, et al. Small noncleaved cell lymphoma in adults: superior results for stages I-III disease. *J Clin Oncol.* 1990;8:615–622.

40. Philip T, Meckenstock R, Deconnick E, et al. Treatment of poor prognosis Burkitt's lymphoma in adults with the SociétéFrançaised'OncologiePédiatrique LMB Protocol—a study of the Federation Nationale des Centres de LutteContre le Cancer (FNLCC). *Eur J Cancer.* 1992;28:1954–1959.

41. Rizzieri DA, Johnson JL, Niedzwiecki D, et al. Intensive chemotherapy with and without cranial radiation for Burkitt leukemia and lymphoma: final results of Cancer and Leukemia Group B Study 9251. *Cancer.* 2004;100:1438–1448.

42. Magrath I, Adde M, Shad A, et al. Adults and children with small non-cleaved-cell lymphoma have a similar excellent outcome when treated with the same chemotherapy regimen. *J Clin Oncol.* 1996;14:925–934.

43. Mead GM, Sydes MR, Walewski J, et al. An international evaluation of CODOX-M and CODOX-M alternating with IVAC in adult Burkitt's lymphoma: results of United Kingdom Lymphoma Group LY06 study. *Ann Oncol.* 2002;13:1264–1274.

44. Mead GM, Barrans SL, Qian W, et al. A prospective clinicopathologic study of dose-modified CODOX-M/IVAC in patients with sporadic Burkitt lymphoma defined using cytogenetic and immunophenotypic criteria (MRC/NCRI LY10 trial). *Blood.* 2008;112:2248–2260.

45. Thomas DA, Cortes J, O'Brien S, et al. Hyper-CVAD program in Burkitt's-type adult acute lymphoblastic leukemia. *J Clin Oncol.* 1999;17:2461–2470.

46. Sparano JA, Lee JY, Kaplan LD, et al. Rituximab plus concurrent infusional EPOCH chemotherapy is highly effective in HIV-associated B-cell non-Hodgkin lymphoma. *Blood.* 2010;115:3008–3016.

47. Norin T, Clifford P, Einhorn J, et al. Conventional and superfractionated radiation therapy in Burkitt's lymphoma. *Acta Radiol Ther Phys Biol.* 1971;10:545–557.

48. Norin T, Onyango J. Radiotherapy in Burkitt's lymphoma: conventional or superfractionated regime–early results. *Int J Radiat Oncol Biol Phys.* 1977;2:399–406.

49. Delecluse HJ, Anagnostopoulos I, Dallenbach F, et al. Plasmablastic lymphomas of the oral cavity: a new entity associated with the human immunodeficiency virus infection. *Blood.* 1997;89:1413–1420.

50. Flaitz CM, Nichols CM, Walling DM, et al. Plasmablastic lymphoma: an HIV-associated entity with primary oral manifestations. *Oral Oncol.* 2002;38:96–102.

51. Castillo JJ, Reagan JL. Plasmablastic lymphoma: a systematic review. *Scientific World J.* 2011;11:687–696.

52. Stein H, Harris N, Campo E. Plasmablastic lymphoma. In: S Swerdlow, E Campo N Harris et al. eds., *Who Classification of Tumours of the Haematopoietic and Lymphoid Tissues.* Lyon, France: IARC; 2008: 256–257.

53. Slack GW, Gascoyne RD. MYC and aggressive B-cell lymphomas. *Adv Anat Pathol.* 2011;18:219–228.

54. Hsi ED, Lorsbach RB, Fend F, et al. Plasmablastic lymphoma and related disorders. *Am J Clin Pathol.* 2011;136:183–194.

55. Thakral C, Thomas L, Gajra A, et al. Plasmablastic lymphoma in an immunocompetent patient. *J Clin Oncol.* 2009;27:e78–e81.

56. Vega F, Chang CC, Medeiros LJ, et al. Plasmablastic lymphomas and plasmablastic plasma cell myelomas have nearly identical immunophenotypic profiles. *Mod Pathol.* 2005;18:806–815.

57. Castillo JJ, Winer ES, Stachurski D, et al. Prognostic factors in chemotherapy-treated patients with HIV-associated plasmablastic lymphoma. *Oncologist.* 2010;15:293–299.

58. Liu JJ, Zhang L, Ayala E, et al. Human immunodeficiency virus (HIV)-negative plasmablastic lymphoma: a single institutional experience and literature review. *Leukemia Res.* 2011;35:1571–1577.

59. Spina M, Gloghini A, Tirelli U, et al. Therapeutic options for HIV-associated lymphomas. *Expert Opin Pharmacother.* 2010;11:2471–2481.

60. Bose P, Thompson C, Gandhi D, et al. AIDS-related plasmablastic lymphoma with dramatic, early response to bortezomib. *Eur J Haematol.* 2009;82:490–492.

61. Bibas M, Grisetti S, Alba L, et al. Patient with HIV-associated plasmablastic lymphoma responding to bortezomib alone and in combination with dexamethasone, gemcitabine, oxaliplatin, cytarabine, and pegfilgrastim chemotherapy and lenalidomide alone. *J Clin Oncol.* 2010;28:e704–e708.

62. Suzuki Y, Yoshida T, Nakamura N, et al. CD3- and CD4-positive plasmablastic lymphoma: a literature review of Japanese plasmablastic lymphoma cases. *Intern Med.* 2010;49:1801–1805.

63. Brahmania M, Sylwesterowic T, Leitch H. Plasmablastic lymphoma in the ano-rectal junction presenting in an immunocompetent man: a case report. *J Med Case Rep.* 2011;5:168.

64. Vieira FO, El Gandour O, Baudi FK, et al. Plasmablastic lymphoma in a previously undiagnosed AIDS patient: a case report. *Head Neck Pathol.* 2008;2:92–96.

65. Tsachouridou O, Christoforidou A, Metallidis S, et al. Plasmablastic lymphoma of the oral cavity, a B cell-derived lymphoma associated with HIV infection: a case series. *Eur Arch Otorhinolaryngol.* 2012;269:1713–1719.

66. Rao DD, Aggarwal N, Anehosur V, et al. Plasmablastic lymphoma of the oral cavity in immunocompetent patients: report of two cases. *Int J Oral Maxillofac Surg.* 2010;39:1036–1039.

67. Sarode SC, Sarode GS, Patil A. Plasmablastic lymphoma of the oral cavity: a review. *Oral Oncol.* 2010;46:146–153.

68. Liebow AA, Carrington CR, Friedman PJ. Lymphomatoid granulomatosis. *Hum Pathol.* 1972;3:457–558.

69. Colby TV. Current histological diagnosis of lymphomatoid granulomatosis. *Mod Pathol.* 2012;25:S39–S42.

70. Katzenstein AL, Carrington CB, Liebow AA. Lymphomatoid granulomatosis: a clinicopathologic study of 152 cases. *Cancer.* 1979;43:360–373.

71. Katzenstein AL, Peiper SC. Detection of Epstein-Barr virus genomes in lymphomatoid granulomatosis: analysis of 29 cases by the polymerase chain reaction technique. *Mod Pathol.* 1990;3:435–441.

72. Guinee Jr D, Jaffe E, Kingma D, et al. Pulmonary lymphomatoid granulomatosis. Evidence for a proliferation of Epstein-Barr virus infected B-lymphocytes with a prominent T-cell component and vasculitis. *Am J Surg Pathol.* 1994;18:753–764.

73. Myers JL, Kurtin PJ, Katzenstein AL, et al. Lymphomatoid granulomatosis. Evidence of immunophenotypic diversity and relationship to Epstein-Barr virus infection. *Am J Surg Pathol.* 1995;19:1300–1312.

74. Pittaluga S, Wilson WH, Jaffe E. Lymphomatoid granulomatosis. In: Swerdlow, S., Campo, E., Harris et al. eds. *WHO Classification of Tumours of the Haematopoietic and Lymphoid Tissues.* Lyon: France: IARC; 2008:247–249.

75. Rezai P, Hart EM, Patel SK. Case 169: Lymphomatoid granulomatosis. *Radiology.* 2011;259:604–609.

76. Jaffe ES, Wilson WH. Lymphomatoid granulomatosis: pathogenesis, pathology and clinical implications. *Cancer Surv.* 1997;30:233–248.

77. Wilson WH, Kingma DW, Raffeld M, et al. Association of lymphomatoid granulomatosis with Epstein-Barr viral infection of B lymphocytes and response to interferon-alpha 2b. *Blood.* 1996;87:4531–4537.

78. Jung KH, Sung HJ, Lee JH, et al. A case of pulmonary lymphomatoid granulomatosis successfully treated by combination chemotherapy with rituximab. *Chemotherapy.* 2009;55:386–390.

79. Jaffre S, Jardin F, Dominique S, et al. Fatal haemoptysis in a case of lymphomatoid granulomatosis treated with rituximab. *Eur Respir J.* 2006;27:644–646.

80. Lemieux J, Bernier V, Martel N, et al. Autologous hematopoietic stem cell transplantation for refractory lymphomatoid granulomatosis. *Hematology.* 2002;7:355–358.

81. Nair BD, Joseph MG, Catton GE, et al. Radiation therapy in lymphomatoid granulomatosis. *Cancer.* 1989;64:821–824.

82. Simard H, LeBlanc P. Radiotherapy: an effective treatment of cerebral involvement by lymphomatoid granulomatosis. *Chest.* 1993;103:650–651.

83. Gupta T, Wadasadawala T, Shet T, et al. Isolated central nervous system involvement by lymphomatoid granulomatosis in an adolescent: a case report and review of literature. *Pediatr Hematol Oncol.* 2010;27:150–159.

84. Shank BB, Kelley CD, Nisce LZ, et al. Radiation therapy in lymphomatoid granulomatosis. *Cancer.* 1978;42:2572–2580.

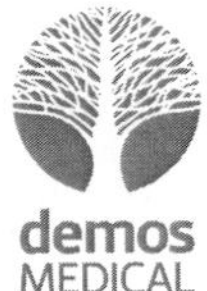

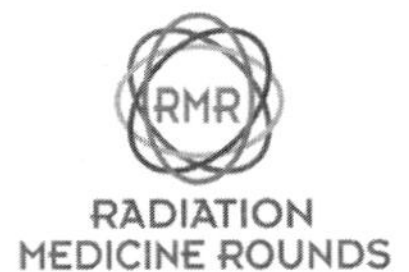

Leukemia Including Lymphoblastic Lymphoma

Chelsea C. Pinnix* and Bouthaina S. Dabaja
The University of Texas MD Anderson Cancer Center, Houston, TX

■ ABSTRACT

Leukemia is a clonal expansion of one of several hematopoietic progenitors that retain the capacity of self-renewal, but are severely limited in their ability to differentiate into functional mature cells. Over the years classification has evolved from being purely based on morphology, to include cytochemistry and number of blasts cells in the FAB (French–American–British) classification (1) to the current WHO classification (2) that includes morphologic, genetic, immunophenotypic features, and clinical syndromes. On the basis of the WHO classification the different subtypes of leukemia will be discussed, including the presentation, diagnosis, treatment and prognosis of acute and chronic leukemias while highlighting the role of radiotherapy in disease management.

Keywords: leukemia, lymphoblastic lymphoma, radiation, acute myeloid leukemia, acute lymphocytic leukemia, chronic lymphocytic leukemia, chronic myeloid leukemia

■ INTRODUCTION

Historically, leukemia was regarded as a neoplastic process that presented with bone marrow and peripheral blood involvement, whereas lymphoma was considered a distinct clinical entity where the abnormal hematopoietic cells formed a mass in organs, soft tissues or lymph nodes. Now, it is appreciated that the distinction is, in fact, blurred, and leukemia can present with a mass lesion, and lymphoma can progress to a leukemic picture. The arrest in maturation along the path of progenitors will ultimately result in the uncontrolled growth of neoplastic cells causing impairment of normal bone marrow cells functions, thus causing the symptomatology appreciated in patients afflicted with leukemias.

Leukemias are typically classified according to the cell of origin. Myeloid neoplasms arise from bone marrow progenitor cells that develop into granulocytes (neutrophils, basophils, and eosinophils), erythrocytes, monocytes, or megakaryocytes. Lymphoid neoplasms arise from cells that normally develop into B- or T-lymphocytes. There is further classification into acute versus chronic types, where acute leukemias are derived from primitive, immature progenitor cells, and chronic leukemias arise from more differentiated, mature cells. It is possible for transformation of a chronic leukemia into a more acute leukemic picture.

The leukemias of myeloid origin include acute myelogenous leukemia (AML), chronic myelogenous leukemia (CML), chronic neutrophilic leukemia, chronic eosinophilic leukemia, and chronic myelomonocytic leukemia. The latter three clinical entities are exceedingly rare and will not be discussed in detail. The leukemias of lymphoid origin include

---

*Corresponding author, The University of Texas MD Anderson Cancer Center, 1515 Holcombe Boulevard, Houston, TX

E-mail address: ccpinnix@mdanderson.org

Radiation Medicine Rounds 3:3 (2012) 459–472.

DOI: 10.5003/2151-4208.3.3.459

demosmedpub.com/rmr

precursor B- and T- cell lymphoblastic leukemia (i.e., acute lymphoblastic leukemia [ALL]), chronic lymphocytic leukemia/small lymphocytic lymphoma (CLL/SLL), and B- and T-cell prolymphocytic leukemia. Lymphoplasmacytic lymphoma, a mature B-cell lymphoid neoplasm, will also be discussed. The classification of leukemia has substantially evolved from being purely morphologic, in which case it was always challenging to differentiate myeloid from lymphoid origin in case of an arrest of maturation at a very early stage, to the modern days, where in addition to morphology, examined by an experienced hematopathologist, immunophenotyping and cytogenetics are used to first differentiate myeloid from lymphoid and then to assign a subtype. Chemotherapy regimens, the need for maintenance chemotherapy, the use of high-dose autologous or allogeneic transplant, and the type of central nervous system prophylaxis to be applied has been all tailored based on subtypes of leukemia.

■ ACUTE MYELOGENOUS LEUKEMIA

AML is the most common acute leukemia in adults, representing 80% of adult cases with a median age of 65 years at diagnosis (3). This is in contrast with the pediatric population, where AML represents less than 10% of acute leukemias in children aged 10 or less. Secondary AML occurs in the setting of an environmental exposure (chemotherapy, benzene exposure, or whole-body ionizing radiation exposure), genetic abnormalities (Trisomy 21, Fanconi anemia, or Bloom syndrome), or other preexisting hematologic disorders (myelodysplastic syndrome) (4–6). De novo AML, on the other hand, occurs in the absence of a preceding event. Patients often present with symptoms related to pancytopenia as the leukemia suppresses normal hematopoiesis such as fatigue, pallor, shortness of breath secondary to anemia; bruising, bleeding secondary to thrombocytopenia/ coagulation defects; or infection secondary to neutropenia. Organomegaly and clinically apparent lymphadenopathy are infrequent. Some patients present with extramedullary disease, often referred to as granulocytic sarcoma or chloroma (7). Common sites of involvement include bone, soft tissue, lymph nodes, and the periosteum.

The gold standard for diagnosis is a bone marrow aspiration and biopsy, although oftentimes, circulating myeloblasts can be appreciated in a peripheral blood smear. On the basis of the WHO criteria (2), the diagnosis is made when at least 20% of nucleated cells in the bone marrow or peripheral blood are myeloid blasts, less than that but more than 5% falls into myelodysplasia. In case translocation such as inv (16) or t(15;17) are present, the number of blasts cells requirement is not needed. The diagnosis of AML is pathologically made based on the identification of the characteristic myeloblast, an immature myeloid cell. Cytochemical reactions to detect myeloperoxidase and nonspecific esterase are used. Finding of Auer Rods (red rod-like granular cytoplasmic structures) can be helpful in case of AML M3–4 subtypes. Immunophenotyping includes a variable combination of CD 11c, CD13, CD 33, CD 34, CD 41, CD 64, CD 68, and CD 117; each combination will be useful to subcategories' myeloid leukemia into its respective WHO category (Table 1). Cytogenetics features are the most powerful predictors of outcome; patients can accordingly be categorized in three risk groups. The favorable cytogenetic risk group includes: inv (16) (p13 q22)/ t(16;16) (13;22)/; t (8;21)(q22;q22); t(15;17)(q22–12–21).

In addition to bone marrow biopsy, workup should include complete blood count (CBC) with differential, PT/PTT, fibrinogen, comprehensive metabolic panel, and baseline virology testing. In the absence of neurologic symptoms, lumbar puncture is not routinely performed out of concern for bleeding risk and contamination of a sanctuary site with neoplastic blasts.

In anticipation of anthracycline therapy, a baseline cardiac scan is often performed, and fertility counseling is administered where appropriate.

There is no standard treatment approach for all patients with AML. Instead, management is guided by cytogenetic and molecular risk group stratification, the patient's age, and performance status. The ultimate goal of therapy is to eliminate the abnormal leukemic cells and restore normal bone marrow function. This is accomplished through the administration of induction therapy to largely reduce the leukemic cell burden, followed by postremission therapy, which aims at eliminating residual blasts that would inevitably lead to relapse in weeks to months after induction therapy. The most common induction regimen is cytarabine (7 days continuous infusion) and an anthracycline (days 1–3, bolus, typically daunorubicin), the so-called "7 + 3" regimen (8). This treatment is toxic and uniformly results in pancytopenia; therefore, transfusion support and antibiotics are often required. Additional side effects of therapy include gastrointestinal toxicity (mucositis, nausea, vomiting, and diarrhea), alopecia, and infertility.

TABLE 1 WHO category of AML

WHO Category of AML	Cell of origin	Cytogenetics	Immunophenotype
AML with t(8;21) (q22;q22)	Myeloid with neutrophil differentiation	T (8;21)	CD34+, CD13+, CD33+
AML with eosinophils and inv(16) or t (16;16)	Potential to differentiate to granulo-monocytic	inv (16) or t(16;16)	CD13+, CD33+, MPO+, CD11c+, CD 64+
AML with t)15;17) (q22;q12)	Granulocytic	t(15;17)	CD33+, CD13+,
AML with 11q23	Multilineage	t(9;11)(p22;q23); t(6;11)(q27,q23); t(11;19)(q23,p13)	CD13+, Cd33+CD14+, Cd11c+,CD36+,CD6+)
AML following MDS, or alkylating agents, or topoisomerase II inhibitors	Hematopoietic	-5/del(5q),-7/del(7q), +8,+11, del(11q); 11q23[(t (9;11), t(6;11), t(11'19)], in therapy related: inversion 16, t(8;16), t(15;17)	CD13+,CD33+,CD34+, CD7+,CD56+
AML minimally differentiated or without maturation	Hematopoietic	No consistent cytogenetic	CD13+,CD33+,CD117+, TDT+ in >1/3 of cases
AML with maturation	Precursor cell with early myeloid development	Deletions translocation of 12p,t(6;9)(p23;q34),T98;16) (p11;p13)	CD13+,CD33+, Cd15+,Cd117+, CD34+,
Acute monoblastic and monocytic	Cells with some monocytic commitment	T(8:16)(p11;p13)	CD13+,CD33+, Cd14+,Cd117+, CD64+,CD68+. Cd34 often negative
Erythroleukemia (myeloid/erythroid) or pure erythroid	Cells with myeloid potential or some degree of commitment to erythroid	-5/del(5q) and -7/del (7q)	Myeloblasts are CD13+,CD33+, Cd34+,Cd117+, MPO+ Erythroblasts lack myeloid associated antigens
Acute megakaryocytic	Cells committed to megakaryocytes	T(1;22)(p13;13)	CD36+,CD41+,Cd61+,CD42+, others may positive CD13+,Cd33+, and Cd34 negative
Others rare leukemias: Acute basophilic, undifferentiated, bilineal, etc.			

Seven to ten days postinduction, unilateral bone marrow biopsy and aspirate is repeated to assess response to therapy and determine the need for a second cycle of induction therapy (which is required in 20%–40% of patients). A complete response is defined as less than 5% blasts appreciated in the bone marrow sample. The options for postremission therapy include consolidation chemotherapy, autologous hematopoietic stem cell transplantation (HSCT), or allogeneic HSCT (9). The choice of treatment is dictated by the cytogenetic/molecular risk and the age/performance status of the patient. For younger patients with high risk disease, allogeneic HSCT with a sibling or HLA matched unrelated donor is preferred. Allogeneic HSCT has the advantage of greater efficacy because of the graft versus leukemia effect; however, the morbidity and mortality is also greater secondary to the risk of graft versus host disease (GVHD). Patients with low-risk disease are appropriate candidates for consolidation chemotherapy, typically with three to four cycles of high-dose Ara-C (HiDAC).

For older patients (age >60), induction and postremission therapy is guided by patient performance status and cytogenetic risk stratification. Treatment options can range from the standard treatment given to younger patients to low-intensity therapy, including subcutaneous cytarabine, 5-azacytidine, and decitabine. Best supportive care with transfusions, prophylactic antibiotics, and antifungal drugs are also an option for more fragile patients.

The role of radiotherapy in the management of patients with AML is diminishing. Historically, radiation has been used as a myeloablative conditioning regimen before allogeneic transplant. In addition to the immune mediated graft versus leukemia effect, the myeloablative high intensity of the conditioning regimen is also thought to contribute to the antileukemic activity of allogeneic HSCT. The most commonly used regimens include cyclophosphamide with fractionated total body irradiation (CYTBI) and oral busulfan and cyclophosphamide (BUCY) (10,11). Concerns with regard to late sequelae (especially in children) that have been deemed to be radiation related, including second malignancies, growth retardation, neuroendocrine dysfunction, pulmonary toxicity, cataracts, and neuropsychologic dysfunction, have resulted in less enthusiasm in radiation-based regimens and a surge in chemotherapy-based approaches. Data with regard to the best myeloablative conditioning regimen before HSCT are mixed. Seven randomized controlled trials have been conducted, comparing CYTBI with BUCY, but they all have less than 200 patients and are underpowered to determine the superior regimen (12–18). The largest meta-analysis to date concluded that transplant-related mortality was significantly less with CYTBI compared with oral BUCY and that the cumulative incidence of complications was no significantly different between the two regimens; however, more severe late toxicity with regard to growth and development was appreciated in children (19).

Radiation therapy is frequently used in the management of symptomatic CNS disease with mass effect in AML and in cases of chloroma. Chloromas rarely present in the absence of marrow involvement but are typically seen in cases of bone marrow biopsy–proven AML. In a recent series from the Memorial Sloan Kettering Cancer Center where 38 patients were treated for chloroma, radiotherapy provided excellent local control (97%) and symptom relief in 95% of cases. Doses of at least 20 Gy are recommended with 24 Gy in 12 fractions proposed as the standard regimen.

Outcomes in AML are heavily influenced by the age at diagnosis. The 5 year survival rate for patients less than 45 years is roughly 45% and drops to 6% for patients older than 65% (20–22). Acute promyelocytic leukemia is a biologically distinct subtype of AML with a cytogenetic hallmark translocation involving the retinoic acid receptor-alpha [t(15;17)] (23). These patients are at early risk of mortality from hemorrhage caused by a characteristic coagulopathy. However, after treatment with all-trans retinoic acid (ATRA) and anthracycline-based chemotherapy, these patients do quite well compared with other AML patients, with CR rates ranging from 80% to 85% and 10 year overall survival rates of 58% to 85%.

■ ACUTE LYMPHOBLASTIC LEUKEMIA

Similar to AML, ALL diagnosis and classification went through major changes. Originally, the FAB classification (24) included three subtypes L1, L2, and L3 based on the pure morphology. Later, the WHO classification introduced the mature B, pre B, and T cell lineage (2) and adverse cytogenetic aberration. Most commonly, ALL is associated with bcr/abl translocation (9;22), t(4;11), and t(8;14)(p24,q32); the latter and its variant are the hallmark of Burkitt leukemia.

Acute leukemia is the most common childhood cancer, comprising roughly 30% of cases (25). ALL is five times more common than AML, with peak incidence between ages 2 and 5 and occurring more frequently in boys than girls (26). There is a higher risk of ALL with certain genetic syndromes, including Trisomy 21, Neurofibromatosis-1 (NF-1), Bloom syndrome and ataxia telangiectasia (27). Children with ALL can present with fever, bone pain, bleeding, infection, or lymphadenopathy (28). Central nervous system involvement (i.e., CNS3 disease, the presence of blasts in the cerebrospinal fluid or radiographically evident CNS disease) at presentation is rare (less than 5% of cases) (29). Clinically apparent lymphadenopathy is frequent (50%–75%), and most patients will have evidence of anemia with or without thrombocytopenia on CBC evaluation. Abnormal lymphoblasts may even be apparent on smear. ALL can also occur in the adult population but is far less frequent. The 5 year overall survival is greater than 85% for children with ALL but, unfortunately, is significantly lower in cases of adult ALL with survival rates of 35% in patients aged 18 to 60 (30,31).

Workup includes CBC with differential, PT/PTT, comprehensive metabolic panel, uric acid levels, and baseline virology, lumbar puncture. Bone marrow biopsy and aspiration should be performed, and appropriate immuno typic, morphologic, molecular, and cytogenetic analyses should be performed on the specimen, because risk stratification is largely based on these features. Seventy to eighty percent of ALL cases are of B-cell precursor origin, expressing CD 10, 19, and 20. T-cell ALL is less common (CD 2, 3, 4, 5, 7, and 8 positive). Specific translocations can heavily influence outcome and, at times, treatment. For example, in 3% to 4% of pediatric ALL patients and 20% to 30% of adult ALL patients that harbor the t(9;22) BCR-ABL translocation, the addition of a tyrosine kinase inhibitor (TKI) such as imatinib or dasatinib should be considered (32,33).

The treatment paradigm for ALL therapy is chemotherapy based on induction, consolidation, and maintenance regimens, typically administered on protocol (34). CNS prophylaxis is typically included with therapy, because up to 80% of children in bone marrow remission after ALL treatment relapse in the CNS with "leukemic meningitis" (35). After induction therapy, more than 95% of patients achieve a CR, regardless of the risk group (36). Most induction protocols include weekly vincristine, daily corticosteroids, and asparaginase. In high-risk patients, anthracyclines may be added. Induction chemotherapy is not without potential fatal toxicity, including tumor lysis syndrome, bleeding, infection, and thrombosis (deep vein thrombosis, pulmonary embolism, or intracranial dural sinus thrombosis with hemorrhage). In the adult ALL population, more dose intensive regimens have been investigated. Kantarjian and colleagues reported on the outcome of 204 newly diagnosed ALL patients treated between 1992 and 1998 with four cycles of Hyper-CVAD alternating with four cycles of high-dose methotrexate and cytarabine coupled with intrathecal CNS prophylaxis. Ninety-one percent of patients experienced complete remission (CR). Compared with 222 patients who were treated with a traditional vincristine, adriamycin, and dexamethasone (VAD) regimen; those treated with hyper-CVAD had improved CR rates and overall survival (37).

Consolidation treatment is administered after induction with the goal of eliminating residual lingering leukemic lymphoblasts. Consolidation lasts between 4 and 6 months, during which a multidrug chemotherapy regimen is given. The choice of drugs is largely influenced by risk assessment, with some high-risk patients even being offered HSCT.

More aggressive chemotherapeutic regimens, however, are accompanied by enhanced long term toxicity, including secondary malignancy and infertility. Maintenance therapy is the last component of therapy. This less intensive regimen of oral 6-mercaptopurine (6-MP) and weekly methotrexate is usually of 24 to 36 months duration.

Radiation therapy for CNS prophylaxis is less frequently used in this pediatric population out of concern for long-term neurologic, cognitive, and endocrine impairments. However, many cooperative groups continue to use cranial radiotherapy in patients with known CNS involvement at diagnosis (CNS3) and in patients with a higher risk of CNS relapse (those with a T cell precursor phenotype and patients with white blood cell counts of 100,000/mcL at the time of diagnosis) (38). The radiation field should cover the entire intracranial meninges with margin on the cribriform plate and the posterior aspect of the orbits and retina. The typical cranial prophylactic dose ranges from 12 to 18 Gy, whereas patients with known CNS involvement should receive does of 18 to 24 Gy (39). Lower doses are usually administered to younger patients.

■ CHRONIC MYELOGENOUS LEUKEMIA

The evolution of treatment for CML is the poster child for bench to bedside medicine at its finest. The prognosis for this hematologic malignancy, which is the cause of 15% to 20% of all leukemias in adults, has remarkably improved over the last decade because of therapy with targeted TKIs. The pathogenesis of CML is related to the constitutive activation of a tyrosine kinase protein, the fusion product that results from a reciprocal translocation of chromosome 9, which harbors the ABL1 gene and chromosome 22, which codes for BCR (40,41). The oncoprotein resulting from the "Philadelphia chromosome" [t(9;22)] was identified as the vital pathophysiological factor in the evolution of the disease(42). Since these key discoveries, treatment has progressed to involve TKIs aimed at impairing the activity of the aberrant protein. As such, CML has transitioned from a highly fatal disease to a chronic disease with 5 year overall survival rates of 89% and disease specific survival rates of 95% (43).

CML is characterized by the unregulated growth of mature granulocytes, particularly neutrophils, but basophils and eosinophils can also be involved. In cases of untreated CML, there are typically three disease phases that resembles acute leukemia: the chronic phase, the accelerated phase, and the terminal blastic phase. Less than half of patients are diagnosed based on abnormalities detected on routine blood work. In symptomatic cases, patients may present with fatigue, weight loss, bleeding, and abdominal fullness (usually do to splenomegaly). Workup requires history and physical with attention paid to spleen size, CBC with differential and smear, comprehensive metabolic panel, and bone marrow biopsy with aspirate. Leukocytosis, predominantly of neutrophil morphology, is appreciated on peripheral blood smear. Blasts usually comprise less than 2% of the sample. The neutrophils seem morphologically normal; however, they are chemically abnormal with low leukocyte alkaline phosphatase (LAP). Often, there is associated absolute basophilia and eosinophilia. Bone marrow evaluation typically reveals granulocytic hyperplasia, and genetic testing is key for the detection of the Philadelphia chromosome, either by karyotyping, fluorescence in situ hybridization, or reverse transcription polymerase chain reaction (RT-PCR).

In the mid 1980s, a prognostic index called the Sokal score was developed based on treatment outcomes of patients who received therapy during the chemotherapy era (44). The Sokal index divides patients into low-, intermediate-, and high-risk groups based on the percentage of blasts in the peripheral blood, platelet count, age, and spleen size. The score remained valid in patients treated with interferon-alpha and was also predictive of outcome in patients receiving TKIs (43,45–47).

In December 2002, based on a randomized trial, the International Randomized Study of Interferon and STI571 (IRIS) demonstrated a dramatic improvement in outcomes with imatinib over interferon-alpha/cytarabine in newly diagnosed chronic phase CML patients, with the Federal Drug Administration (FDA)-approved imatinib (STI571) as the first-line therapy in this patient population (48). With the exciting advent of this novel successful therapy, this trial also established new endpoints to define therapy response, including complete cytogenetic response (CCyR) and major molecular response (MMR), which is defined as a 3-log reduction in BCR-ABL transcript levels. CCyR is the most significant endpoint and has been associated with prolonged survival (46).

Although treatment with front-line imatinib undoubtedly revolutionized therapy for CML patients, the recognition of a patient population who ultimately failed imatinib treatment because of imatinib resistant mutants was sobering. Two second-generation TKIs, dasatinib and nilotinib, with enhanced potency inhibition of BCR-ABL and activity against imatinib resistant cells, were initially FDA approved for salvage therapy in patients who failed prior treatment, including imatinib. Recently, however, these agents have individually been compared in head-to-head phase three trials versus imatinib as initial treatment in newly diagnosed chronic phase patients (Dasatinib versus Imatinib Study In Treatment-naive CML, DASISION and Evaluating Nilotinib Efficacy and Safety in Clinical Trials-Newly Diagnosed Patients, ENESTnd) (49,50). In both studies imatinib was inferior. Nilotinib has actually been shown to have a modest progression free survival benefit. These trials prompted FDA approval for both drugs as front-line therapy in 2010. These second-generation TKIs seem to be more effective than imatinib as initial therapy, but longer follow-up of these trials is required.

The current recommendation for newly diagnosed patients in chronic phase is imatinib, nilotinib, or dasatinib. Patients should be evaluated for treatment response via serial hematologic evaluations of peripheral blood, as well as molecular and cytogenetic analyses of bone marrow. Patients with minimal response should be switched to a different TKI or considered for HSCT. Patients who present with accelerated phase disease, if not eligible for a clinical trial, can be given first-line dasatinib or nilotinib. HSCT can also be considered if a matched donor is available. Last, in patients with blast crisis, ALL- or AML-type induction chemotherapy should be given with a TKI based on whether the CML blasts are of lymphoid or myeloid differentiation. This should be followed by HSCT if feasible.

There is little role for radiotherapy in the management of CML. Historically, when HSCT was a more integral aspect of treatment for CML, total body irradiation was often used as a conditioning regimen before transplant. Now, HSCT is generally reserved for patients who have failed first and second like TKI therapy and patients with more advanced disease. Typically, when HSCT is indicated, chemotherapy has largely replaced radiotherapy for conditioning.

■ CHRONIC LYMPHOCYTIC LEUKEMIA/SMALL LYMPHOCYTIC LYMPHOMA

CLL and SLL represent different points on the spectrum of the same disease process. This disease entity is a B-cell neoplasm characterized by the accumulation of abnormally functioning monoclonal lymphocytes. It is the most common adult leukemia in Western countries, representing 30% of all leukemias in the United States (51). CLL and SLL largely affect an older adult population with a median diagnosis of 70 years; however, younger adults can also be affected (52). The most common presentation is painless peripheral lymphadenopathy (50%–90% of patients) (53). Patients less frequently present with splenomegaly (25%–55%) and hepatomegaly (15%–25%). B symptoms are uncommon, present in roughly 5% to 10% of patients (54). Median survival is 8 to 10 years (55).

CLL and SLL are distinguished clinically and hematogically. The diagnosis of CLL is made in patients with greater than 5,000 clonal B lymphocytes per mcL in a peripheral blood specimen. Patients with SLL have less than 5,000 B cells per mcL in the presence of lymphadenopathy and/or splenomegaly. When these criteria are not met, with less than 5,000 B cells in the absence of organomegaly, patients are deemed to have a lymphoproliferative disorder called monoclonal B lymphocytosis (MBL) that can progress to CLL in small fraction of patients (56).

In addition to CBC with differential and smear analysis, workup should include history and physical with lymph node and spleen evaluation, comprehensive metabolic panel, LDH and $\beta_2$microglobulin. Bone marrow biopsy and aspirate are not required for diagnosis. In the setting of peripheral lymphadenopathy, CT imaging of the neck, chest, abdomen and pelvis should be performed. Immunophenotypic analysis is essential for diagnosis and typically reveals small lymphocytes that express B cell–associated antigens CD19 and CD20, although CD20 expression is usually weak. CD 23 is positive. They also express CD5, a T cell–associated antigen. They are CD10–, CD43± and cyclin D1–. It is important to distinguish CLL/SLL from the B-cell CD5+ neoplasm, mantle cell lymphoma.

CLL is a heterogenous disease process with variable prognosis. Recently, increased understanding of the molecular mechanisms underlying CLL has shed light on the disease heterogeneity. Thus, cytogenetic analysis should be conducted (typically with fluorescence in situ hybridization) to search for chromosomal abnormalities, because this information affects prognosis and management decisions. Patients found to have deletions of chromosome 11 [del(11q23)] or chromosome 17 [del(17p13)] have loss of tumor suppression genes ATM and TP53, respectively, and have

been shown to have aggressive disease and poorer response to therapy with resultant inferior survival (57). Mutational status of the immunoglobulin heavy chain variable region genes (IGVH) should be determined, because patients without mutations in IGVH have worse survival when compared their counterparts with the gene mutated (58).

Because studies have demonstrated no improvement in survival with early versus delayed treatment and because most therapies are not curative, not all patients receive therapy at the time of diagnosis and observation is an option (59). Early stage asymptomatic CLL patients are often observed and followed with serial CBCs and clinical examinations. There is no standard approach to the management of patients with symptomatic CLL or advanced stage CLL and SLL. Therapy can include purine analogs (usually fludarabine), alkylating agents (chlorambucil or bendamustine), monoclonal antibodies (anti CD-20 rituximab or anti CD-52 alemtuzumab) or combination therapy.

Radiation is the mainstay of therapy for localized Ann Arbor stage I SLL. A series of 54 patients treated at Standford for all stages of SLL between 1963 and 1983 demonstrated excellent local control with primary radiotherapy. In the subset of patients treated with stage I and IE disease that were treated with involved field or extended field radiotherapy, the 10 year freedom from relapse was 80%, with doses between 40 and 44 Gy. Patients with disseminated CLL and SLL can effectively be palliated with low-dose radiotherapy (usually 2 Gy in 2 fractions) to bulky adenopathy, causing discomfort, compression neuropathy, or vital organ compromise (60,61). Radiation therapy is also effective as palliative treatment for splenomegaly, causing compressive symptoms or cytopenias (62–64). Doses administered range from 1 to 10 Gy in fraction sizes of 25 to 100 cGy.

■ LYMPHOBLASTIC LYMPHOMA

B- and T-cell lymphoblastic lymphoma (LBL) can be considered an extramedullary presentation of B- and T-cell ALL. There is a significant clinical and biological overlap between LBL and ALL; as such, the treatment strategy for both diseases is similar. By definition, LBL is diagnosed in patients who have a mass lesion (often in the mediastinum) in the setting of 25% or fewer blast cells in the bone marrow. It is a rare diagnosis in adults, representing roughly 2% of all NHL in the adult population (65). Most cases of

LBL are T cell derived (90%), with B-cell LBL occurring 10% of the time.

The most common presentation of T-cell LBL is in a young adult male, because the median patient age is 16, with a 2:1 male to female predominance. Fifty to seventy percent of patients will present with a symptomatic mediastinal mass, which results in obstructive-type symptoms (superior vena cava syndrome, tracheal obstruction, pericardial effusion with or without tamponade). Another common finding is cervical, supraclavicular, or axillary lymphadenopathy at the time of diagnosis, which occurs in 50% of patients (66). Advanced disease is not infrequent with bone marrow involvement in roughly half of cases at the time of presentation. If there is abdominal involvement, the liver and spleen are sites that can harbor metastatic disease. As the disease progresses, patients experience a leukemic phase, which is often indistinguishable from T-cell ALL (67).

B-cell LBL has a clinical picture distinct from T-cell LBL. These patients often have primary skin involvement, because mediastinal masses and peripheral lymphadenopathy is rare (68). There is no male predominance in B-cell LBL, and the disease is often less aggressive, although aggressive variants of B-cell LBL can occur.

The diagnosis of LBL should be established in an incisional or excisional biopsy specimen. Histochemical analysis and flow cytometry evaluation is necessary for diagnosis. Blasts can be present in tissue biopsy specimen, peripheral blood or bone marrow. Histochemical analysis and flow cytometry evaluation is necessary for diagnosis. The differential diagnosis in the adult population includes ALL, Burkitt's lymphoma, thymoma, diffuse large cell lymphoma, neuroendocrine tumor, germ cell tumors, and sarcoma. To distinguish T- and C-cell linage of LBL, immunotyping is often used, because rearrangement of the antigen receptor genes may not be specific to lineage (69).

Historically, radiation with extended field radiotherapy was the primary treatment modality for children with LBL, but survival rates were extremely poor, with less than 10% of patients surviving because of swift progression of disease (70). Combined modality therapy with an aggressive chemotherapy regiment and local radiotherapy offered improved outcomes; however, the chemotherapeutic agents used were often those used for other aggressive NHLs and failure rates were still unacceptably high (71). In an effort to improve patient outcomes, pediatric oncologists adopted ALL treatment approaches for children with LBL and results were promising (72). On the basis of the success of ALL therapeutic strategies in the pediatric population, the oncology community followed suit, offering adult LBL patients similar regiments with encouraging results.

The primary strategy in the management of LBL is centered at aggressive chemotherapy with an induction phase, consolidation/intensification and long-term maintenance. Tumor lysis syndrome is common and should be anticipated. In cases of relapse or persistent disease after chemotherapy, allogeneic HSCT is preferred. In cases of mediastinal involvement, radiotherapy should be administered, especially in cases where there is residual disease after systemic therapy.

Between 1989 and 1998,, the German multicenter study group for adult ALL (GMALL) treated 45 adult patients with T-LBL according to a protocol based on ALL therapy (73). The regimen included an eight drug induction treatment, followed by consolidation, reinduction, and maintenance. CNS prophylaxis included intrathecal methotrexate, prophylactic cranial irradiation (PCI) to 24 Gy (during phase II induction after CR), and intrathecal triple chemotherapy with methotrexate, cytarabine, and dexamethasone (during reinduction). Prophylactic radiotherapy to the mediastinum to 24 Gy was recommended, regardless of tumor response in the mediastinum. Ninety three percent of patients achieved a CR. Unfortunately, 36% patients relapsed in the first 12 months, with almost half (47%) of recurrences in the mediastinum despite mediastinal radiotherapy in six of seven patients. This study demonstrated that a high CR rate can be achieved in these patients; however, mediastinal recurrences can be challenging, arguing for treatment intensification by the way of dose escalation or increased chemotherapy.

A study from MD Anderson conducted between 1992 and 2001 also reported favorable CR rates in 33 patients with LBL treated with an intensive chemotherapy regimen, hyper-CVAD (fractionated cyclophosphamide, vincristine, adriamycin, and dexamethasone), either standard or modified (74). In this cohort study, CNS prophylaxis included alternating intrathecal treatment with methotrexate and cytarabine. No PCI was given, but radiotherapy was permitted to 24 to 30 Gy for known CNS disease at presentation. All patients with mediastinal disease were recommended to have involved field radiotherapy to 30 to 39 Gy over 4 to 5 weeks before maintenance treatment. Ninety one percent of patients achieved a CR with 30% of patients relapsing or progressing within a median of 13 months. This regimen was associated with improved local control in the mediastinum, with only 7% of patients relapsing in the mediastinum. In an earlier retrospective study from MDACC between 1980 and 1998 evaluating the role of mediastinal radiotherapy for adult patients with T-cell LBL treated predominantly with hyper-CVAD, local radiation to 26 to 39 Gy significantly decreased the risk of mediastinal recurrence (75). In an analysis of patients with mediastinal T-cell LBL comparing 19 patients who received radiotherapy with 24 patients who did not, 0% of patients who were irradiated experience a mediastinal recurrence, compared with 33% of patients not receiving radiation therapy who did relapse in the mediastinum. However, there was no difference in overall survival rates. Taken together, these studies suggest a critical role in consolidative radiotherapy in patients with mediastinal LBL.

■ LYMPHOPLASMACYTIC LYMPHOMA/WALDENSTRÖM MACROGLOBULINEMIA

Lymphoplasmacytic lymphoma (LPL) is a diagnosis of exclusion. The 2008 WHO classification describes LPL as a neoplasm of small B lymphocytes, plasma cells and plasmacytoid lymphocytes involving the bone marrow, occasionally the lymph nodes and spleen and not meeting criteria for any other small B cell lymphoid neoplasm. Waldenström macroglobulinemia (WM) is defined as an LPL with bone marrow involvement and IgM monoclonal gammopathy of any concentration. In 1958, Jan Waldenström described WM in two patients who presented with oronasal epistaxis, lymphadenopathy, cytopenias, and increased sedimentation rate (76). Patients are diagnosed with 'smoldering' WM when they meet the diagnostic criteria for WM but are asymptomatic with no evidence of anemia, lymphadenopathy, organomegaly, or hyperviscosity. These patients do not require therapy and, instead, can be monitored for disease progression.

LPL is rare, comprising 1% of hematologic neoplasms in the United States and Western Europe (77). Most patients with LPL may present with symptoms related to anemia, including weakness and fatigue. Organomegaly and lymphadenopathy are also presenting symptoms in 20% of patients (78). Still one third of patients are asymptomatic at the time of diagnosis (79). Those with WM may have hyperviscosity symptoms related to the serum presence of the IgM monoclonal protein in 30% of presenting cases (79). If the serum viscosity is <4 centipoises (cP)

however there are rarely hyperviscosity clinical manifestations (normal value is ≤1.8 cP). When clinically relevant, hyperviscosity does cause symptoms; they are typically manifested neurologically with headache, vision changes, tinnitus, deafness, vertigo, and ataxia. Circulating IgM may also result in amyloidosis (because of tissue deposition), peripheral neuropathy, and cryoglobulinemia (because of cold-induced macroglobulin precipitation) (80,81).

Bone marrow biopsy with aspirate and serum blood samples is necessary for diagnosis. An infiltrative lymphoplasmacytic cell population is appreciated in the bone marrow, as evidenced by the presence of small lymphocytes with plasmacytoid/plasma cell differentiation. Immunophenotypic studies are essential. The infiltrate should express pan B-cell markers CD 19, 20, and 22 and are typically negative for CD3 and CD 103 (82). The most common genetic aberration is a deletion of chromosome 6q21, which is present in 42% to 63% of cases and is associated with poor prognosis (83–85). The immunoglobulin M serum protein is a monoclonal pentamer that is responsible for the hyperviscosity symptoms that typically occur at serum viscosity levels of 4.0 cP. Quantitative immunoglobulin analysis and serum protein electrophoresis (SPEP) are included in the workup for WM. Other diagnostic evaluations include CBC with differential, comprehensive metabolic panel, β_2 microglobulin, serum viscosity and CT imaging of the chest, abdomen, and pelvis. If the IgM levels are greater than 3.0 g/L or if hyperviscosity is suspected, then retinal examination should be performed. Other considerations include cold agglutinins and cryocrit in patients with suspected cryoglobulinemia.

Patients with symptomatic hyperviscosity should be treated with emergent plasmapheresis. There is no standard therapy for WM, and unfortunately, current treatments are not curative. Treatment options include the monoclonal antibody rituximab, nucleoside analogs (fludarabine or cladribine), and alkylating agents (chlorambucil and cyclophosphamide). HSCT may be an option for some patients; however, if stem cell transplant is being considered, then oral alkylator therapy and nucleoside analogs should not be administered, because these agents can interfere with stem cell collection. Furthermore, nucleoside analogs have been shown to be associated with an increased risk of disease transformation and AML (86).

Because of the low toxicity of rituximab and phase II studies revealing good response rates, it is advisable to include rituximab in the initial therapeutic regimen for patients with LPL and WM (87–89). Caution should be used, however, because rituximab can cause a serum IgM flare with secondary hyperviscosity; therefore, patients should closely be monitored. The NCCN recommends prophylactic plasmapheresis in patients with IgM greater than 5,000 mg/dL before rituximab therapy. Rituximab can be administered as single-agent therapy or as part of combination therapy. Other regimens with minimal stem cell toxicity include bortezomib, a reversible proteosome inhibitor that acts on the 20S core of the proteosome. It has also demonstrated acceptable response rates in phase II trials (90,91). The most common side effect of bortezomib therapy is neuropathy. Potentially, stem cell toxic regimens include nucleoside analogs with or without rituximab. Cyclophosphamide and chlorambucil containing regimens are also an option.

There is no established role for radiotherapy in the treatment of LDL and WM. There have been a few cases reports of splenic radiotherapy in patients with symptomatic splenomegaly in the setting of WM where palliative radiotherapy provided symptomatic relief and good local control within the field (92,93). Palliative radiotherapy has also been used as a treatment modality in rare cases of CNS infiltration of neoplastic WM cells (Bing–Neel syndrome) (94).

■ CONCLUSION

Genomic research has revolutionized patient stratification and treatment in leukemia. The role of radiation therapy in the management of acute and chronic leukemias has diminished over the last few decades, because chemotherapy-based conditioning regimens have replaced total body irradiation as preparation for stem cell transplantation. Palliative radiotherapy, however, is quite effective and is often used in several settings.

■ REFERENCES

1. Bennett JM, Catovsky D, Daniel MT, et al. Proposals for the classification of the acute leukaemias. French-American-British (FAB) co-operative group. *Br J Haematol.* 1976;33:451–458.

2. Jaffe ES, Stein H, Vardiman JW. *Classification of Tumours of Haematopoietic and Lymphoid Tissues.* 3rd ed. Lyon, France: International Agency for Research on Cancer. Lyon; 2001.

3. Yamamoto JF, Goodman MT. Patterns of leukemia incidence in the United States by subtype and demographic characteristics, 1997–2002. *Cancer Causes Control.* 2008;19:379–390.

4. Preston DL, Kusumi S, Tomonaga M, et al. Cancer incidence in atomic bomb survivors. Part III. Leukemia, lymphoma and multiple myeloma, 1950–1987. *Radiat Res.* 1994;137:S68–S97.

5. Hasle H, Clemmensen IH, Mikkelsen M. Risks of leukaemia and solid tumours in individuals with Down's syndrome. *Lancet.* 2000;355:165–169.

6. Taylor AM. Chromosome instability syndromes. *Best Pract Res Clin Haematol.* 2001;14:631–644.

7. Byrd JC, Edenfield WJ, Shields DJ, et al. Extramedullary myeloid cell tumors in acute nonlymphocytic leukemia: a clinical review. *J Clin Oncol.* 1995;13:1800–1816.

8. Yates J, Glidewell O, Wiernik P, et al. Cytosine arabinoside with daunorubicin or adriamycin for therapy of acute myelocytic leukemia: a CALGB study. *Blood.* 1982;60:454–462.

9. Smith M, Barnett M, Bassan R, et al. Adult acute myeloid leukaemia. *Crit Rev Oncol Hematol.* 2004;50:197–222.

10. Brochstein JA, Kernan NA, Groshen S, et al. Allogeneic bone marrow transplantation after hyperfractionated total-body irradiation and cyclophosphamide in children with acute leukemia. *N Engl J Med.* 1987;317:1618–1624.

11. Santos GW, Tutschka PJ, Brookmeyer R, et al. Marrow transplantation for acute nonlymphocytic leukemia after treatment with busulfan and cyclophosphamide. *N Engl J Med.* 1983;309:1347–1353.

12. Blaise D, Maraninchi D, Michallet M, et al. Long-term follow-up of a randomized trial comparing the combination of cyclophosphamide with total body irradiation or busulfan as conditioning regimen for patients receiving HLA-identical marrow grafts for acute myeloblastic leukemia in first complete remission. *Blood.* 2001;97:3669–3671.

13. Blume KG, Kopecky KJ, Henslee-Downey JP, et al. A prospective randomized comparison of total body irradiation-etoposide versus busulfan-cyclophosphamide as preparatory regimens for bone marrow transplantation in patients with leukemia who were not in first remission: a Southwest Oncology Group study. *Blood.* 1993;81:2187–2193.

14. Clift RA, Radich J, Appelbaum FR, et al. Long-term follow-up of a randomized study comparing cyclophosphamide and total body irradiation with busulfan and cyclophosphamide for patients receiving allogenic marrow transplants during chronic phase of chronic myeloid leukemia. *Blood.* 1999;94:3960–3962.

15. Ringden O, Remberger M, Ruutu T, et al. Increased risk of chronic graft-versus-host disease, obstructive bronchiolitis, and alopecia with busulfan versus total body irradiation: long-term results of a randomized trial in allogeneic marrow recipients with leukemia. Nordic Bone Marrow Transplantation Group. *Blood.* 1999;93:2196–2201.

16. Dusenbery KE, Daniels KA, McClure JS, et al. Randomized comparison of cyclophosphamide-total body irradiation versus busulfan-cyclophosphamide

conditioning in autologous bone marrow transplantation for acute myeloid leukemia. *Int J Radiat Oncol Biol Phys.* 1995;31:119–128.

17. Devergie A, Blaise D, Attal M, et al. Allogeneic bone marrow transplantation for chronic myeloid leukemia in first chronic phase: a randomized trial of busulfan-cytoxan versus cytoxan-total body irradiation as preparative regimen: a report from the French Society of Bone Marrow Graft (SFGM). *Blood.* 1995;85:2263–2268.

18. Bunin N, Aplenc R, Kamani N, et al. Randomized trial of busulfan vs total body irradiation containing conditioning regimens for children with acute lymphoblastic leukemia: a Pediatric Blood and Marrow Transplant Consortium study. *Bone Marrow Transplant.* 2003;32:543–548.

19. Gupta T, Kannan S, Dantkale V, et al. Cyclophosphamide plus total body irradiation compared with busulfan plus cyclophosphamide as a conditioning regimen prior to hematopoietic stem cell transplantation in patients with leukemia: a systematic review and meta-analysis. *Hematol Oncol Stem Cell Ther.* 2011;4:17–29.

20. Lowenberg B, Downing JR, Burnett A. Acute myeloid leukemia. *N Engl J Med.* 1999;341:1051–1062.

21. Abou-Jawde RM, Sobecks R, Pohlman B, et al. The role of post-remission chemotherapy for older patients with acute myelogenous leukemia. *Leuk Lymphoma.* 2006;47:689–695.

22. Kantarjian H, Ravandi F, O'Brien S, et al. Intensive chemotherapy does not benefit most older patients (age 70 years or older) with acute myeloid leukemia. *Blood.* 2010;116:4422–4429.

23. de The H, Chomienne C, Lanotte M, et al. The t(15;17) translocation of acute promyelocytic leukaemia fuses the retinoic acid receptor alpha gene to a novel transcribed locus. *Nature.* 1990;347:558–561.

24. Brearley RL, Johnson SA, Lister TA. Acute lymphoblastic leukaemia in adults: clinicopathological correlations with the French-American-British (FAB) co-operative group classification. *Eur J Cancer.* 1979;15:909–914.

25. National Cancer Institute. *SEER Cancer Statistic Review, 1973–1999.* Bethesda, MD: Author; 2000.

26. Svendsen AL, Feychting M, Klaeboe L, et al. Time trends in the incidence of acute lymphoblastic leukemia among children 1976–2002: a population-based Nordic study. *J Pediatr.* 2007;151:548–550.

27. Buffler PA, Kwan ML, Reynolds P, et al. Environmental and genetic risk factors for childhood leukemia: appraising the evidence. *Cancer Invest.* 2005;23:60–75.

28. Margolin JF, Steuber CF, Poplack DG. *Principles and Practice of Pediatric Oncology.* 4th ed. Philadelphia, PA: Lippincott-Raven; 2001.

29. Bleyer WA. Central nervous system leukemia. *Pediatr Clin North Am.* 1988;35:789–814.

30. Pui CH, Robison LL, Look AT. Acute lymphoblastic leukaemia. *Lancet.* 2008;371:1030–1043.

31. Pulte D, Gondos A, Brenner H. Improvement in survival in younger patients with acute lymphoblastic leukemia from the 1980s to the early 21st century. *Blood.* 2009;113:1408–1411.

32. Ottmann OG, Hoelzer D. The ABL tyrosine kinase inhibitor STI571 (Glivec) in Philadelphia positive acute lymphoblastic leukemia—promises, pitfalls and possibilities. *Hematol J.* 2002;3:2–6.

33. Ohanian M, Cortes J, Kantarjian H, et al. Tyrosine kinase inhibitors in acute and chronic leukemias. *Expert Opin Pharmacother.* 13:927–938.

34. Pui CH, Evans WE. Treatment of acute lymphoblastic leukemia. *N Engl J Med.* 2006;354:166–178.

35. Evans AE, Gilbert ES, Zandstra R. The increasing incidence of central nervous system leukemia in children. (Children's Cancer Study Group A). *Cancer.* 1970;26:404–409.

36. Stanulla M, Schrappe M. Treatment of childhood acute lymphoblastic leukemia. *Semin Hematol.* 2009;46:52–63.

37. Kantarjian HM, O'Brien S, Smith TL, et al. Results of treatment with hyper-CVAD, a dose-intensive regimen, in adult acute lymphocytic leukemia. *J Clin Oncol.* 2000;18:547–561.

38. Pui CH, Howard SC. Current management and challenges of malignant disease in the CNS in paediatric leukaemia. *Lancet Oncol.* 2008;9:257–268.

39. Schrappe M, Reiter A, Ludwig WD, et al. Improved outcome in childhood acute lymphoblastic leukemia despite reduced use of anthracyclines and cranial radiotherapy: results of trial ALL-BFM 90. German-Austrian-Swiss ALL-BFM Study Group. *Blood.* 2000;95:3310–3322.

40. Nowell P HD. A minute chromosome in human granulocytic leukemia. *Science.* 1960;132:1497.

41. Shtivelman E, Lifshitz B, Gale RP, et al. Fused transcript of abl and bcr genes in chronic myelogenous leukaemia. *Nature.* 1985;315:550–554.

42. Goldman JM, Melo JV. Targeting the BCR-ABL tyrosine kinase in chronic myeloid leukemia. *N Engl J Med.* 2001;344:1084–1086.

43. Druker BJ, Guilhot F, O'Brien SG, et al. Five-year follow-up of patients receiving imatinib for chronic myeloid leukemia. *N Engl J Med.* 2006;355:2408–2417.

44. Sokal JE, Cox EB, Baccarani M, et al. Prognostic discrimination in "good-risk" chronic granulocytic leukemia. *Blood.* 1984;63:789–799.

45. Milojkovic D, Nicholson E, Apperley JF, et al. Early prediction of success or failure of treatment with second-generation tyrosine kinase inhibitors in patients with chronic myeloid leukemia. *Haematologica.* 2010;95:224–231.

46. de Lavallade H, Apperley JF, Khorashad JS, et al. Imatinib for newly diagnosed patients with chronic myeloid leukemia: incidence of sustained responses in an intention-to-treat analysis. *J Clin Oncol.* 2008;26:3358–3363.

47. Marin D, Marktel S, Bua M, et al. Prognostic factors for patients with chronic myeloid leukaemia in chronic phase treated with imatinib mesylate after failure of interferon alfa. *Leukemia.* 2003;17:1448–1453.

48. O'Brien SG, Guilhot F, Larson RA, et al. Imatinib compared with interferon and low-dose cytarabine for newly diagnosed chronic-phase chronic myeloid leukemia. *N Engl J Med.* 2003;348:994–1004.

49. Saglio G, Kim DW, Issaragrisil S, et al. Nilotinib versus imatinib for newly diagnosed chronic myeloid leukemia. *N Engl J Med.* 2010;362:2251–2259.

50. Kantarjian H, Shah NP, Hochhaus A, et al. Dasatinib versus imatinib in newly diagnosed chronic-phase chronic myeloid leukemia. *N Engl J Med.* 2010;362:2260–2270.

51. Siegel R, Naishadham D, Jemal A. Cancer statistics, 2012. *CA Cancer J Clin.* 2012;62:10–29.

52. Smith A, Howell D, Patmore R, et al. Incidence of haematological malignancy by sub-type: a report from the Haematological Malignancy Research Network. *Br J Cancer,* 2011;105:1684–1692.

53. Binet JL. New data on the prognosis of chronic lymphoid leukemia: anatomo-clinical classification. *Acquis Med Recent.* 1981;198:191–200.

54. Hallek M, Cheson BD, Catovsky D, et al. Guidelines for the diagnosis and treatment of chronic lymphocytic leukemia: a report from the International Workshop on Chronic Lymphocytic Leukemia updating the National Cancer Institute-Working Group 1996 guidelines. *Blood.* 2008;111:5446–5456.

55. Molica S, Levato D. What is changing in the natural history of chronic lymphocytic leukemia? *Haematologica.* 2001;86:8–12.

56. Rawstron AC, Bennett FL, O'Connor SJ, et al. Monoclonal B-cell lymphocytosis and chronic lymphocytic leukemia. *N Engl J Med.* 2008;359:575–583.

57. Dohner H, Stilgenbauer S, Benner A, et al. Genomic aberrations and survival in chronic lymphocytic leukemia. *N Engl J Med.* 2000;343:1910–1916.

58. Hamblin TJ, Davis Z, Gardiner A, et al. Unmutated Ig V(H) genes are associated with a more aggressive form of chronic lymphocytic leukemia. *Blood.* 1999;94:1848–1854.

59. Chemotherapeutic options in chronic lymphocytic leukemia: a meta-analysis of the randomized trials. CLL Trialists' Collaborative Group. *J Natl Cancer Inst.* 1999;91:861–868.

60. Rossier C, Schick U, Miralbell R, et al. Low-dose radiotherapy in indolent lymphoma. *Int J Radiat Oncol Biol Phys.* 2011;81:e1–e6.

61. Chan EK, Fung S, Gospodarowicz M, et al. Palliation by low-dose local radiation therapy for indolent non-Hodgkin lymphoma. *Int J Radiat Oncol Biol Phys.* 2011;81:e781–e786.

62. Chisesi T, Capnist G, Dal Fior S. Splenic irradiation in chronic lymphocytic leukemia. *Eur J Haematol.* 1991;46:202–204.

63. Guiney MJ, Liew KH, Quong GG, et al. A study of splenic irradiation in chronic lymphocytic leukemia. *Int J Radiat Oncol Biol Phys.* 1989;16:225–229.

64. Lavrenkov K, Krepel-Volsky S, Levi I, et al. Low dose palliative radiotherapy for splenomegaly in hematologic disorders. *Leuk Lymphoma.* 2012;53:430–434.

65. Ohno H, Fukuhara S. Significance of rearrangement of the BCL6 gene in B-cell lymphoid neoplasms. *Leuk Lymphoma.* 1997;27:53–63.

66. Streuli RA, Kaneko Y, Variakojis D, et al. Lymphoblastic lymphoma in adults. *Cancer.* 1981;47:2510–2516.

67. Copelan EA, McGuire EA. The biology and treatment of acute lymphoblastic leukemia in adults. *Blood.* 1995;85:1151–1168.

68. Shafer D, Wu H, Al-Saleem T, et al. Cutaneous precursor B-cell lymphoblastic lymphoma in 2 adult patients: clinicopathologic and molecular cytogenetic studies with a review of the literature. *Arch Dermatol.* 2008;144:1155–1162.

69. Szczepanski T, Pongers-Willemse MJ, Langerak AW, et al. Ig heavy chain gene rearrangements in T-cell acute lymphoblastic leukemia exhibit predominant DH6–19 and DH7–27 gene usage, can result in complete V-D-J rearrangements, and are rare in T-cell receptor alpha beta lineage. *Blood.* 1999;93:4079–4085.

70. Glatstein E, Kim H, Donaldson SS, et al. Non-Hodgkin's lymphomas. VI. Results of treatment in childhood. *Cancer.* 1974;34:204–211.

71. Le Gouill S, Lepretre S, Briere J, et al. Adult lymphoblastic lymphoma: a retrospective analysis of 92 patients under 61 years included in the LNH87/93 trials. *Leukemia.* 2003;17:2220–2224.

72. Reiter A, Schrappe M, Ludwig WD, et al. Intensive ALL-type therapy without local radiotherapy provides a 90% event-free survival for children with T-cell lymphoblastic lymphoma: a BFM group report. *Blood.* 2000;95:416–421.

73. Hoelzer D, Gokbuget N, Digel W, et al. Outcome of adult patients with T-lymphoblastic lymphoma treated according to protocols for acute lymphoblastic leukemia. *Blood.* 2002;99:4379–4385.

74. Thomas DA, O'Brien S, Cortes J, et al. Outcome with the hyper-CVAD regimens in lymphoblastic lymphoma. *Blood.* 2004;104:1624–1630.

75. Dabaja BS, Ha CS, Thomas DA, et al. The role of local radiation therapy for mediastinal disease in adults with T-cell lymphoblastic lymphoma. *Cancer.* 2002;94:2738–2744.

76. Waldenstrom J. Macroglobulinaemia. *Acta Haematol.* 1958;20:33–39.

77. Morton LM, Wang SS, Devesa SS, et al. Lymphoma incidence patterns by WHO subtype in the United States, 1992–2001. *Blood.* 2006;107:265–276.

78. Vitolo U, Ferreri AJ, Montoto S. Lymphoplasmacytic lymphoma—Waldenstrom's macroglobulinemia. *Crit Rev Oncol Hematol.* 2008;67:172–185.

79. Garcia-Sanz R, Montoto S, Torrequebrada A, et al. Waldenstrom macroglobulinaemia: presenting features and outcome in a series with 217 cases. *Br J Haematol.* 2001;115:575–582.

80. Treon SP. How I treat Waldenstrom macroglobulinemia. *Blood.* 2009;114:2375–2385.

81. Vijay A, Gertz MA. Waldenstrom macroglobulinemia. *Blood.* 2007;109:5096–5103.

82. Morice WG, Chen D, Kurtin PJ, et al. Novel immunophenotypic features of marrow lymphoplasmacytic lymphoma and correlation with Waldenstrom's macroglobulinemia. *Mod Pathol.* 2009;22:807–816.

83. Chang H, Qi C, Trieu Y, et al. Prognostic relevance of 6q deletion in Waldenstrom's macroglobulinemia: a multicenter study. *Clin Lymphoma Myeloma.* 2009;9:36–38.

84. Cook JR, Aguilera NI, Reshmi S, et al. Deletion 6q is not a characteristic marker of nodal lymphoplasmacytic lymphoma. *Cancer Genet Cytogenet.* 2005;162:85–88.

85. Schop RF, Kuehl WM, Van Wier SA, et al. Waldenstrom macroglobulinemia neoplastic cells lack immunoglobulin heavy chain locus translocations but have frequent 6q deletions. *Blood.* 2002;100:2996–3001.

86. Leleu X, Soumerai J, Roccaro A, et al. Increased incidence of transformation and myelodysplasia/acute leukemia in patients with Waldenstrom macroglobulinemia treated with nucleoside analogs. *J Clin Oncol.* 2009;27:250–255.

87. Ansell SM, Kyle RA, Reeder CB, et al. Diagnosis and management of Waldenstrom macroglobulinemia: Mayo stratification of macroglobulinemia and risk-adapted therapy (mSMART) guidelines. *Mayo Clin Proc.* 2010;85:824–833.

88. Fonseca R. Strategies for risk-adapted therapy in myeloma. *Hematology Am Soc Hematol Educ Program.* 2007:304–310.

89. Dimopoulos MA, Gertz MA, Kastritis E, et al. Update on treatment recommendations from the Fourth International Workshop on Waldenstrom's Macroglobulinemia. *J Clin Oncol.* 2009;27:120–126.

90. Chen CI, Kouroukis CT, White D, et al. Bortezomib is active in patients with untreated or relapsed Waldenstrom's macroglobulinemia: a phase II study of the National Cancer Institute of Canada Clinical Trials Group. *J Clin Oncol.* 2007;25:1570–1575.

91. Dimopoulos MA, Anagnostopoulos A, Kyrtsonis MC, et al. Treatment of relapsed or refractory Waldenstrom's macroglobulinemia with bortezomib. *Haematologica.* 2005;90:1655–1658.

92. Cavanna L, Berte R, Lazzaro A, et al. Advanced Waldenstrom's macroglobulinemia: a case of possible cure after systemic chemotherapy, splenic radiation and splenectomy. *Acta Haematol.* 2002;108:97–101.

93. Davda R, Davies S, Kumaran T. Splenic irradiation in the management of Waldenstrom macroglobulinemia. *Leuk Lymphoma.* 2009;50:1047–1049.

94. Delgado J, Canales MA, Garcia B, et al. Radiation therapy and combination of cladribine, cyclophosphamide, and prednisone as treatment of Bing-Neel syndrome: Case report and review of the literature. *Am J Hematol.* 2002;69:127–131.

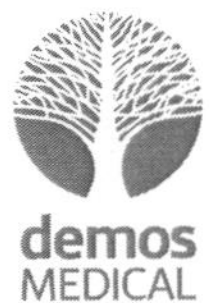

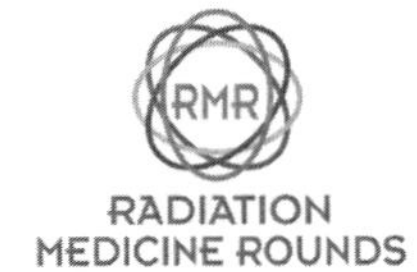

Plasma Cell Dyscrasias

Andrew J. Yee,[1]* Karen M. Winkfield,[2] and Noopur S. Raje[1]

[1]Center for Multiple Myeloma, Massachusetts General Hospital Cancer Center, Boston, MA

[2]Hematologic Malignancy Service, Department of Radiation Oncology, Massachusetts General Hospital Cancer Center, Boston, MA

■ ABSTRACT

Plasma cell dyscrasias are characterized by a neoplastic proliferation of plasma cells. Multiple myeloma is the archetypal plasma cell disorder; monoclonal gammopathy of unknown significance is a precursor condition to multiple myeloma. Multiple myeloma is the second most common hematologic malignancy with a median age at diagnosis of 66. The last 2 decades have witnessed dramatic advances in the treatment of myeloma with the introduction of autologous stem cell transplant, proteasome inhibition, and immunomodulatory agents. The incorporation of novel agents in myeloma treatment has led to significant improvements in overall survival.

Keywords: multiple myeloma, monoclonal gammopathy of unknown significance, plasma cell dyscrasia

■ INTRODUCTION

Plasma cell disorders are a group of related diseases where there is proliferation of malignant plasma cells in the bone marrow and accompanied by the presence of a monoclonal immunoglobulin (Ig) or Ig fragment in the serum and/or urine of patients (1). Multiple myeloma (MM) and its precursor condition, monoclonal gammopathy of unknown significance (MGUS) are the principal plasma cell disorders. Other plasma cell disorders include Waldenström's macroglobulinemia, primary amyloidosis, and heavy chain diseases. This chapter will focus on MGUS and MM.

■ MONOCLONAL GAMMOPATHY OF UNKNOWN SIGNIFICANCE

Monoclonal gammopathy of unknown significance is an asymptomatic clonal plasma cell disorder defined by a serum monoclonal protein <3 g/dL and <10% plasma cells in the bone marrow (2). MGUS is a common condition seen with increasing age and is observed in 3.2% of individuals 50 years old or older and 5.3% among individuals 70 years or older (3). By the time a monoclonal protein can be detected by serum electrophoresis, an expansion of clonal plasma cells to roughly one billion cells is already present (4).

---

*Corresponding author, Massachusetts General Hospital Cancer Center, 275 Cambridge Street, Boston, MA

E-mail address: ayee1@partners.org

Radiation Medicine Rounds 3:3 (2012) 473–488.

DOI: 10.5003/2151–4208.3.3.473

MGUS is a premalignant condition, with a risk of progression to MM or related disorders such as lymphoma or amyloidosis of about 1% per year or 25% at 20 years (5). Additional longitudinal studies in other cohorts have shown that MGUS consistently precedes MM, for example, when serum samples obtained 2 to 9.8 years before diagnosis have been studied in the Prostate, Lung, Colorectal, and Ovarian Cancer Screening Trial (6) and similarly, in the Department of Defense Serum Repository (7). Risk factors for progression include high-serum monoclonal protein (≥1.5 g/dL), non-IgG MGUS, and abnormal serum-free light chain ratio (8). In some patients, an intermediate, more advanced stage, smoldering MM, may be identified before the onset of MM, when end organ involvement becomes manifest (9). At this time, treatment for MGUS and smoldering MM consists of risk stratification and close observation (2).

produce circulating monoclonal antibodies. It is the second most common hematologic malignancy (more than 10% of all hematologic malignancies) and responsible for nearly 2% of all cancer deaths. There were an estimated 21,700 new cases of MM and 10,710 deaths from MM in the United States in 2012 (10). MM is a disease of older patients. In one series, the median age at diagnosis was 66; 2% were younger than 40 years old, and 38% were 70 years old or older (11). African-Americans have twofold to threefold higher incidence of MM compared with Caucasians (12).

The cause of MM is unknown. Epidemiology studies have found an association between exposures associated with farming but not necessarily with tobacco or diet (13). Rare familial clusters of MM have been reported (14), and an increased risk of MGUS and MM has been reported in family members of patients with plasma cell dyscrasias, suggesting a genetic susceptibility or shared environmental factors that remain poorly understood (15,16).

■ MULTIPLE MYELOMA

Epidemiology

MM is a plasma cell dyscrasia characterized by a clonal expansion of antibody-producing plasma cells that infiltrate the bone marrow at multiple sites and

Biology

The development of MM is a multistep process reflecting an accumulation of genetic changes in conjunction with changes in the bone marrow milieu

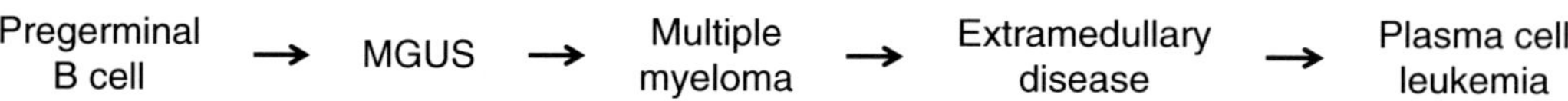

FIGURE 1 Pathogenesis of plasma cell dyscrasia. The initial events in the transformation from a normal pregerminal B cell to ultimately multiple myeloma include IgH translocations and hyperdiploidy. Dysregulation of cyclin D is also a common early event. Monoclonal gammopathy (MGUS) of unknown significance is a malignant precursor condition to multiple myeloma. Mutations in *NRAS*, *KRAS*, and *FGFR3* are associated with the evolution of MGUS to multiple myeloma. *MYC* dysregulation, p18 deletion, and p53 deletion are later events and associated with more aggressive disease.

Source: Adapted from Ref. (4) and (128).

that support the progression of disease (Figure 1). It arises from a precursor state of MGUS that progresses to bone marrow involvement, and then in advanced cases, to an extramedullary stage from where MM cell lines can be derived (4). One of the initiating events in the pathogenesis of MM includes aberrant chromosomal translocations from normally physiological B cell recombination, resulting in the dysregulation of an oncogene. Five recurrent IgH translocations have been identified in MM: 4p16 (*MMSET* and *FGFR3*), 6p21 (*CCND3*), 11q13 (*CCND1*), 16q23 (*MAF*), and 20q11 (*MAFB*) (4). Furthermore, MM tumor cells uniformly have high levels of cyclin D1, D2, and D3, suggesting a unifying early event in the pathogenesis of MM (4,17). Later events include copy number alterations, translocations, hyperdiploidy, and mutations resulting in dysregulation of genes such as *NRAS* and *KRAS* (18).

Interactions between the MM cells and the bone marrow microenvironment also play a critical role in the pathogenesis of the disease (19). The bone marrow microenvironment forms a supportive niche for the proliferation of tumor cells, which in turn symbiotically shapes the microenvironment to create a permissive niche. In MM, the balance between osteoclasts and osteoblasts is shifted in favor of osteoclast activity, favoring bone resorption and leading to disease-defining osteolytic lesions (20).

Recently, whole genome and whole exome sequencing of 38 MM patients identified mutations in genes involved in protein translation (e.g., with mutations in *DIS3* (also known as *RRP44*) and *FAM46C*), histone methylation, blood coagulation, and members of the NF-κB signaling (21). Four percent of patients had activating mutations in the BRAF kinase, suggesting a potential role for BRAF inhibitors in clinical use.

Clinical and Laboratory Features

The hallmark of MM is a malignant, clonal proliferation of plasma cells that produce a monoclonal protein (M-protein or immunoglobulin or paraprotein), with bone marrow infiltration and destruction. This leads to end organ involvement, with hypercalcemia, anemia, renal dysfunction, and lytic bone lesions (also remembered by its mnemonic, "CRAB").

In a Mayo Clinic survey of 1027 newly diagnosed patients, anemia (hemoglobin ≤12 g/dL) was present in the majority of patients (73%).

Hypercalcemia (calcium ≥11 mg/dL) was present in 13% of patients, and renal impairment (defined as creatinine of 2 mg/dL or more) was present in 19% of patients (11). At the time of diagnosis, bone pain was present in 58% of patients; 79% had a bony abnormality on conventional radiographs (i.e., 67% had lytic lesions, and 20% had osteoporosis) (Figure 2).

Causes of renal dysfunction include direct toxicity to the kidney from light chain aggregation and tubular obstruction, leading to cast nephropathy, as well as dehydration and hypercalcemia (22). Renal dysfunction is more common in patients with light chain MM (35% of patients present with creatinine ≥2 mg/dL) compared with 19% for the MM population as a whole (11). Extramedullary disease or soft tissue involvement is uncommon at presentation, ranging from 0.4% in the Mayo Clinic series (11) to 7% in an Italian series of 1003 patients and is associated with worse outcome (23).

Monoclonal Protein

Nearly all patients with MM (97%) have an M-protein that may be detected in the serum or urine by protein electrophoresis (Figure 3) or immunofixation; 7% of patients do not have a detectable serum monoclonal protein (11).Roughly half of the patients have an IgG monoclonal protein, 20% have an IgA monoclonal protein. In 16% of patients, the

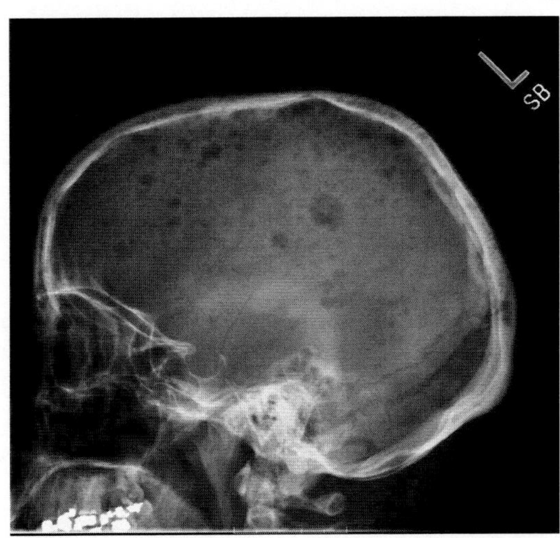

FIGURE 2 Lytic lesions in multiple myeloma. Multiple lytic lesions are seen in the calvarium of this 48-year-old woman with IgG kappa multiple myeloma.

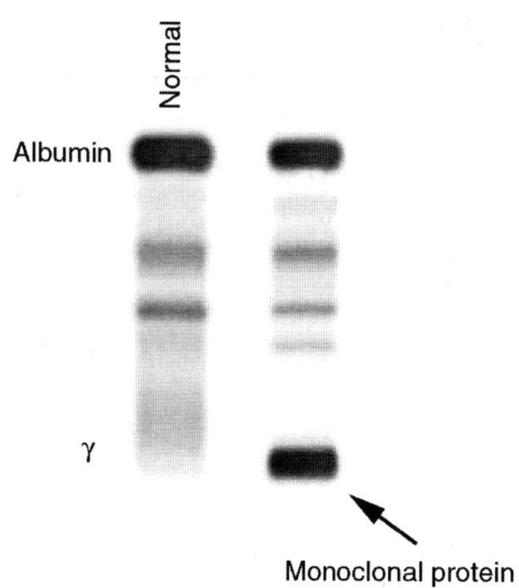

FIGURE 3 Serum protein electrophoresis. Comparison of normal serum protein electrophoresis versus presence of monoclonal protein in the γ region. The majority of the serum protein is albumin. Immunoglobulins are present in the γ band of the electrophoresis.

monoclonal protein is only a free light chain (also known as Bence Jones protein) not bound to a heavy chain (11).

The serum free light chain assay has emerged in the past decade as a new method that may obviate the need for traditionally relying on urine studies to identify and monitor patients with light chain only disease. A significant majority of patients with plasma cell disorders have an excess involved free light chain or abnormal free light chain ratio (of note, 14% of patients have a normal serum free light chain ratio) (24,25). Given its increased sensitivity, for example, in one study, 19 out of 28 patients who were classified as non-secretory MM were found to have measurably increased concentrations of light chain (and abnormal kappa/lambda ratio) with this approach (26).

Of note, in the Mayo Clinic series, over a third of patients had a known plasma cell proliferative process (e.g., MGUS or solitary plasmacytoma) before diagnosis with MM (11). More recent work has shown that nearly all cases of MM are preceded by an MGUS state (6,7).

Diagnostic Workup

Consensus guidelines recommend history and physical examination, a complete blood cell count, a metabolic panel, and measurement of β_2-microglobulin

(27,28). The level of serum β_2-microglobulin correlates with the burden of disease and is used for staging (29). The monoclonal protein can be detected with serum and urine protein electrophoresis with immunofixation and serum free light chains. Quantitative levels of IgG, IgA, and IgM are also measured. In 91% of patients at diagnosis, one or more involved immunoglobulin levels are depressed (11). To evaluate for bone marrow involvement, bone marrow aspiration for cytogenetics and FISH analysis and biopsy is generally recommended.

To evaluate for lytic bone lesions, a skeletal survey involving conventional radiographs of the spine, pelvis, skull, humeri, and femurs, is traditionally used. MRI and positron emission tomography (PET) are more sensitive than conventional radiography and should be considered at symptomatic sites that do not have a correlate on plain films (30). Traditional bone scintigraphy using technetium, although useful for detecting metastatic bone lesions from solid tumors, has a lower detection rate compared with conventional radiography (31). The lower sensitivity of technetium bone scintigraphy has been attributed to osteoblast dysfunction in MM.

Diagnostic Criteria and Prognostic Factors

The International Myeloma Working Group has established diagnostic criteria for MM and other plasma cell disorders such as Waldenström's macroglobulinemia and amyloidosis in 2003 and then updated in 2009 (Table 1) (28,32). The hallmarks of diagnosing MM include bone marrow involvement, the presence of a monoclonal protein in serum or urine (except in rare patients with non-secretory MM), *and* evidence of end organ involvement, manifested as hypercalcemia, renal insufficiency, anemia, or bone lesions.

Patients with an elevated monoclonal protein (>3 g/dL) or bone marrow involvement (clonal bone marrow plasma cells over 10%) *without* end organ involvement are classified as smoldering (asymptomatic) multiple myeloma (2). These patients have a significantly higher risk of progression to myeloma or related disorder compared with MGUS.

Classically, MM has been staged according to the Durie–Salmon system that was reported nearly 4 decades ago (Table 2) (33). The Durie–Salmon system correlated total MM tumor burden with clinical factors such as number of bone lesions and the amount of monoclonal protein. However, a limitation of the Durie–Salmon system is the subjectivity of determining the number of lytic lesions. The

TABLE 1   Diagnostic criteria for plasma cell disorders

Disorder	Disease definition
Monoclonal gammopathy of unknown significance	All three criteria must be met: • Serum monoclonal protein <3 g/dL • Clonal bone marrow plasma cells <10% • Absence of end-organ damage such as hypercalcemia, renal insufficiency, anemia, and bone lesions that can be attributed to the plasma cell disorder
Smoldering multiple myeloma (asymptomatic multiple myeloma)	Both criteria must be met: • Serum monoclonal protein (IgG or IgA) ≥ 3 g/dL and/or clonal bone marrow plasma cells ≥ 10% • Absence of end-organ damage such as lytic bone lesions, anemia, hypercalcemia, or renal failure that can be attributed to the plasma cell disorder
Multiple myeloma	All three criteria must be met except as noted: • Clonal bone marrow plasma cells ≥10% • Presence of serum or urinary monoclonal protein (except in patients with true nonsecretory multiple myeloma) • Evidence of end-organ damage attributed to plasma cell disorder: ○ Hypercalcemia, calcium ≥11.5 mg/dL ○ Renal insufficiency, serum creatinine >2 mg/dL ○ Anemia: normochromic, normocytic with a hemoglobin >2 g/dL below the lower limit of normal or a hemoglobin value <10 g/dL ○ Bone lesions; lytic lesions, severe osteopenia, or pathologic fractures

Source: Adapted from Ref. (28).

International Staging System was later devised to be based on objective criteria, and it stratifies patients into three groups based on serum β_2-microglobulin and albumin levels (29). Patients with stage I disease have a median overall survival of 62 months; stage II disease, median survival 44 months; and stage III disease 29 months. Of note, this staging system was developed before use of newer therapies such as bortezomib or lenalidomide was increasingly adopted.

FISH and conventional karyotype may be used to risk-stratify patients and guide therapy (Table 3) (34–36). Gene expression profiling may also be used to identify patients with high-risk disease, though is not widely available for clinical use (37).

A quarter of newly diagnosed patients will have intermediate to high-risk disease, including patients with deletion 17p (leading to loss of tumor suppressor p53), t(4;14), or t(14;16) by FISH. The majority, 75% of patients, will have standard risk disease, including patients with hyperdiploid karyotype. Patients with standard risk disease have an expected median survival of over 6–7 years, whereas patients with high-risk disease have a median survival of roughly 3 years (38).

Treatment

The past 2 decades have seen dramatic advances in the treatment of MM, beginning with the publication of a randomized trial investigating the use of high dose melphalan and autologous stem cell transplant in 1996 (39), followed by the introduction of immunomodulatory drugs thalidomide (40) and lenalidomide (41), and the proteasome inhibitor bortezomib (42). With these new treatments, the 5 year relative survival rate has increased in the Surveillance Epidemiology and End Results (SEER) database from 28.8% from the period of 1990–1992 to 34.7% in 2002 to 2004 to 40.3% in 2003 to

TABLE 2 Durie–Salmon Staging System And International Staging System

Stage	Durie–Salmon Stage	ISS Stage

I	All of the following:
	• Hemoglobin value >10 g/dL
	• Serum calcium value normal or ≤12 mg/dL
	• Bone x-ray, 0–1 lesion or solitary bone plasmacytoma only
	• Low M-component production rate:
	  ○ IgG value <5 g/dL
	  ○ IgA value <3 g/dL
	  ○ Urine light chain M-component on electrophoresis < 4 g/24 h
		Serum β_2-microglobulin <3.5 mg/L
		AND
		Serum albumin ≥3.5 g/dL

II	Neither stage I nor stage III	Serum β_2-microglobulin <3.5 mg/L, but serum albumin <3.5 g/dL OR Serum β_2-microglobulin 3.5 to <5.5 mg/L, irrespective of serum albumin

III	One or more of the following:
	• Hemoglobin value <8.5 g/dL
	• Serum calcium value >12 mg/dL
	• Advanced lytic bone lesions (≥ 3 lesions)
	• High M-component production rate
	  ○ IgG value >7 g/dL
	  ○ IgA value >5 g/dL
	  ○ Urine light chain M-component >12 g/24 h
		Serum β_2-microglobulin ≥5.5 mg/L

Source: Adapted from Ref. (29) and (33).

TABLE 3 Risk stratification of multiple myeloma

Risk	Karyotype
Standard risk	Hyperdiploidy t(11;14) t(6;14)
Intermediate risk	t(4;14) Deletion 13 or hypodiploidy by conventional karyotyping
High risk	17p deletion t(14;16) t(14;20) High-risk gene expression profiling signature

Source: Adapted from Ref. (36).

2007 (43,44). Previously, most of the survival benefit observed was in younger patients, but a more recent analysis showed that older patients over the age of 70 were deriving benefit as well (43,44).

Patients with symptomatic MM require treatment. Without treatment, survival ranges from 6 to 7 months from time of diagnosis (45,46). Treatment generally consists of an induction phase to treat symptoms and reduce disease burden followed by a maintenance phase. In patients who are medically fit, the induction phase is typically followed by stem cell harvest and consolidation with high dose chemotherapy with melphalan and autologous stem cell transplant. Conventionally, clinical trials of high dose chemotherapy autologous stem cell transplantation in MM have focused on patients 65 years of age or younger. In the United States, greater emphasis is placed on the patient's "physiologic" age and co-morbidities than chronologic age. Allogeneic stem cell transplant remains investigational in the initial treatment of patients.

Induction Therapy for Transplant-Eligible Patients

The goal of induction in newly diagnosed transplant-eligible patients is to palliate symptoms and achieve a deep response before stem cell collection and high dose therapy. Responses to treatment (e.g., complete response and very good partial response [VGPR]) have been categorized according to decline in monoclonal protein and other criteria by the International Myeloma Working Group (47).

The practice of using high dose chemotherapy with melphalan and later paired with autologous stem cell transplantation was introduced in the early 1980s (48,49). Furthermore, the association between the magnitude of response and long-term outcomes is best established for response assessment after autologous transplant, though there is a trend toward a similar association with response assessments measured before transplant (50–52). On the other hand, others have argued that the benefit of complete response is limited to high-risk subgroups identified by gene expression profiling (53).

Historically, beginning in the 1980s, the combination of vincristine, doxorubicin, and dexamethasone (VAD) was used for induction (54). However, highly active regimens using lenalidomide and/or bortezomib have supplanted VAD. Examples of modern regimens in use include doublet combinations of bortezomib and dexamethasone (55) and lenalidomide and dexamethasone (56), as well as triplet combinations of lenalidomide, bortezomib, dexamethasone (RVD) (57) and cyclophosphamide, bortezomib, dexamethasone (CyBorD) (58). A quadruplet combination where cyclophosphamide is added to RVD has been studied in the EVOLUTION trial, though no substantial advantage over three drug combinations was noted in a phase II trial (59). The choice of regimen may vary depending on drug availability from country to country.

After four cycles of RVD, 75% of patients in a phase II trial achieved a partial response or better (as defined by a reduction in the monoclonal protein by 50% or more); this increased to 100% with additional cycles (57). Drugs with potential for stem cell toxicity such as melphalan are generally not used during induction (60). The number of cycles of treatment, especially with lenalidomide-containing regimens is limited to roughly four cycles, as additional cycles may compromise the ability to collect stem cells (61,62).

Autologous Stem Cell Transplant

The main goal of autologous stem cell transplant is to achieve complete remission in patients with residual disease after induction as well as to consolidate and increase the duration of complete remission. In the Medical Research Council VII Trial, the median overall survival was increased by 1 year with autologous stem cell transplant compared with chemotherapy (63), and similar findings have been reported in other randomized trials with long-term follow-up (64). A limitation of most of these trials is that they were performed before the widespread use of newer agents such as bortezomib or immunomodulatory drugs such as lenalidomide.

Stem cells conventionally are mobilized with chemotherapy (cyclophosphamide) and growth factor simulation with filgrastim, and collected peripherally (65). High dose melphalan at 200 mg/m² is the most commonly used conditioning regimen; total body irradiation is no longer used (66).

Induction Therapy for Transplant-Ineligible Patients

In patients who are not considered eligible for transplant because of age or comorbidities, the same principles of palliation of symptoms and achieving a deep response also apply. Although the same regimens for induction in transplant-eligible patients may be used, melphalan-based therapies or lenalidomide with dexamethasone are also commonly given, owing to better tolerability in this typically older patient population.

In the past, in the absence of autologous transplant, achieving a complete response was unusual with the traditional combination of the oral alkylating agent melphalan and prednisone. However, in recent years, achieving a complete response with newer combinations using immunomodulatory drugs and/or bortezomib has now been possible, including older patients (67). For example, the VISTA trial compared the regimen of bortezomib, melphalan, and prednisone (VMP) with melphalan and prednisone (MP) in patients who were not candidates for autologous stem cell transplant (68). Overall survival was significantly improved in the VMP group versus MP group, with 3 year overall survival of 68.5% versus 54%, respectively (69).

Strategies aimed at improving the tolerability of treatment and decreasing risk of adverse events include using a lower dose of dexamethasone (56), decreasing the frequency of bortezomib to weekly (70,71), and changing the mode of administration from intravenous to subcutaneous (72). These changes have maintained the efficacy of treatment and allowed for longer duration of exposure to therapy.

Maintenance Therapy

To extend the duration of complete remission after autologous stem cell transplant, maintenance regimens have been proposed. The increased tolerability and efficacy of newer anti-MM agents has increased the attractiveness and the applicability of this approach; previous attempts at maintenance therapy with older conventional chemotherapy agents such as melphalan or interferon were not beneficial (73).

Lenalidomide

Three randomized trials have explored the use of lenalidomide as maintenance therapy, with two of the trials after autologous stem cell transplant (74,75) and one trial after 9 months of melphalan-based therapy in patients ineligible for high dose treatment (76). In all three trials, there was a near doubling in progression free survival with lenalidomide maintenance, for example, from 27 to 46 months in the CALGB 100104 study (75). Furthermore, the CALGB study showed an overall survival benefit with lenalidomide: 15% of the lenalidomide group had died compared with 23% in the placebo group ($P < .03$) and at 3 years, the overall survival was 88% in the lenalidomide group compared with 80% in the placebo group.

Risk of Secondary Malignancy

However, a significant concern with maintenance therapy is the risk of secondary malignancy. The risk of second primary cancers was roughly double in the maintenance group (7%–7.7%) compared with the placebo group (2.6%–3%). The secondary cancers observed included both hematological malignancies such as acute myelogenous leukemia as well as solid tumors. This increased risk of secondary malignancies has been seen in other settings, in patients with relapsed or refractory MM who were treated with lenalidomide. The incidence of secondary malignancy in this population was 3.98% compared with 1.38% in control patients in an analysis of clinical trials with lenalidomide (77). The overall risk-benefit of lenalidomide maintenance therapy vs. later use of lenalidomide at relapse awaits further elaboration.

Bortezomib

Bortezomib has also been studied as maintenance therapy. In the HOVON-65/GMMG-HD4 study, bortezomib was given every 2 weeks and was associated with increasing the near CR and CR rate from 31% to 49% (78).

Supportive care

Modern treatments for MM are generally well-tolerated. There are several key side effects. Peripheral neuropathy is one of the principal side effects of bortezomib and can be managed with prompt dose reduction (79,80) and administering it once/week instead of the traditional twice/week schedule (70,71). Changing the route of administration from intravenous to subcutaneous is another means for mitigating the risk of peripheral neuropathy. A study in patients with relapsed MM found that the grade 2 or worse peripheral neuropathy was 24% in the subcutaneous group compared with 41% in the intravenous group (72). Herpes zoster is seen with increased frequency in patients treated with bortezomib, and prophylaxis with acyclovir is generally given (81,82). Lenalidomide is associated with thromboembolic events, especially when given with high dose dexamethasone (56). Aspirin is recommended for prophylaxis in lenalidomide-containing regimens (83).

Bone disease

Bone involvement is one of the defining characteristics of MM, either as lytic lesions or diffuse osteopenia. Bisphosphonates such as pamidronate and zoledronic acid inhibit osteoclast activity and can palliate pain and prevent bone-related complications (84–86). Hypercalcemia is associated with increased bone resorption in MM, and bisphosphonates also play a key role in the treatment of hypercalcemia. Zoledronic acid, which is more potent than pamidronate, is superior to pamidronate for treating hypercalcemia (87).

In addition to playing an important supportive role, bisphosphonates may have a direct antitumor effect. The MRC Myeloma IX trial compared zoledronic acid with oral clodronic acid and found that zoledronic acid reduced mortality by 16% and increased median overall survival from 44.5 months to 50 months (88). The benefit of zoledronic acid on skeletal morbidity was also seen in patients without bone lesions at baseline (89).

A key concern with bisphosphonates, especially zoledronic acid, is the risk of osteonecrosis of the jaw (ONJ) (90). In the MRC Myeloma IX trial, the rate of ONJ was 4% (88). Attention to dental hygiene and minimizing invasive procedures may reduce the risk of ONJ (91).

Denosumab is a monoclonal antibody to RANK ligand that also inhibits osteoclasts and showed promising activity in MM in a phase II trial (92). Although denosumab was superior to zoledronic acid in patients with solid tumors and bone metastases, denosumab was inferior in a subset analysis of MM patients in a phase III trial (93). However, interpretation is limited based on the small numbers in the trial. A larger phase III study (NCT01345019) focusing on patients with MM is ongoing.

Vertebroplasty (injection of methyl methacrylate or bone cement) and kyphoplasty (use of an inflatable balloon followed by instillation of bone cement) are percutaneous procedures for treating compression fractures, and have been used in the setting of MM (94,95).

Palliative Radiation Therapy
Radiation also plays a key role for palliation of painful bony lesions in MM. An estimated 38% of patients are expected to receive radiation over the course of their illness (96). The primary indication for the use of radiation therapy is palliation of bone pain. However, other indications include impending fracture, cord compression, or relief of symptoms associated with a mass (i.e., cranial nerve palsies, cosmesis, or organ or joint dysfunction) (Figure 4). Doses of 20 to 35 Gy can be used, but it is essential to consider ability to retreat when designing treatment fields, particularly of the spine. In our experience, we have found that doses of 20 Gy delivered in either 5 or 10 fractions provide adequate symptom relief.

Areas of investigation

Timing of transplant
Conventional practice is to perform autologous stem cell transplant in patients who are eligible after four cycles of induction therapy. However, given the increasing effectiveness of induction treatment, a key question in MM treatment is the timing of transplant. Prior studies using older, historical chemotherapy regimens demonstrated no significant survival advantage with autologous transplant upfront (97,98). The IFM/DFCI 2009 trial (NCT01191060) is an ongoing phase III trial that will help clarify, in the era of novels drugs, the benefit and role of autologous stem cell transplant. This trial, started in 2010, randomizes patients after induction with RVD chemotherapy to autologous stem cell transplant versus additional cycles of RVD treatment. It is expected to complete data collection in 2018.

Tandem transplant refers to a planned second autologous stem cell transplant within 6 months of the first transplant. In two trials, IFM 94 and Bologna 96, a second autologous transplant was associated with improved outcomes compared with a single transplant, with the IFM 94 trial showing improvement in overall survival (99,100). However, on subset analysis, most of the benefit with a second transplant was seen in patients who did not achieve a CR or VGPR after the first autologous transplant.

Allogeneic Stem Cell Transplant
Allogeneic stem cell transplantation has also been considered, in light of the improved tolerability of non-myeloablative regimens compared with myeloablative regimens (which were associated with prohibitively high treatment-related mortality) as well as to take advantage of the graft v. MM effect of the allograft (101,102). However, with the advent of more effective anti-MM regimens, the magnitude of the benefit of reduced intensity myeloablative transplant is less pronounced, as was recently described in the HOVON-50 study (103).

Future Therapies
There continues to be burgeoning development in new anti-MM therapies with promising activity. These include next generation proteasome inhibitors such as carfilzomib, MLN 9708, and marizomib (104), as well as new immunomodulatory drugs such as pomalidomide (105). Carfilzomib was recently approved by the FDA in July 2012 for patients who have progressive disease after at least two prior therapies, including bortezomib and an immunomodulatory agent.

Novel targets

Newer targets for treatment include CS1, a cell surface glycoprotein that is highly expressed in MM cells. CS1 is neutralized by the monoclonal antibody elotuzumab (106). Another target is B-cell activating factor (BAFF), a growth factor for B cells, and serum levels of BAFF are increased in MM patients (107–109). BAFF inhibition is also being used in autoimmune disorders; belimumab is approved for treatment of systemic lupus erythematosus (110). Tabalumab (LY2127399) is a monoclonal antibody targeting BAFF under clinical development for MM (111). The aggresome, which similar to the proteasome, also degrades misfolded and unfolded proteins, is also another novel target for anti-MM therapy through inhibition of histone deacetylase 6 (HDAC6) (112,113). Other agents under development include cyclin dependent kinase (CDK) (114), aurora kinase (115), mTOR (116), and activin inhibitors (117), which have promising activity in vitro and in early phase clinical trials (118,119).

■ SOLITARY PLASMACYTOMA

Solitary plasmacytomas are plasma cell disorders where there is an isolated clonal tumor of plasma cells involving bone in the absence of systemic involvement (i.e., no anemia, hypercalcemia, renal insufficiency, or multiple bone lesions). When these tumors arise out of soft tissue instead of the bone marrow, they are classified as extramedullary or extraosseous plasmacytomas. Solitary plasmacytomas are uncommon and constitute about 5% of all patients with plasma cell dyscrasias (120). Extraosseous plasmacytomas most commonly are located in the upper respiratory tract, in the head and neck region. Extramedullary plasmacytomas are generally associated with improved survival compared with solitary bone plasmacytomas, suggesting a different biology or earlier detection (121).

Radiation Therapy

Radiation therapy with curative intent is the treatment of choice for both solitary plasmacytoma of bone (SPB) and extramedullary plasmacytoma (122). Median time to progression to MM in patients with SPB is 2–3 years, with a median overall survival of roughly 10 years (123). There is no standard of care with respect to treatment field and dose requirements for these rare entities because of the lack of prospective clinical trials. Several retrospective reports show excellent local control with doses of 40 to 50 Gy delivered over 4 to 5 weeks (124–126).

At our institution, we obtain either a PET/CT scan or an MRI to help delineate the full tumor extent. In most cases, we avoid treating the entire bone, particularly if the lesion is involving a long bone. The clinical target volume (CTV) for SPB includes the gross tumor with a generous margin (2 cm or more) (Figure 5A). For extramedullary plasmacytomas, regional nodal irradiation is no longer advised for all patients. The inclusion of regional nodes in the CTV is based on clinical expertise and is more apropos for extramedullary plasmacytomas that involve lymphoid tissue or sites that have a rich lymphatic drainage pattern (e.g., Waldeyer ring, base of tongue). Small extraosseous tumors can occasionally be treated with surgery alone.

There may be no significant change in the radiographic appearance of bony lesions, so radiographic surveillance for SPB looks for evidence of local progression or new lesions outside of the treatment field that would signal a progression to MM. For all patients, it is important to consider the amount of bone marrow involved in the treatment field (Figure 5B), because the majority of patients with SPB will eventually develop MM and likely require systemic therapy and/or stem cell transplantation (120,127).

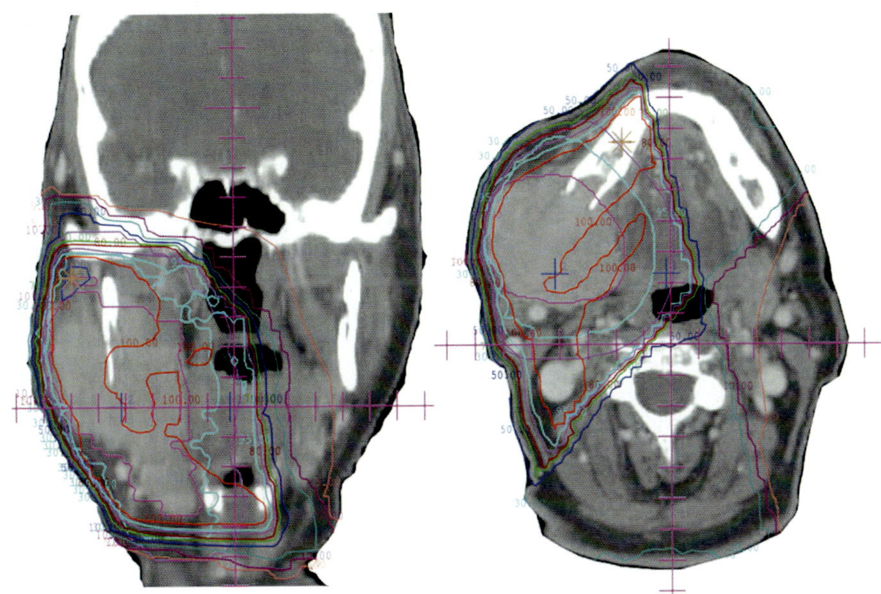

FIGURE 4 Palliative radiation therapy for symptomatic facial mass. Patient presented with facial swelling, facial numbness, and trismus. Coronal and axial images from radiation treatment plan showing large mass originating from maxilla and involving muscles of mastication. A wedged pair was used to treat the mass along with a 1cm clinical target volume (CTV) expansion plus an additional 5 mm for planning target volume (PTV). Symptoms improved after 20 Gy of radiation.

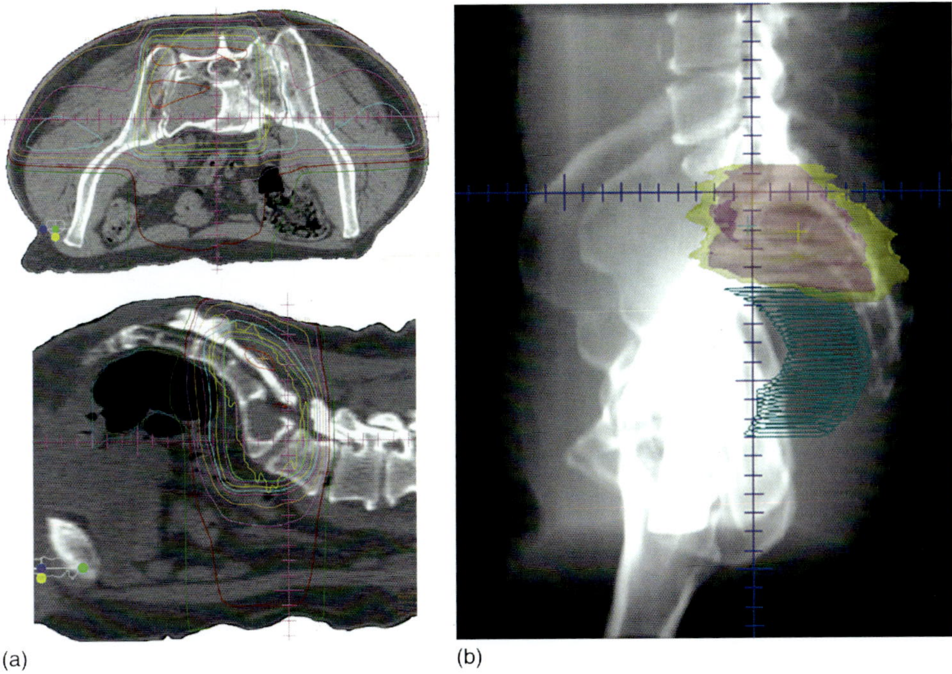

(a)   (b)

FIGURE 5 Definitive radiation therapy for solitary plasmacytoma of bone. (a) Axial and sagittal images from radiation treatment plan showing a large lytic lesion involving the left hemi-sacrum. A 3 field plan is designed to treat the lesion with a generous margin. Iliac wings are spared. (b) Digitally reconstructed radiograph showing pelvic bones in relation to tumor.

■ REFERENCES

1. Rajkumar SV, Kyle RA. Multiple myeloma: diagnosis and treatment. *Mayo Clin Proc.* 2005;80(10):1371–82.

2. Kyle RA, Durie BG, Rajkumar SV, et al. Monoclonal gammopathy of undetermined significance (MGUS) and smoldering (asymptomatic) multiple myeloma: IMWG consensus perspectives risk factors for progression and guidelines for monitoring and management. *Leukemia.* 2010;24(6):1121–7.

3. Kyle RA, Therneau TM, Rajkumar SV, et al. Prevalence of monoclonal gammopathy of undetermined significance. *N Engl J Med.* 2006;354(13):1362–9.

4. Bergsagel PL, Kuehl WM. Molecular pathogenesis and a consequent classification of multiple myeloma. *J Clin Oncol.* 2005;23(26):6333–8.

5. Kyle RA, Therneau TM, Rajkumar SV, et al. A long-term study of prognosis in monoclonal gammopathy of undetermined significance. *N Engl J Med.* 2002;346(8):564–9.

6. Landgren O, Kyle RA, Pfeiffer RM, et al. Monoclonal gammopathy of undetermined significance (MGUS) consistently precedes multiple myeloma: a prospective study. *Blood.* 2009;113(22):5412–7.

7. Weiss BM, Abadie J, Verma P, Howard RS, Kuehl WM. A monoclonal gammopathy precedes multiple myeloma in most patients. *Blood.* 2009;113(22):5418–22.

8. Rajkumar SV, Kyle RA, Therneau TM, et al. Serum free light chain ratio is an independent risk factor for progression in monoclonal gammopathy of undetermined significance. *Blood.* 2005;106(3):812–7.

9. Kyle RA, Remstein ED, Therneau TM, et al. Clinical course and prognosis of smoldering (asymptomatic) multiple myeloma. *N Engl J Med.* 2007;356(25):2582–90.

10. Siegel R, Naishadham D, Jemal A. Cancer statistics, 2012. *CA Cancer J Clin.* 2012;62(1):10–29.

11. Kyle RA, Gertz MA, Witzig TE, et al. Review of 1027 patients with newly diagnosed multiple myeloma. *Mayo Clin Proc.* 2003;78(1):21–33.

12. Waxman AJ, Mink PJ, Devesa SS, et al. Racial disparities in incidence and outcome in multiple myeloma: a population-based study. *Blood.* 2010;116(25):5501–6.

13. Kyle RA, Rajkumar SV. Epidemiology of the plasma-cell disorders. *Best Pract Res Clin Haematol.* 2007;20(4):637–64.

14. Lynch HT, Ferrara K, Barlogie B, et al. Familial myeloma. *N Engl J Med.* 2008;359(2):152–7.

15. Landgren O, Kristinsson SY, Goldin LR, et al. Risk of plasma cell and lymphoproliferative disorders among 14621 first-degree relatives of 4458 patients with monoclonal gammopathy of undetermined significance in Sweden. *Blood.* 2009;114(4):791–5.

16. Vachon CM, Kyle RA, Therneau TM, et al. Increased risk of monoclonal gammopathy in first-degree relatives of patients with multiple myeloma or monoclonal gammopathy of undetermined significance. *Blood.* 2009;114(4):785–90.

17. Shaughnessy JD, Jr., Barlogie B. Using genomics to identify high-risk myeloma after autologous stem cell transplantation. *Biol Blood Marrow Transplant.* 2006;12(Suppl 1):77–80.

18. Morgan GJ, Walker BA, Davies FE. The genetic architecture of multiple myeloma. *Nat Rev Cancer.* 2012;12(5):335–48.

19. Raje N, Roodman GD. Advances in the biology and treatment of bone disease in multiple myeloma. *Clin Cancer Res.* 2011;17(6):1278–86.

20. Hideshima T, Mitsiades C, Tonon G, Richardson PG, Anderson KC. Understanding multiple myeloma pathogenesis in the bone marrow to identify new therapeutic targets. *Nat Rev Cancer.* 2007;7(8):585–98.

21. Chapman MA, Lawrence MS, Keats JJ, et al. Initial genome sequencing and analysis of multiple myeloma. *Nature.* 2011;471(7339):467–72.

22. Dimopoulos MA, Kastritis E, Rosinol L, Blade J, Ludwig H. Pathogenesis and treatment of renal failure in multiple myeloma. *Leukemia.* 2008;22(8):1485–93.

23. Varettoni M, Corso A, Pica G, Mangiacavalli S, Pascutto C, Lazzarino M. Incidence, presenting features and outcome of extramedullary disease in multiple myeloma: a longitudinal study on 1003 consecutive patients. *Ann Oncol.* 2010;21(2):325–30.

24. Dispenzieri A, Kyle R, Merlini G, et al. International Myeloma Working Group guidelines for serum-free light chain analysis in multiple myeloma and related disorders. *Leukemia.* 2009;23(2):215–24.

25. Katzmann JA, Dispenzieri A, Kyle RA, et al. Elimination of the need for urine studies in the screening algorithm for monoclonal gammopathies by using serum immunofixation and free light chain assays. *Mayo Clin Proc.* 2006;81(12):1575–8.

26. Drayson M, Tang LX, Drew R, Mead GP, Carr-Smith H, Bradwell AR. Serum free light-chain measurements for identifying and monitoring patients with nonsecretory multiple myeloma. *Blood.* 2001;97(9):2900–2.

27. Anderson KC, Alsina M, Bensinger W, et al. Multiple myeloma. *J Natl Compr Canc Netw.* 2011;9(10):1146–83.

28. Kyle RA, Rajkumar SV. Criteria for diagnosis, staging, risk stratification and response assessment of multiple myeloma. *Leukemia.* 2009;23(1):3–9.

29. Greipp PR, San Miguel J, Durie BG, et al. International staging system for multiple myeloma. *J Clin Oncol.* 2005;23(15):3412–20.

30. Terpos E, Moulopoulos LA, Dimopoulos MA. Advances in imaging and the management of myeloma bone disease. *J Clin Oncol.* 2011;29(14):1907–15.

31. Dimopoulos M, Terpos E, Comenzo RL, et al. International myeloma working group consensus statement and guidelines regarding the current role of imaging techniques in the diagnosis and monitoring of multiple Myeloma. *Leukemia.* 2009;23(9):1545–56.

32. International Myeloma Working Group. Criteria for the classification of monoclonal gammopathies, multiple myeloma and related disorders: a report of the

International Myeloma Working Group. *Br J Haematol.* 2003;121(5):749–57.

33. Durie BGM, Salmon SE. A clinical staging system for multiple myeloma. Correlation of measured cell mass with presenting clinical features, response to treatment and survival. *Cancer.* 1975;36:842–54.

34. Fonseca R, Bergsagel PL, Drach J, et al. International Myeloma Working Group molecular classification of multiple myeloma: spotlight review. *Leukemia.* 2009;23(12):2210–21.

35. Kumar SK, Mikhael JR, Buadi FK, et al. Management of newly diagnosed symptomatic multiple myeloma: updated Mayo Stratification of Myeloma and Risk-Adapted Therapy (mSMART) consensus guidelines. *Mayo Clin Proc.* 2009;84(12):1095–110.

36. Rajkumar SV. Multiple myeloma: 2012 update on diagnosis, risk-stratification, and management. *Am J Hematol.* 2012;87(1):78–88.

37. Zhou Y, Barlogie B, Shaughnessy JD, Jr. The molecular characterization and clinical management of multiple myeloma in the post-genome era. *Leukemia.* 2009;23(11):1941–56.

38. Rajkumar SV. Treatment of multiple myeloma. *Nat Rev Clin Oncol.* 2011;8(8):479–91.

39. Attal M, Harousseau JL, Stoppa AM, et al. A prospective, randomized trial of autologous bone marrow transplantation and chemotherapy in multiple myeloma. Intergroupe Francais du Myelome. *N Engl J Med.* 1996;335(2):91–7.

40. Singhal S, Mehta J, Desikan R, et al. Antitumor activity of thalidomide in refractory multiple myeloma. *N Engl J Med.* 1999;341(21):1565–71.

41. Dimopoulos M, Spencer A, Attal M, et al. Lenalidomide plus dexamethasone for relapsed or refractory multiple myeloma. *N Engl J Med.* 2007;357(21):2123–32.

42. Richardson PG, Barlogie B, Berenson J, et al. A phase 2 study of bortezomib in relapsed, refractory myeloma. *N Engl J Med.* 2003;348(26):2609–17.

43. Brenner H, Gondos A, Pulte D. Recent major improvement in long-term survival of younger patients with multiple myeloma. *Blood.* 2008;111(5):2521–6.

44. Pulte D, Gondos A, Brenner H. Improvement in survival of older adults with multiple myeloma: results of an updated period analysis of SEER data. *Oncologist.* 2011;16(11):1600–3.

45. McArthur JR, Athens JW, Wintrobe MM, Cartwright GE. Melphalan and myeloma. Experience with a low-dose continuous regimen. *Ann Intern Med.* 1970;72(5):665–70.

46. Osgood EE. The survival time of patients with plasmocytic myeloma. *Cancer Chemother Rep.* 1960;9:1–10.

47. Rajkumar SV, Harousseau JL, Durie B, et al. Consensus recommendations for the uniform reporting of clinical trials: report of the International Myeloma Workshop Consensus Panel 1. *Blood.* 2011;117(18):4691–5.

48. Barlogie B, Hall R, Zander A, Dicke K, Alexanian R. High-dose melphalan with autologous bone marrow transplantation for multiple myeloma. *Blood.* 1986;67(5):1298–301.

49. McElwain TJ, Powles RL. High-dose intravenous melphalan for plasma-cell leukaemia and myeloma. *Lancet.* 1983;2(8354):822–4.

50. Lahuerta JJ, Mateos MV, Martinez-Lopez J, et al. Influence of pre- and post-transplantation responses on outcome of patients with multiple myeloma: sequential improvement of response and achievement of complete response are associated with longer survival. *J Clin Oncol.* 2008;26(35):5775–82.

51. Harousseau JL, Attal M, Avet-Loiseau H. The role of complete response in multiple myeloma. *Blood.* 2009;114(15):3139–46.

52. Chanan-Khan AA, Giralt S. Importance of achieving a complete response in multiple myeloma, and the impact of novel agents. *J Clin Oncol.* 2010;28(15):2612–24.

53. Haessler J, Shaughnessy JD, Jr., Zhan F, et al. Benefit of complete response in multiple myeloma limited to high-risk subgroup identified by gene expression profiling. *Clin Cancer Res.* 2007;13(23):7073–9.

54. Rajkumar SV. Multiple myeloma: the death of VAD as initial therapy. *Blood.* 2005;106(1):2–3.

55. Harousseau JL, Attal M, Avet-Loiseau H, et al. Bortezomib plus dexamethasone is superior to vincristine plus doxorubicin plus dexamethasone as induction treatment prior to autologous stem-cell transplantation in newly diagnosed multiple myeloma: results of the IFM phase III trial. *J Clin Oncol.* 2010;28(30):4621–9.

56. Rajkumar SV, Jacobus S, Callander NS, et al. Lenalidomide plus high-dose dexamethasone versus lenalidomide plus low-dose dexamethasone as initial therapy for newly diagnosed multiple myeloma: an open-label randomised controlled trial. *Lancet Oncol.* 2010;11(1):29–37.

57. Richardson PG, Weller E, Lonial S, et al. Lenalidomide, bortezomib, and dexamethasone combination therapy in patients with newly diagnosed multiple myeloma. *Blood.* 2010;116(5):679–86.

58. Reeder CB, Reece DE, Kukreti V, et al. Cyclophosphamide, bortezomib and dexamethasone induction for newly diagnosed multiple myeloma: high response rates in a phase II clinical trial. *Leukemia.* 2009;23(7):1337–41.

59. Kumar S, Flinn I, Richardson PG, et al. Randomized, multicenter, phase 2 study (EVOLUTION) of combinations of bortezomib, dexamethasone, cyclophosphamide, and lenalidomide in previously untreated multiple myeloma. *Blood.* 2012;119(19):4375–82.

60. Prince HM, Imrie K, Sutherland DR, et al. Peripheral blood progenitor cell collections in multiple myeloma: predictors and management of inadequate collections. *Br J Haematol.* 1996;93(1):142–5.

61. Kumar S, Dispenzieri A, Lacy MQ, et al. Impact of lenalidomide therapy on stem cell mobilization and engraftment post-peripheral blood stem cell transplantation in patients with newly diagnosed myeloma. *Leukemia.* 2007;21(9):2035–42.

62. Paripati H, Stewart AK, Cabou S, et al. Compromised stem cell mobilization following induction therapy with lenalidomide in myeloma. *Leukemia*. 2008;22(6):1282–4.

63. Child JA, Morgan GJ, Davies FE, et al. High-dose chemotherapy with hematopoietic stem-cell rescue for multiple myeloma. *N Engl J Med*. 2003;348:1875–83.

64. Barlogie B, Attal M, Crowley J, et al. Long-term follow-up of autotransplantation trials for multiple myeloma: update of protocols conducted by the intergroupe francophone du myelome, southwest oncology group, and university of arkansas for medical sciences. *J Clin Oncol*. 2010;28(7):1209–14.

65. Mark T, Stern J, Furst JR, et al. Stem cell mobilization with cyclophosphamide overcomes the suppressive effect of lenalidomide therapy on stem cell collection in multiple myeloma. *Biol Blood Marrow Transplant*. 2008;14(7):795–8.

66. Moreau P, Facon T, Attal M, et al. Comparison of 200 mg/m2 melphalan and 8 Gy total body irradiation plus 140 mg/m^2 melphalan as conditioning regimens for peripheral blood stem cell transplantation in patients with newly diagnosed multiple myeloma: final analysis of the Intergroupe Francophone du Myelome 9502 randomized trial. *Blood*. 2002;99(3):731–5.

67. Gay F, Larocca A, Wijermans P, et al. Complete response correlates with long-term progression-free and overall survival in elderly myeloma treated with novel agents: analysis of 1175 patients. *Blood*. 2011;117(11):3025–31.

68. San Miguel JF, Schlag R, Khuageva NK, et al. Bortezomib plus melphalan and prednisone for initial treatment of multiple myeloma. *N Engl J Med*. 2008;359(9):906–17.

69. Mateos MV, Richardson PG, Schlag R, et al. Bortezomib plus melphalan and prednisone compared with melphalan and prednisone in previously untreated multiple myeloma: updated follow-up and impact of subsequent therapy in the phase III VISTA trial. *J Clin Oncol*. 2010;28(13):2259–66.

70. Bringhen S, Larocca A, Rossi D, et al. Efficacy and safety of once-weekly bortezomib in multiple myeloma patients. *Blood*. 2010;116(23):4745–53.

71. Reeder CB, Reece DE, Kukreti V, et al. Once- versus twice-weekly bortezomib induction therapy with CyBorD in newly diagnosed multiple myeloma. *Blood*. 2010;115(16):3416–7.

72. Moreau P, Pylypenko H, Grosicki S, et al. Subcutaneous versus intravenous administration of bortezomib in patients with relapsed multiple myeloma: a randomised, phase 3, non-inferiority study. *Lancet Oncol*. 2010;12(5):431–40.

73. Ludwig H, Durie BG, McCarthy P, et al. IMWG consensus on maintenance therapy in multiple myeloma. *Blood*. 2012;119(13):3003–15.

74. Attal M, Lauwers-Cances V, Marit G, et al. Lenalidomide maintenance after stem-cell transplantation for multiple myeloma. *N Engl J Med*. 2012;366(19):1782–91.

75. McCarthy PL, Owzar K, Hofmeister CC, et al. Lenalidomide after stem-cell transplantation for multiple myeloma. *N Engl J Med*. 2012;366(19):1770–81.

76. Palumbo A, Hajek R, Delforge M, et al. Continuous lenalidomide treatment for newly diagnosed multiple myeloma. *N Engl J Med*. 2012;366(19):1759–69.

77. Dimopoulos MA, Richardson PG, Brandenburg N, et al. A review of second primary malignancy in patients with relapsed or refractory multiple myeloma treated with lenalidomide. *Blood*. 2012;119(12):2764–7.

78. Sonneveld P, Schmidt-Wolf IG, van der Holt B, et al. Bortezomib induction and maintenance treatment in patients with newly diagnosed multiple myeloma: results of the randomized phase III HOVON-65/ GMMG-HD4 trial. *J Clin Oncol*. 2012;30(24):2946–55

79. Richardson PG, Briemberg H, Jagannath S, et al. Frequency, characteristics, and reversibility of peripheral neuropathy during treatment of advanced multiple myeloma with bortezomib. *J Clin Oncol*. 2006;24(19):3113–20.

80. Richardson PG, Sonneveld P, Schuster MW, et al. Reversibility of symptomatic peripheral neuropathy with bortezomib in the phase III APEX trial in relapsed multiple myeloma: impact of a dose-modification guideline. *Br J Haematol*. 2009;144(6):895–903.

81. Chanan-Khan A, Sonneveld P, Schuster MW, et al. Analysis of herpes zoster events among bortezomib-treated patients in the phase III APEX study. *J Clin Oncol*. 2008;26(29):4784–90.

82. Vickrey E, Allen S, Mehta J, Singhal S. Acyclovir to prevent reactivation of varicella zoster virus (herpes zoster) in multiple myeloma patients receiving bortezomib therapy. *Cancer*. 2009;115(1):229–32.

83. Snowden JA, Ahmedzai SH, Ashcroft J, et al. Guidelines for supportive care in multiple myeloma 2011. *Br J Haematol*. 2011;154(1):76–103.

84. Berenson JR, Lichtenstein A, Porter L, et al. Efficacy of pamidronate in reducing skeletal events in patients with advanced multiple myeloma. Myeloma Aredia Study Group. *N Engl J Med*. 1996;334(8):488–93.

85. Rosen LS, Gordon D, Kaminski M, et al. Zoledronic acid versus pamidronate in the treatment of skeletal metastases in patients with breast cancer or osteolytic lesions of multiple myeloma: a phase III, double-blind, comparative trial. *Cancer J*. 2001;7(5):377–87.

86. Terpos E, Sezer O, Croucher PI, et al. The use of bisphosphonates in multiple myeloma: recommendations of an expert panel on behalf of the European Myeloma Network. *Ann Oncol*. 2009;20(8):1303–17.

87. Major P, Lortholary A, Hon J, et al. Zoledronic acid is superior to pamidronate in the treatment of hypercalcemia of malignancy: a pooled analysis of two randomized, controlled clinical trials. *J Clin Oncol*. 2001;19(2):558–67.

88. Morgan GJ, Davies FE, Gregory WM, et al. First-line treatment with zoledronic acid as compared with clodronic acid in multiple myeloma (MRC Myeloma IX): a randomised controlled trial. *Lancet*. 2010;376(9757):1989–99.

89. Morgan GJ, Child JA, Gregory WM, et al. Effects of zoledronic acid versus clodronic acid on skeletal morbidity in

patients with newly diagnosed multiple myeloma (MRC Myeloma IX): secondary outcomes from a randomised controlled trial. *Lancet Oncol.* 2011;12(8):743–52.

90. Woo SB, Hellstein JW, Kalmar JR. Systematic review: bisphosphonates and osteonecrosis of the jaws. *Ann Intern Med.* 2006;144(10):753–61.

91. Dimopoulos MA, Kastritis E, Bamia C, et al. Reduction of osteonecrosis of the jaw (ONJ) after implementation of preventive measures in patients with multiple myeloma treated with zoledronic acid. *Ann Oncol.* 2009;20(1):117–20.

92. Vij R, Horvath N, Spencer A, et al. An open-label, phase 2 trial of denosumab in the treatment of relapsed or plateau-phase multiple myeloma. *Am J Hematol.* 2009;84(10):650–6.

93. Henry DH, Costa L, Goldwasser F, et al. Randomized, double-blind study of denosumab versus zoledronic acid in the treatment of bone metastases in patients with advanced cancer (excluding breast and prostate cancer) or multiple myeloma. *J Clin Oncol.* 2011;29(9):1125–32.

94. Dudeney S, Lieberman IH, Reinhardt MK, Hussein M. Kyphoplasty in the treatment of osteolytic vertebral compression fractures as a result of multiple myeloma. *J Clin Oncol.* 2002;20(9):2382–7.

95. Fourney DR, Schomer DF, Nader R, et al. Percutaneous vertebroplasty and kyphoplasty for painful vertebral body fractures in cancer patients. *J Neurosurg.* 2003;98(Suppl 1):21–30.

96. Featherstone C, Delaney G, Jacob S, Barton M. Estimating the optimal utilization rates of radiotherapy for hematologic malignancies from a review of the evidence: part II-leukemia and myeloma. *Cancer.* 2005;103(2):393–401.

97. Fermand JP, Katsahian S, Divine M, et al. High-dose therapy and autologous blood stem-cell transplantation compared with conventional treatment in myeloma patients aged 55 to 65 years: long-term results of a randomized control trial from the Group Myelome-Autogreffe. *J Clin Oncol.* 2005;23(36):9227–33.

98. Barlogie B, Kyle RA, Anderson KC, et al. Standard chemotherapy compared with high-dose chemoradiotherapy for multiple myeloma: final results of phase III US Intergroup Trial S9321. *J Clin Oncol.* 2006;24(6):929–36.

99. Attal M, Harousseau JL, Facon T, et al. Single versus double autologous stem-cell transplantation for multiple myeloma. *N Engl J Med.* 2003;349(26):2495–502.

100. Cavo M, Tosi P, Zamagni E, et al. Prospective, randomized study of single compared with double autologous stem-cell transplantation for multiple myeloma: Bologna 96 clinical study. *J Clin Oncol.* 2007;25(17):2434–41.

101. Crawley C, Lalancette M, Szydlo R, et al. Outcomes for reduced-intensity allogeneic transplantation for multiple myeloma: an analysis of prognostic factors from the Chronic Leukaemia Working Party of the EBMT. *Blood.* 2005;105(11):4532–9.

102. Bruno B, Rotta M, Patriarca F, et al. A comparison of allografting with autografting for newly diagnosed myeloma. *N Engl J Med.* 2007;356(11):1110–20.

103. Lokhorst HM, van der Holt B, Cornelissen JJ, et al. Donor versus no-donor comparison of newly diagnosed myeloma patients included in the HOVON-50 multiple myeloma study. *Blood.* 2012;119(26):6219–25.

104. Moreau P, Richardson PG, Cavo M, et al. Proteasome inhibitors in multiple myeloma: ten years later. *Blood.* 2012.

105. Lacy MQ, Tefferi A. Pomalidomide therapy for multiple myeloma and myelofibrosis: an update. *Leuk Lymphoma.* 2011;52(4):560–6.

106. Lonial S, Vij R, Harousseau JL, et al. Elotuzumab in combination with lenalidomide and low-dose dexamethasone in relapsed or refractory multiple myeloma. *J Clin Oncol.* 2012;30(16):1953–9.

107. Moreaux J, Legouffe E, Jourdan E, et al. BAFF and APRIL protect myeloma cells from apoptosis induced by interleukin 6 deprivation and dexamethasone. *Blood.* 2004;103(8):3148–57.

108. Neri P, Kumar S, Fulciniti MT, et al. Neutralizing B-cell activating factor antibody improves survival and inhibits osteoclastogenesis in a severe combined immunodeficient human multiple myeloma model. *Clin Cancer Res.* 2007;13(19):5903–9.

109. Tai YT, Li XF, Breitkreutz I, et al. Role of B-cell-activating factor in adhesion and growth of human multiple myeloma cells in the bone marrow microenvironment. *Cancer Res.* 2006;66(13):6675–82.

110. Liu Z, Davidson A. BAFF and selection of autoreactive B cells. *Trends Immunol.* 2011;32(8):388–94.

111. Raje NS, Hohl RJ, Faber EA, et al. Phase I study of LY2127399, a human anti-BAFF antibody, and bortezomib in patients with previously treated multiple myeloma. *J Clin Oncol.* 2011;29:Abstract 8012.

112. Hideshima T, Bradner JE, Wong J, et al. Small-molecule inhibition of proteasome and aggresome function induces synergistic antitumor activity in multiple myeloma. *Proc Natl Acad Sci U S A.* 2005;102(24):8567–72.

113. Santo L, Hideshima T, Kung AL, et al. Preclinical activity, pharmacodynamic, and pharmacokinetic properties of a selective HDAC6 inhibitor, ACY-1215, in combination with bortezomib in multiple myeloma. *Blood.* 2012;119(11):2579–89.

114. Santo L, Vallet S, Hideshima T, et al. AT7519, A novel small molecule multi-cyclin-dependent kinase inhibitor, induces apoptosis in multiple myeloma via GSK-3beta activation and RNA polymerase II inhibition. *Oncogene.* 2010;29(16):2325–36.

115. Gorgun G, Calabrese E, Hideshima T, et al. A novel Aurora-A kinase inhibitor MLN8237 induces cytotoxicity and cell-cycle arrest in multiple myeloma. *Blood.* 2010;115(25):5202–13.

116. Cirstea D, Hideshima T, Rodig S, et al. Dual inhibition of akt/mammalian target of rapamycin pathway by

nanoparticle albumin-bound-rapamycin and perifosine induces antitumor activity in multiple myeloma. *Mol Cancer Ther.* 2010;9(4):963–75.

117. Vallet S, Mukherjee S, Vaghela N, et al. Activin A promotes multiple myeloma-induced osteolysis and is a promising target for myeloma bone disease. *Proc Natl Acad Sci U S A.* 2010;107(11):5124–9.

118. Cirstea D, Vallet S, Raje N. Future novel single agent and combination therapies. *Cancer J.* 2009;15(6):511–8.

119. Mahindra A, Laubach J, Raje N, Munshi N, Richardson PG, Anderson K. Latest advances and current challenges in the treatment of multiple myeloma. *Nat Rev Clin Oncol.* 2012;9(3):135–43.

120. Soutar R, Lucraft H, Jackson G, et al. Guidelines on the diagnosis and management of solitary plasmacytoma of bone and solitary extramedullary plasmacytoma. *Br J Haematol.* 2004;124(6):717–26.

121. Dores GM, Landgren O, McGlynn KA, Curtis RE, Linet MS, Devesa SS. Plasmacytoma of bone, extramedullary plasmacytoma, and multiple myeloma: incidence and survival in the United States, 1992–2004. *Br J Haematol.* 2009;144(1):86–94.

122. Dimopoulos MA, Goldstein J, Fuller L, Delasalle K, Alexanian R. Curability of solitary bone plasmacytoma. *J Clin Oncol.* 1992;10(4):587–90.

123. Dimopoulos MA, Moulopoulos LA, Maniatis A, Alexanian R. Solitary plasmacytoma of bone and asymptomatic multiple myeloma. *Blood.* 2000;96:2037–44.

124. Dagan R, Morris CG, Kirwan J, Mendenhall WM. Solitary plasmacytoma. *Am J Clin Oncol.* 2009;32(6):612–7.

125. Ozsahin M, Tsang RW, Poortmans P, et al. Outcomes and patterns of failure in solitary plasmacytoma: a multicenter Rare Cancer Network study of 258 patients. *Int J Radiat Oncol Biol Phys.* 2006;64(1):210–7.

126. Tsang RW, Gospodarowicz MK, Pintilie M, et al. Solitary plasmacytoma treated with radiotherapy: impact of tumor size on outcome. *Int J Radiat Oncol Biol Phys.* 2001;50(1):113–20.

127. Frassica DA, Frassica FJ, Schray MF, Sim FH, Kyle RA. Solitary plasmacytoma of bone: Mayo Clinic experience. *Int J Radiat Oncol Biol Phys.* 1989;16(1):43–8.

128. Landgren O, Waxman AJ. Multiple myeloma precursor disease. *JAMA.* 2010;304(21):2397–404.

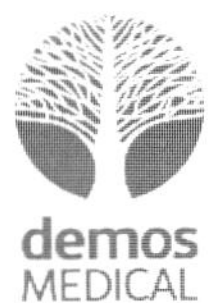

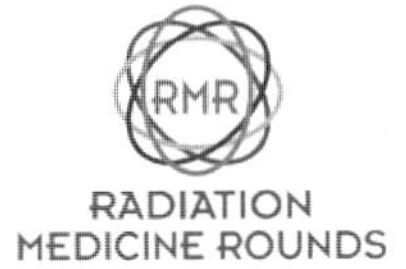

Role of FDG-PET Scans in Management of Lymphoma

Jeremy S. Abramson[*1] and Victorine V. Muse[2]

[1]*Center for Lymphoma, Massachusetts General Hospital Cancer Center, Boston, MA*

[2]*Department of Radiology, Massachusetts General Hospital, Boston, MA*

■ ABSTRACT

FDG-PET scanning has emerged as a vital tool in the initial staging, interim restaging, and end of treatment response assessment in lymphoma. Compared to CT scans alone, PET evaluation at diagnosis of diffuse large B-cell lymphoma (DLBCL) and Hodgkin lymphoma (HL) increases the sensitivity for disease detection, particularly in extranodal sites of disease, and will upstage patients in approximately 15% of cases. At interim restaging during chemotherapy, PET scans have proven an important prognostic tool in the setting of HL, where a negative interim PET scan predicts for a high cure rate compared to patients with persistent increased FDG activity. Interim PET scans in DLBCL, however, appear less reproducibly predictive of prognosis due to increased false positives when the scan is performed shortly after chemoimmunotherapy. At the end of treatment, PET scans enhance the ability to determine complete remission, especially in the setting of residual masses, which often represents benign sclerosis, and have thus been incorporated into standard response criteria for DLBCL and HL. Beyond achievement of complete remission, PET scans have no role currently in the long-term follow up of patients where CT scans alone appear sufficient. While having a critical role in staging and restaging of high-grade B-cell lymphomas and HL, there is presently no clearly defined role in the evaluation of low-grade histologies such as follicular lymphoma, small lymphocytic lymphoma, or marginal zone lymphoma. Active areas of investigation include using interim PET scans to guide intensification or deintensification of therapy, as well as incorporation of PET imaging into the design of radiation treatment fields.

Keywords: PET, FDG, Hodgkin lymphoma, diffuse large B-cell lymphoma, non-Hodgkin lymphoma, response, staging

■ INTRODUCTION

Advances in molecular biology and genetics have led to improved diagnostic and therapeutic strategies for lymphoma. The growing number of chemotherapy agents and targeted regimens for lymphoma therapy makes it increasingly important to not only accurately stage but to precisely monitor treatment response both during and after therapy. Combined Positron Emission Tomography with [18F] fluoro-2-deoxy-D-glucose (FDG-PET) coregistered with a computed tomography (CT) scan (PET/CT) has

---

*Corresponding author, Massachusetts General Hospital Cancer Center, 55 Fruit Street, Boston, MA

E-mail address: jabramson@partners.org

Radiation Medicine Rounds 3:3 (2012) 489–502.

DOI: 10.5003/2151–4208.3.3.489

emerged as the most accurate tool currently available in the evaluation of Hodgkin lymphoma and aggressive subtypes of non-Hodgkin lymphoma. This chapter will review the current role for PET/CT in the initial diagnosis and staging, interval re-staging, end-of-treatment restaging, and long-term follow up of lymphoid malignancies.

Perspective

Contrast-enhanced computed tomography has been the dominant tool for the last 30 years and still remains, to a large degree, the first line imaging technique because of its wide availability, low cost and easy reproducibility. Although CT provides accurate localization of organs and lesions, interpretation is limited because nodal involvement is based on size criteria, whereas delineation of extranodal disease and bone marrow is suboptimal.

The first molecular imaging agent for lymphoma assessment, gallium-67 citrate ($_{67}$GA), improved the accuracy of treatment response assessment in patients with lymphoma, where patients achieving a negative gallium scan demonstrated a significant improvement in progression-free survival compared with those with a persistently positive scan. There are a number of technical and clinical factors that have limited the use gallium, such as the lack of accessibility, low spatial resolution, low sensitivity (nodal disease: 44%–48%; extranodal disease: 42%–52%) and its limited use for imaging intra-abdominal disease because of its physiologic bowel uptake (1).

Gallium imaging has largely been replaced by FDG, which is a radiolabeled isomer of glucose and serves as a biomarker for glucose metabolism. FDG-PET is superior to $_{67}$GA in terms of sensitivity for the detection and specificity of lymphoma. The use of PET/CT can upstage patients because of the detection of additional sites of lymphomatous involvement such as the liver, spleen (Figure 1) and lung, which may result in a change of treatment strategy (2).

FDG-PET complements the standard anatomic imaging modalities of computed tomography and magnetic

resonance imaging. CT provides accurate anatomic detail whereas PET demonstrates both normal and abnormal tissue function. When combined, the two modalities have increased sensitivity and specificity in identifying and localizing functional abnormalities than either alone (2–4).

Technique

Integrated PET/CT scanners have been available since 2000 and have replaced the stand-alone machines, which are no longer manufactured; a positive byproduct of this is a dramatic decrease in time of combined acquisition. The PET/CT machine

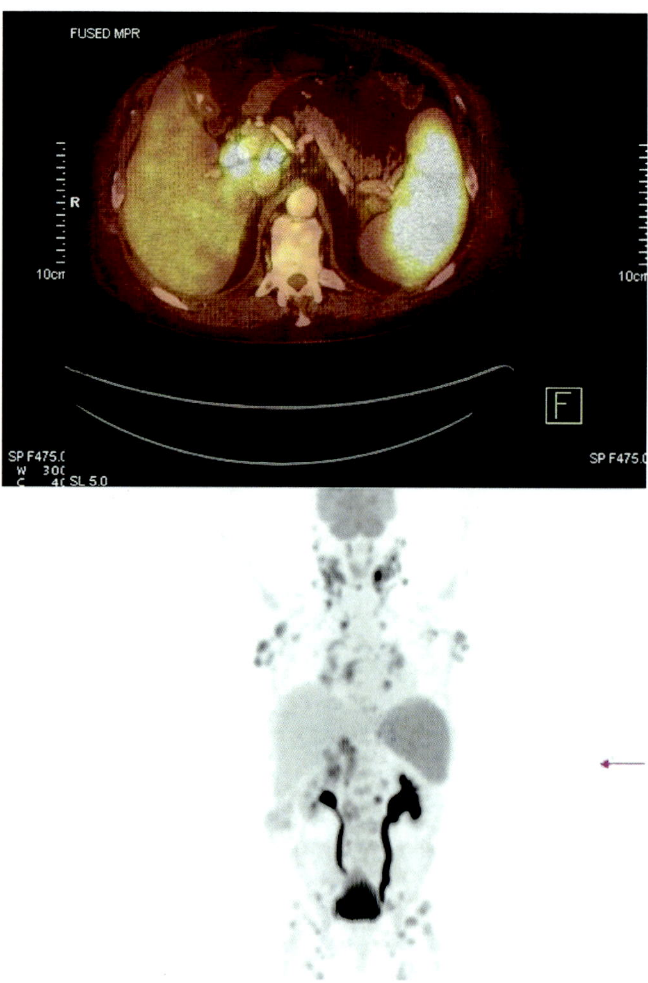

FIGURE 1 Axial fused PET/CT image demonstrates marked FDG uptake in a spleen normal by CT scan alone. Whole body PET image demonstrates nodal extent of disease in peripheral T-cell lymphoma.

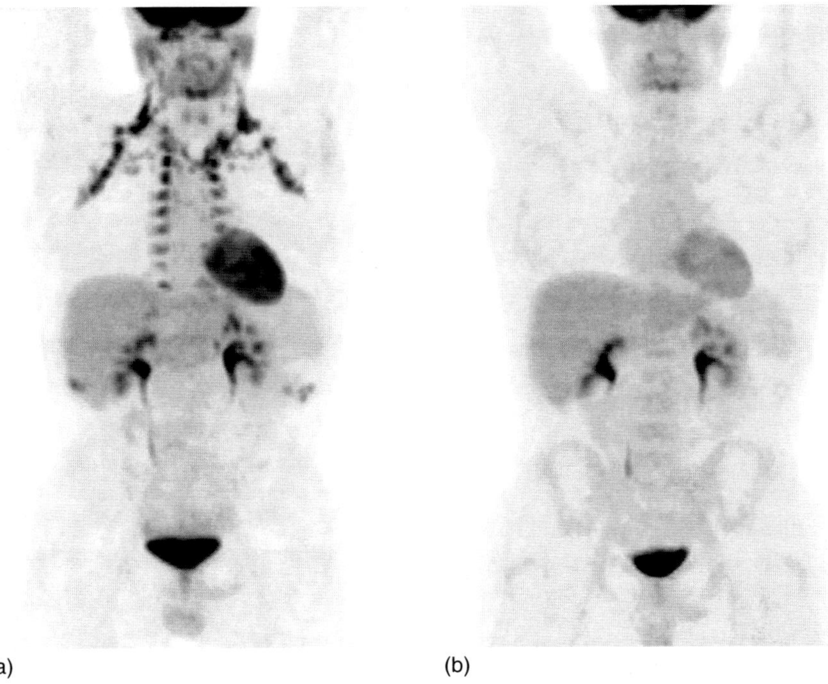

(a)   (b)

FIGURE 2   (a) Whole body PET image of a patient with treated HL demonstrating marked FDG uptake in the neck and paraspinal regions, which correlated to regions of fat density on CT (b) complete resolution after 6 months during warm weather.

combines a multidetector CT scanner with a high-resolution PET scanner, which allows the acquisition of three-dimensional images. Axial whole body images are routinely obtained from base of skull to upper thigh, the ideal parameters for a systemic disease such as lymphoma (5,6).

PET/CT protocols continue to evolve, but all have similar guidelines with the goal being the acquisition of accurately coregistered anatomic and functional images by minimizing FDG uptake in normal tissue (skeletal muscle, brown fat, kidneys, bladder, and myocardium) to maximize concentration in the target lesion(s). Preliminary steps include checking a fasting blood glucose level, which ideally is less than 140 mg/dl, keeping the patient warm to limit brown fat activity (Figure 2) and limiting physical activity. Low-density oral contrast is also usually given. After an IV dose of FDG is administered, the patient is instructed to limit physical activity and refrain from speaking. Imaging is typically performed 1 hour after injection to allow a steady state. A low-dose noncontrast CT is obtained first for attenuation correction and anatomic correlation.

PET images are obtained using overlapping bed positions, time varying with patient size and FDG activity. A diagnostic CT scan can be obtained with or without IV contrast last. The fused PET/CT images can be viewed in any plane for interpretation. CT attenuation value (Hounsfield units) and standard uptake values (SUV) are calculated at the workstation. PET images can be viewed fused with the attenuation-corrected CT scan (CT-AC) or the diagnostic CT scan. Both the CT-AC and the PET images are acquired during quiet breathing, whereas the diagnostic CT requires a single breath hold, so manual adjustments to the fused data may be needed (5,6).

There are conflicting studies on the value of IV contrast and obtaining a diagnostic quality CT scan during the combined exam (the CT-AC cannot be used for CT interpretation). Some author feel the increased sensitivity in the liver and spleen and the detection of extranodal sites reduce the number of indeterminate PET findings whereas others have shown little value of the full contrast-enhanced CT scan when combined with PET, thus allowing reduction in the total radiation dose of the study (7,8). With the recent advent of routine diagnostic CT low-dose protocols available, this should become less of an issue.

Interpretation

In addition to patient variables, technical parameters such as tube current, field of view, image reconstruction, data analysis and quality control can make it difficult to compare studies even at the same institution. The presence or absence of abnormal FDG accumulation in the PET images in combination with their size and intensity are evaluated. Visual assessment uses mediastinal blood pool uptake as the reference background activity to define abnormal FDG accumulation. Defined visual criteria have been addressed by the International Harmonization Criteria (IHP) and are delineated in a future section (9). Standardized uptake values (SUV) represent calculated estimates of tissue metabolic activity and can be used for semiquantitative analysis on PET/CT scans. Measurement and application of the SUV in interpretation may allow more accurate comparison of lesions between exams, however until PET/CT parameters and protocols become as uniform as those for CT alone, qualitative visual assessment remains the standard (9,10).

■ INITIAL STAGING

Incorporation of PET scans into the staging of aggressive lymphomas has improved accuracy compared with CT scans alone. In diffuse large B-cell lymphoma (DLBCL) and Hodgkin lymphoma (HL), PET may upstage patients because of detection of disease that was occult on CT scans, particularly disease involving extranodal sites such as bone, liver and spleen, mucosal disease, or disease involving otherwise normal sized lymph nodes (Figure 3) (11–13). Initial reports comparing PET and CT staging for lymphoma found sensitivity of 65%-84% with CT scans, compared with 82% to 99% with PET (14–18), and sensitivity and specificity of PET has continued to improve since that time because of improved technology with combined PET/CT scanners. Improved sensitivity of PET scans results in disease upstaging in approximately 15% of patients with DLBCL (Figure 4) and Hodgkin lymphoma, and downstaging in 5% or less of cases (11,19–22).

Perspective

Despite alteration of clinical stage on the bases of PET/CT scans, these staging differences usually do not result in changes in therapy. Given that the Ann Arbor staging system used to guide prognosis and treatment selection was not designed to include PET scans, it is difficult to know whether the stage identified by PET scan improves prognostication compared with stage determined purely by CT scans. It may, in fact, result in a stage migration whereby patients who are upstaged from limited to advanced stage because of disease that had been occult by CT will make the advanced stage cohort of patients seem to fare better by including patients with only a minimal amount of advanced disease, whereas limited stage patients will also seem to fare better based on removal of these relatively favorable low-burden advanced stage patients from the limited-stage population.

Imaging Considerations Based on Histology

Although PET/CT is now routinely included in the initial staging of high-grade lymphomas such as DLBCL, Burkitt lymphoma and HL, it is not recommended for routine staging in low-grade non-Hodgkin lymphomas outside of the context of a clinical trial. This includes follicular lymphoma, marginal zone lymphomas, small lymphocytic lymphoma, lymphoplasmacytic lymphoma, and others. In general, higher grade diseases have higher uptake based on SUV compared with lower grade histologies, but significant overlap limits this approach for grading, and certainly does not replace a histopathologic diagnosis on biopsy tissue (23). One reason is the lack of sensitivity by PET in certain subsets, such as extranodal marginal zone and small lymphocytic lymphomas which may be minimally FDG-avid or negative by PET scan, but this does not apply to others such as follicular lymphoma, which is nearly always FDG-avid (24–28). T-cell lymphomas, though generally high-grade diseases, demonstrate significant variability in FDG-avidity with the majority being intensely FDG-avid, but they should not be assumed to be FDG-avid for the purposes of staging (29). Given that indolent lymphoma histologies should not be staged with PET scans, complete radiographic staging is not recommended until a tissue diagnosis is obtained to best guide optimal use of imaging modalities.

There is generally no role for PET in the initial staging of indolent histologies because of the lack of effect of FDG-avidity on prognosis and management

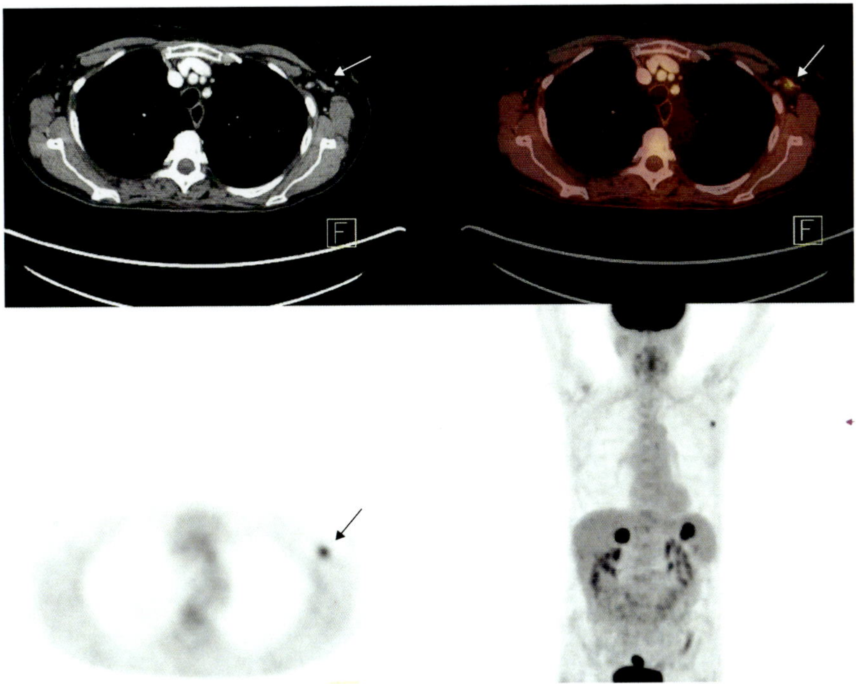

FIGURE 3 PET/CT images show a PET positive 7 mm left axillary lymph node, which would have been normal by CT criteria alone.

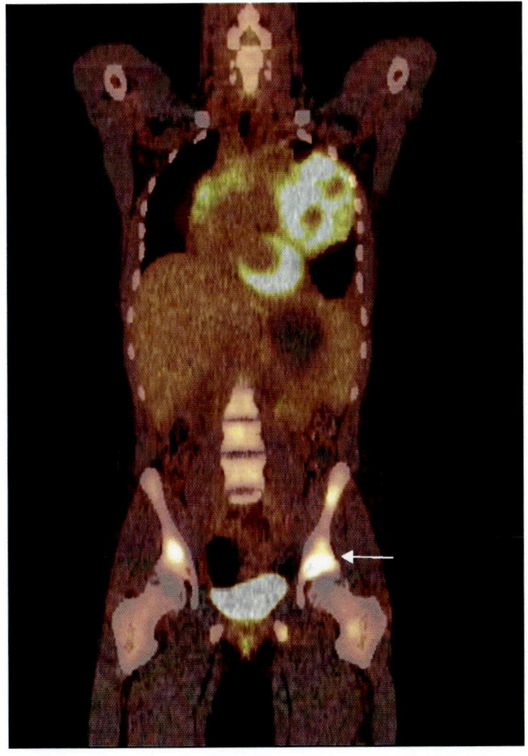

FIGURE 4 Coronal fused PET/CT in what was thought to be limited stage primary mediastinal B-cell lymphoma demonstrates bone lesions seen by FDG uptake alone, upstaging the patient to stage IV.

in these incurable diseases with lengthy natural histories. In DLBCL, Burkitt lymphoma, and HL, goal of treatment is cure, and failure to eradicate all sites of disease is associated with a significant risk of mortality. Optimal identification of all sites of disease to direct therapy and insure complete remission after treatment is therefore essential. In follicular lymphoma, on the other hand, nearly 90% of patients are identified at advanced stage and are considered incurable with standard therapies. The goal of treatment is to manage the disease as needed over time to prolong life and preserve quality of life, but early initiation of therapy in asymptomatic patients does not improve overall survival. Treatment, then, is only used if the disease is causing local or systemic symptoms, is bulky or rapidly progressive, or is impairing healthy bone marrow or organ function; PET scans do not add value to CT scans alone in informing these treatment decisions, so their use is not routinely recommended. There are, however, two select scenarios in follicular lymphoma where PET imaging may be considered. One is in the uncommon scenario where follicular lymphoma seems to be localized and thus involved field radiation therapy (IFRT) is being considered with curative intent. PET scanning in this scenario, in concert with bone marrow aspiration and biopsy, may help confirm the disease is indeed localized and optimally target the use of radiation, where doses for curative intent have historically been 30 to 36 Gy, but recent data suggest that 24 Gy offers similar efficacy (30). In the setting of advanced stage disease, palliative therapy to a discrete region can be treated to a significantly lower dose of 4 Gy (2 Gy × 2), with less associated toxicity (31). A second scenario where PET may be informative in an indolent lymphoma is where high-grade transformation is suspected. Heterogeneity may be seen within lymphomas, and so presence of discordant areas of uptake cannot be assumed to denote transformation, but it may be used to direct the biopsy to the area of highest FDG-avidity to increase the diagnostic yield in identifying transformed disease (32,33).

Bone Marrow Assessment

Routine initial staging of lymphoma patients often includes bone marrow aspiration and biopsy because of low sensitivity of CT scans for identifying marrow involvement. Incorporation of functional imaging raises the question of whether PET/CT can identify marrow disease and thus spare patients an invasive staging technique. Several studies have evaluated this question in DLBCL and HL and found improved sensitivity of PET/CT compared with bone marrow biopsy in the staging of Hodgkin lymphoma and, to a slightly lesser extent, aggressive NHL (34–36). Bone marrow involvement in Hodgkin lymphoma and aggressive NHL may be patchy, and so PET/CT may perform better in these scenarios over a blind bone marrow biopsy which may miss disease because of sampling (Figure 5). When diffuse uptake is noted on PET scan, however, caution must be used in interpretation, because false positives may occur because of inflammatory uptake or marrow rebound. In these scenarios, bone marrow biopsy is required for assessment. In HL and DLBCL, the negative predictive value of PET/CT for bone marrow involvement is quite high, approaching 100% in some series (10,34–40). On the basis of these data, one may consider omitting bone marrow sampling in high-grade histologies with a negative PET scan. In patients with positive uptake on PET imaging, however, bone marrow biopsy can provide complementary information, and is recommended. PET scans are not sensitive for the detection of indolent lymphomas in the bone marrow, where needle sampling is still required when bone marrow staging is indicated (38,41,42). General recommendations on role of PET scans in lymphoma assessment are listed in Table 1.

■ INTERIM RESTAGING

In HL, interim PET performed after 2 cycles of therapy has been shown to be powerfully predictive of outcome (Figure 6), particularly in advanced stage disease where interim PET negative patients were reported to have a progression-free survival (PFS) of 95%, compared with only 13% in interim PET positive patients (43). The prognostic value seems more muted in limited stage disease where interim PET was not as predictive, with both interim PET positive and negative patients demonstrating encouraging outcomes (44).

In DLBCL patients treated with R-CHOP (rituximab, cyclophosphamide, doxorubicin, vincristine and prednisone), a negative PET scan after 2 cycles predicts a PFS of 85% compared with 47% to 72% in patients with positive interim scans, so a positive interim PET scan in DLBCL may not be as powerfully predictive of outcome as was observed in advanced HL (45–47). Studies including patients treated before the introduction of rituximab demonstrated a higher predictive

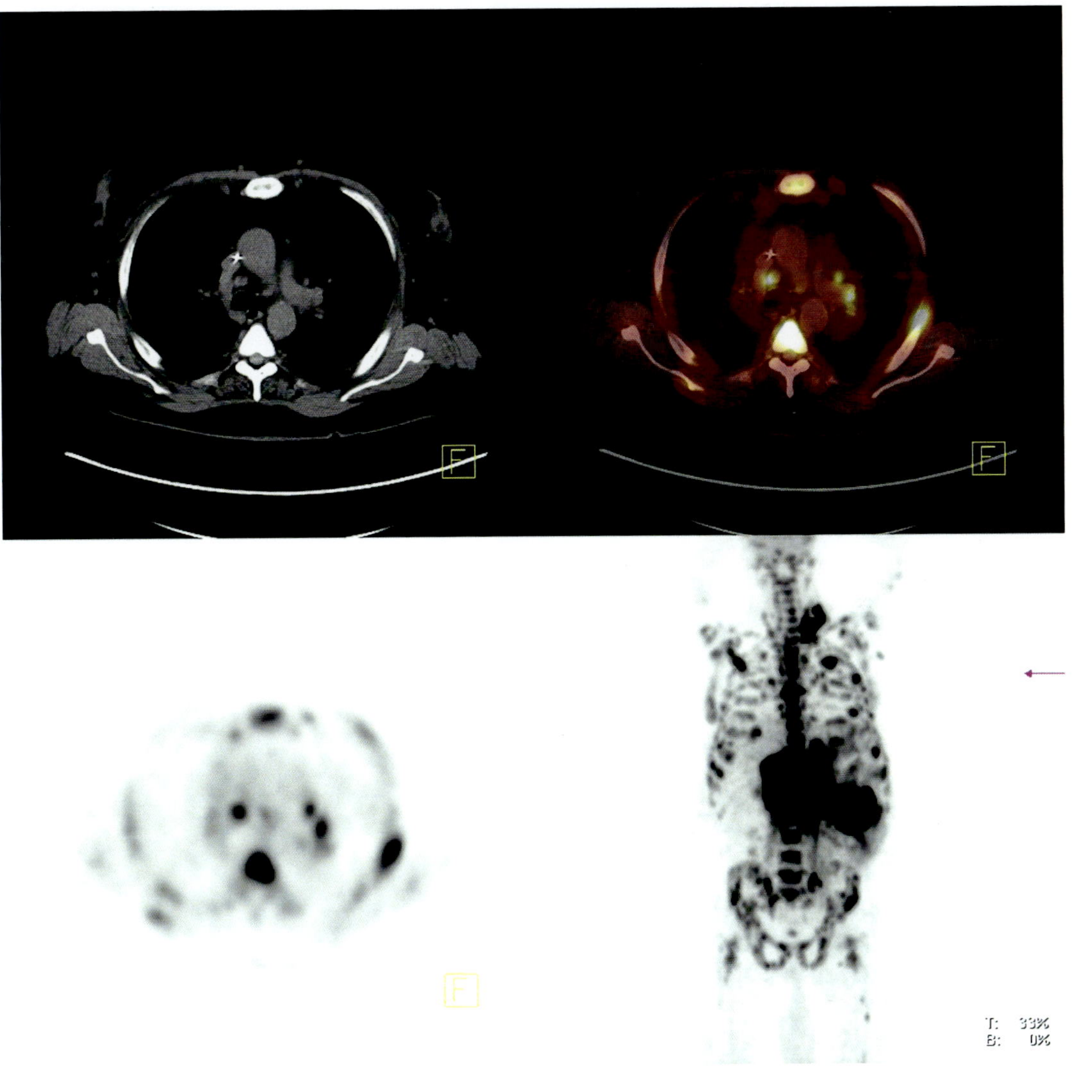

FIGURE 5 DLBCL PET/CT demonstrates patchy but diffuse marrow involvement, disease could be missed by sampling error.

TABLE 1 Recommendations for PET/CT in lymphoma care

	Hodgkin lymphoma	Aggressive non-Hodgkin lymphomas	Indolent non-Hodgkin lymphomas
Initial Staging	Recommended	Recommended	Not recommended, except when high-grade transformation is suspected or for confirmation of localized disease
Interim Restaging	Recommended, and may guide use of radiotherapy in limited stage disease	Controversial	Not recommended
End-of-Treatment Restaging	Recommended	Recommended	Not recommended
Routine Surveillance in Remission	Not recommended	Not recommended	Not recommended

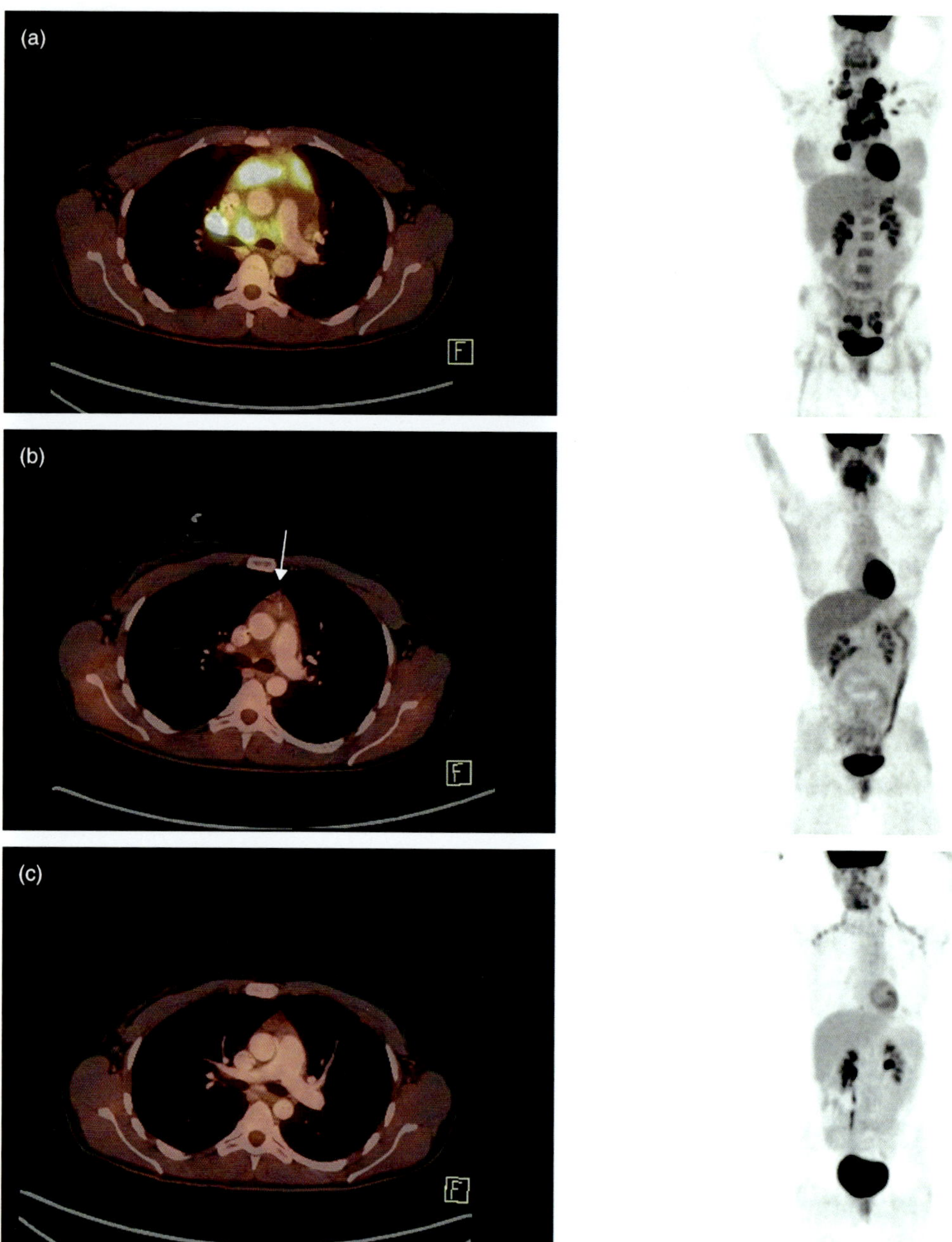

FIGURE 6 (a) Baseline PET/CT for HL demonstrates stage IV disease. (b) After three cycles of treatment interim PET/CT shows residual mass (arrow) but is PET negative. (c) At the end of treatment, PET/CT demonstrates PET-negative residual mass consistent with CR (notice FDG uptake in brown fat in supraclavicular regions).

power (48–50), suggesting that rituximab may decrease the accuracy of interim imaging in aggressive NHL, perhaps by increasing intratumoral inflammation through mechanisms of antibody-dependent cell-mediated toxicity and complement activation. One prospective study found that interim PET in DLBCL was not a reliable predictor of persistent disease. In fact, among 38 patients with a positive interim PET scan who underwent biopsy for confirmation, 33 proved negative, and had an identical PFS compared with those patients with negative interim PET scans (51).

Imaging Considerations

PET imaging has been extensively explored as an early biomarker of treatment response in lymphoma. Overall, the sensitivity and specificity for interim PET has ranged from 50% to 100% and 73% to 100% in DLBCL, and 65% to 100% and 94% to 100% in HL (52). Variability across studies derives, in part, from nonuniform timing of the interim scans, as well as lack of uniform criteria for response assessment during treatment. For example, low-level uptake may be interpreted as positive by some readers, though such low-level uptake, dubbed minimal residual uptake, has been shown to predict similar outcomes as a negative PET scan (53). The definition of what constitutes minimal residual uptake, has likewise not been uniform across studies. This led to a consensus conference in Deauville France with the goal of producing simple reproducible criteria for interpretation of interim PET scans in HL and DLBCL (54). The resulting criteria use a 5-point qualitative scale based on degree of uptake of target lesions compared with the mediastinal blood pool and liver (Table 2). These criteria, dubbed the "Deauville Criteria", have been subsequently validated with the definition of a positive PET scan being scores of 4 or 5, meaning uptake in target lesions greater than uptake in the healthy liver. A high negative predictive value of 92% was observed in advanced stage HL, and was independent of the clinical risk score (55). The 5-point criteria was less well validated in a prospective DLBCL study, however, where instead calculating the percent change in SUV and defining a negative scan as a greater than 66% reduction in maximal SUV performed better (56,57). This remains a source of ongoing investigation, and presently quantitative value of SUV uptake cannot be routinely recommended because of a number of factors affecting reproducibility and variability in this figure, including timing between injection and scanning, scanner calibration, reconstruction parameters, partial volume effect and blood glucose level, among others (55).

Perspective

A vital question is whether interim PET scans can be used to alter therapy in DLBCL and HL, with the goals of intensifying therapy and improving outcomes in interim PET-positive patients while potentially decreasing treatment intensity and associated toxicity in interim PET-negative patients. Such studies are currently underway, but no prospective study has yet demonstrated that altering therapy based on interim PET scan results in improves outcome, so treatment modification based on interim PET result alone cannot be recommended outside of a clinical trial. Ultimately, PET may be useful in guiding chemotherapy intensification and the use of consolidative radiation therapy (RT) in patients with limited stage disease, but this has not been prospectively validated. There are suggestive retrospective data that PET may be used to guide RT in limited stage disease. By province-wide policy in British Columbia, patients with limited stage HL receive 2 cycles of ABVD followed by interim PET scan. Patients who achieve a negative interim PET scan, which occurs in approximately 80% or patients, receive 2 additional cycles and no further therapy. Patients with an interim positive scan, however, go on to receive consolidative radiation. Retrospective analysis of this strategy shows a 4 year failure-free survival of 96%, with no difference between interim PET positive and negative patients (58). The ongoing RAPID trial is seeking to address this question prospectively by administering three cycles of ABVD in limited-stage HL, followed by PET-CT. Interim PET negative patients are randomized to observation versus consolidative radiation, and these data are eagerly anticipated.

In the treatment of nonbulky limited-stage HL and DLBCL, randomized trials have demonstrated no overall survival benefit favoring combined modality therapy over chemotherapy alone (59–62). Given that either combined modality therapy or chemotherapy alone are acceptable treatment approaches

TABLE 2 Deauville 5-point scale for interim PET interpretation

Score	Definition
1	No FDG uptake in tumor
2	FDG uptake in tumor less than the mediastinal blood pool
3	FDG uptake in tumor greater than the mediastinal blood pool but less than the liver
4	FDG uptake in tumor greater than the liver
5	Markedly increased uptake at any site or new sites of disease

in these patients, PET scans may be used to guide the application of RT only to the small proportion of patients who have positive interim PET scans and are likeliest to derive benefit, thereby avoiding the potential late toxicities in the majority of patients who will be cured with chemotherapy alone. The retrospective British Columbia data validate this approach presently, and prospective data are forthcoming for confirmation.

END-OF-TREATMENT RESTAGING

Multiple studies confirm that PET/CT clearly enhances the restaging accuracy of HL and aggressive NHL by confirming complete remission, particularly in the setting of residual masses (9,23,63–72). The negative predictive value ranges from 89% to 100% in HL, and approaches 100% in DLBCL. Recognition of the value offered by negative PET scans led to the revised response criteria for clinical trials in lymphoma where a patient with aggressive lymphoma is now considered in complete remission if the PET scan is negative, regardless of the size of a residual mass (73). Positive predictive values are lower in both HL and DLBCL, averaging between 50% and 90%, demonstrating the occurrence of false positive PET scans at end of therapy, reinforcing the need for biopsy confirmation of persistent disease before embarking on further treatments. As with interim scans, the heterogeneity in accuracy of PET scans across studies speaks to the need for uniform criteria for interpretation of end-of-treatment PET/CT scans. Such criteria were proposed in 2007 by the International Harmonization Project (IHP), and are now routinely used in clinical trials to guide end-of-treatment assessments (74).

Imaging Considerations

In an effort to reduce the number of false positives, several recommendations were made by the IHP including waiting 3 weeks after chemotherapy and 8 to 12 weeks after RT before obtaining the PET/CT. Residual masses >2 cm are positive for residual disease if their FDG avidity exceeds that of the mediastinal blood pool; <2 cm lesions are considered positive if they are greater than background (74).

PET scans are not recommended as end-of-treatment assessments in low-grade histologies such as follicular lymphoma, small lymphocytic lymphomas and marginal zone lymphomas, where PET/CT scans have not been demonstrated to offer value in guiding therapy compared with CT scans alone. There

is, however, early evidence that PET scans serve as an independent prognostic factor at the end of treatment in follicular lymphoma (75,76). Performance of PET scans in this indication and modification of therapy based on those results, however, have not yet been demonstrated to offer value, and so PET scans in these indications should presently be reserved for clinical trials.

PET restaging is routinely recommended in curable diseases that are FDG-avid, given that findings of minimal residual disease not evident by PET scan would significantly affect prognosis and management. Biopsy is encouraged to confirm persistent disease before altering or intensifying therapy because of the existence of false positives.

USE OF PET/CT IN RADIATION TREATMENT PLANNING

Radiation therapy plays a critical role in the modern management of lymphoma. Current applications include use as monotherapy for curative intent in localized indolent lymphomas, nodular lymphocyte-predominant Hodgkin lymphoma, and cutaneous lymphomas; as a component of combined modality therapy in limited-stage classical Hodgkin lymphoma and aggressive NHL; and as a palliative therapy for symptomatic sites of advanced stage or relapsed/refractory disease. Radiation treatment fields have evolved significantly over the years, reducing from extended-field techniques to involved-field techniques with preserved efficacy and decreased toxicity (77–79). More recently, further reduction to an involved nodal technique, with radiation administered only to clearly involved nodes as opposed to the entire nodal region, has demonstrated encouraging findings in retrospective analysis and is being explored in prospective studies (80) Given that PET imaging enhances the sensitivity and specificity in defining involved nodal sites of disease, use of PET scans in treatment planning may facilitate tailoring of treatment volumes to insure inclusion of all involved nodes and decrease exposure to uninvolved tissues. Retrospective studies have shown that incorporation of PET imaging does change treatment volumes in a large proportion of patients with some fields being reduced compared with CT planning alone, and other patients having fields increased to include FDG-avid nodes or regions that were of normal size on traditional CT (81–83). A prospective study also demonstrated a significant effect on the treatment volume in certain patients, though it caused no change compared with CT planning in 85% of cases. This technique represents an appealing addition to current treatment planning, particularly when using an involved-nodal approach, though clinical trials are needed to validate effects of PET-guided planning on local disease control and toxicity before recommending widespread application over existing techniques (84).

■ SURVEILLANCE IMAGING IN REMISSION

PET scans are not recommended for surveillance imaging once patients have achieved a complete remission. Incorporation of PET in this setting does not seem to add value to CT scans, and in fact leads to an unacceptably high rate of false positive scans with resultant unnecessary biopsies and treatment, as well as anxiety, increased cost and radiation exposure (85,86). Recurrences detected by routine imaging have not been associated with improved survival compared with those detected clinically, further decreasing enthusiasm in this approach (87–89). Accordingly, PET scans in aggressive lymphomas should not be used for surveillance after complete remission has been confirmed.

■ CONCLUSIONS

PET scans have increased the sensitivity in the initial staging of aggressive lymphomas, where it is now standard of care. Interim restaging offers prognostic information in HL, particularly in patients with advanced stage disease, but is less well validated in other histologies. Treatment intensification or de-intensification based on interim PET result has not yet been prospectively validated, and is currently under investigation in clinical trials. In nonbulky limited stage HL and DLBCL where either combined modality therapy or chemotherapy alone are considered acceptable treatment approaches, there are some data to support avoiding radiation therapy in patients with negative interim PET scans given the exquisite chemosensitivity this demonstrates, and the excellent prognosis of this group without consolidative radiation. At end-of-treatment, PET should be used in the final restaging to confirm complete remission in aggressive lymphomas, but positive scans should generally be confirmed with tissue biopsy before proceeding with salvage therapy. Inclusion of PET/CT into treatment planning for consolidative radiation has been shown to alter treatment volumes compared with traditional CT planning, and requires ongoing validation in prospective clinical trials. Once

complete remission has been demonstrated, PET does not have a role in routine radiographic surveillance where it increases cost and radiation exposure without apparent clinical benefit to the patient.

■ REFERENCES

1. Okada M, Sato N, Ishii K, Matsumura K, Hosono M, Murakami T. FDG PET/CT versus CT, MR imaging, and 67Ga scintigraphy in the posttherapy evaluation of malignant lymphoma. *Radiographics.*2010;30(4):939–957.

2. Tsukamoto N, Kojima M, Hasegawa M, et al. The usefulness of (18)F-fluorodeoxyglucose positron emission tomography ((18)F-FDG-PET) and a comparison of (18) F-FDG-pet with (67)gallium scintigraphy in the evaluation of lymphoma: relation to histologic subtypes based on the World Health Organization classification. *Cancer.* 2007;110(3):652–659.

3. Paes FM, Kalkanis DG, Sideras PA, Serafini AN. FDG PET/CT of extranodal involvement in non-Hodgkin lymphoma and Hodgkin disease. *Radiographics.* 2010;30(1):269–291.

4. Baba S, Abe K, Isoda T, Maruoka Y, Sasaki M, Honda H. Impact of FDG-PET/CT in the management of lymphoma. *Ann Nucl Med.* 2011;25(10):701–716.

5. Blodgett TM, Meltzer CC, Townsend DW. PET/CT: form and function. *Radiology.* 2007;242(2):360–385.

6. Boellaard R, O'Doherty MJ, Weber WA, et al. FDG PET and PET/CT: EANM procedure guidelines for tumour PET imaging: version 1.0. *Eur J Nucl Med Mol Imaging.* 2010;37(1):181–200.

7. Elstrom RL, Leonard JP, Coleman M, Brown RK. Combined PET and low-dose, noncontrast CT scanning obviates the need for additional diagnostic contrast-enhanced CT scans in patients undergoing staging or restaging for lymphoma. *Ann Oncol.* 2008;19(10):1770–1773.

8. Rodriguez-Vigil B, Gomez-Leon N, Pinilla I, et al. PET/CT in lymphoma: prospective study of enhanced full-dose PET/CT versus unenhanced low-dose PET/CT. *J Nucl Med.* 2006;47(10):1643–1648.

9. Spaepen K, Stroobants S, Dupont P, et al. Prognostic value of positron emission tomography (PET) with fluorine-18 fluorodeoxyglucose ([18F]FDG) after first-line chemotherapy in non-Hodgkin's lymphoma: is [18F] FDG-PET a valid alternative to conventional diagnostic methods? *J Clin Oncol.* 15 2001;19(2):414–419.

10. Richardson SE, Sudak J, Warbey V, Ramsay A, McNamara CJ. Routine bone marrow biopsy is not necessary in the staging of patients with classical Hodgkin lymphoma in the 18F-fluoro-2-deoxyglucose positron emission tomography era. *Leuk Lymphoma.* 2012;53(3):381–385.

11. Hutchings M, Loft A, Hansen M, et al. Position emission tomography with or without computed tomography in the primary staging of Hodgkin's lymphoma. *Haematologica.* 2006;91(4):482–489.

12. Schaefer NG, Hany TF, Taverna C, et al. Non-Hodgkin lymphoma and Hodgkin disease: coregistered FDG PET and CT at staging and restaging—do we need contrast-enhanced CT? *Radiology.* 2004;232(3):823–829.

13. Moog F, Bangerter M, Diederichs CG, et al. Extranodal malignant lymphoma: detection with FDG PET versus CT. *Radiology.* 1998;206(2):475–481.

14. Sasaki M, Kuwabara Y, Koga H, et al. Clinical impact of whole body FDG-PET on the staging and therapeutic decision making for malignant lymphoma. *Ann Nucl Med.* 2002;16(5):337–345.

15. Stumpe KD, Urbinelli M, Steinert HC, Glanzmann C, Buck A, von Schulthess GK. Whole-body positron emission tomography using fluorodeoxyglucose for staging of lymphoma: effectiveness and comparison with computed tomography. *Eur J Nucl Med.* 1998;25(7):721–728.

16. Weihrauch MR, Re D, Bischoff S, et al. Whole-body positron emission tomography using 18F-fluorodeoxyglucose for initial staging of patients with Hodgkin's disease. *Ann Hematol.* 2002;81(1):20–25.

17. Wirth A, Seymour JF, Hicks RJ, et al. Fluorine-18 fluoro-deoxyglucose positron emission tomography, gallium-67 scintigraphy, and conventional staging for Hodgkin's disease and non-Hodgkin's lymphoma. *Am J Med.* 2002;112(4):262–268.

18. Jerusalem G, Beguin Y, Fassotte MF, et al. Whole-body positron emission tomography using 18F-fluorodeoxyglucose compared to standard procedures for staging patients with Hodgkin's disease. *Haematologica.* 2001;86(3):266–273.

19. Buchmann I, Reinhardt M, Elsner K, et al. 2-(fluorine-18) fluoro-2-deoxy-D-glucose positron emission tomography in the detection and staging of malignant lymphoma. A bicenter trial. *Cancer.* 2001;91(5):889–899.

20. Munker R, Glass J, Griffeth LK, et al. Contribution of PET imaging to the initial staging and prognosis of patients with Hodgkin's disease. *Ann Oncol.* 2004;15(11):1699–1704.

21. Pelosi E, Pregno P, Penna D, et al. Role of whole-body [18F] fluorodeoxyglucose positron emission tomography/computed tomography (FDG-PET/CT) and conventional techniques in the staging of patients with Hodgkin and aggressive non Hodgkin lymphoma. *Radiol Med.* 2008;113(4):578–590.

22. Rigacci L, Vitolo U, Nassi L, et al. Positron emission tomography in the staging of patients with Hodgkin's lymphoma. A prospective multicentric study by the Intergruppo Italiano Linfomi. *Ann Hematol.* 2007;86(12):897–903.

23. Schoder H, Noy A, Gonen M, et al. Intensity of 18fluorodeoxyglucose uptake in positron emission tomography distinguishes between indolent and aggressive non-Hodgkin's lymphoma. *J Clin Oncol.* 2005;234643–4651.

24. Weiler-Sagie M, Bushelev O, Epelbaum R, et al. (18)F-FDG avidity in lymphoma readdressed: a study of 766 patients. *J Nucl Med.* 2010;51(1):25–30.

25. Beal KP, Yeung HW, Yahalom J. FDG-PET scanning for detection and staging of extranodal marginal zone lymphomas of the MALT type: a report of 42 cases. *Ann Oncol.* 2005;16(3):473–480.

26. Elstrom R, Guan L, Baker G, et al. Utility of FDG-PET scanning in lymphoma by WHO classification. *Blood.* 2003;101(10):3875–3876.

27. Jerusalem G, Beguin Y, Najjar F, et al. Positron emission tomography (PET) with 18F-fluorodeoxyglucose (18F-FDG) for the staging of low-grade non-Hodgkin's lymphoma (NHL). *Ann Oncol.* 2001;12(6):825–830.

28. Wohrer S, Jaeger U, Kletter K, et al. 18F-fluoro-deoxyglucose positron emission tomography (18F-FDG-PET) visualizes follicular lymphoma irrespective of grading. *Ann Oncol.* 2006;17(5):780–784.

29. Kako S, Izutsu K, Ota Y, et al. FDG-PET in T-cell and NK-cell neoplasms. *Ann Oncol.* 2007;18(10):1685–1690.

30. Lowry L, Smith P, Qian W, et al. Reduced dose radiotherapy for local control in non-Hodgkin lymphoma: a randomised phase III trial. *Radiother Oncol.* 2011;100(1):86–92.

31. Haas RL, Poortmans P, de Jong D, et al. High response rates and lasting remissions after low-dose involved field radiotherapy in indolent lymphomas. *J Clin Oncol.* 2003;21(13):2474–2480.

32. Bruzzi JF, Macapinlac H, Tsimberidou AM, et al. Detection of Richter's transformation of chronic lymphocytic leukemia by PET/CT. *J Nucl Med.* 2006;47(8):1267–1273.

33. Noy A, Schoder H, Gonen M, et al. The majority of transformed lymphomas have high standardized uptake values (SUVs) on positron emission tomography (PET) scanning similar to diffuse large B-cell lymphoma (DLBCL). *Ann Oncol.* 2009;20(3):508–512.

34. Muzahir S, Mian M, Munir I, et al. Clinical utility of 18F FDG-PET/CT in the detection of bone marrow disease in Hodgkin's lymphoma. *Brit J Radiol.* 2012;85(1016):e490–6.

35. Pelosi E, Penna D, Deandreis D, et al. FDG-PET in the detection of bone marrow disease in Hodgkin's disease and aggressive non-Hodgkin's lymphoma and its impact on clinical management. *Quart Nucl Med Mole Imag.* 2008;52(1):9–16.

36. Moulin-Romsee G, Hindie E, Cuenca X, et al. (18)F-FDG PET/CT bone/bone marrow findings in Hodgkin's lymphoma may circumvent the use of bone marrow trephine biopsy at diagnosis staging. *Eur J Nucl Med Mol Imaging.* 2010;37(6):1095–1105.

37. Purz S, Mauz-Korholz C, Korholz D, et al. [18F] Fluorodeoxyglucose positron emission tomography for detection of bone marrow involvement in children and adolescents with Hodgkin's lymphoma. *J Clin Oncol.* 2011;29(26):3523–3528.

38. Mittal BR, Manohar K, Malhotra P, et al. Can fluorodeoxyglucose positron emission tomography/computed tomography avoid negative iliac crest biopsies in evaluation of marrow involvement by lymphoma at time of initial staging? *Leuk Lymphoma.* 2011;52(11):2111–2116.

39. Ngeow JY, Quek RH, Ng DC, et al. High SUV uptake on FDG-PET/CT predicts for an aggressive B-cell lymphoma in a prospective study of primary FDG-PET/CT staging in lymphoma. *Ann Oncol.* 2009;20(9):1543–1547.

40. Hong J, Lee Y, Park Y, et al. Role of FDG-PET/CT in detecting lymphomatous bone marrow involvement in

patients with newly diagnosed diffuse large B-cell lymphoma. *Ann Hematol.* 2012;91(5):687–695.

41. Chen YK, Yeh CL, Tsui CC, Liang JA, Chen JH, Kao CH. F-18 FDG PET for evaluation of bone marrow involvement in non-Hodgkin lymphoma: a meta-analysis. *Clin Nucl Med.* 2011;36(7):553–559.

42. Pakos EE, Fotopoulos AD, Ioannidis JP. 18F-FDG PET for evaluation of bone marrow infiltration in staging of lymphoma: a meta-analysis. *J Nucl Med.* 2005;46(6):958–963.

43. Gallamini A, Hutchings M, Rigacci L, et al. Early interim 2-[18F]fluoro-2-deoxy-D-glucose positron emission tomography is prognostically superior to international prognostic score in advanced-stage Hodgkin's lymphoma: a report from a joint Italian-Danish study. *J Clin Oncol.* 2007;25(24):3746–3752.

44. Barnes JA, LaCasce AS, Zukotynski K, et al. End-of-treatment but not interim PET scan predicts outcome in nonbulky limited-stage Hodgkin's lymphoma. *Ann Oncol.* 2011;22(4):910–915.

45. Horning SJ, Juweid ME, Schoder H, et al. Interim positron emission tomography scans in diffuse large B-cell lymphoma: an independent expert nuclear medicine evaluation of the Eastern Cooperative Oncology Group E3404 study. *Blood.* 2010;115(4):775–777; quiz 918.

46. Pregno P, Chiappella A, Bello M, et al. Interim 18-FDG-PET/CT failed to predict the outcome in diffuse large B-cell lymphoma patients treated at the diagnosis with rituximab-CHOP. *Blood.* 2012;119(9):2066–2073.

47. Safar V, Dupuis J, Itti E, et al. Interim [18F]fluoro-deoxyglucose positron emission tomography scan in diffuse large B-cell lymphoma treated with anthracycline-based chemotherapy plus rituximab. *J Clin Oncol.* 2012;30(2):184–190.

48. Haioun C, Itti E, Rahmouni A, et al. [18F]fluoro-2-deoxy-D-glucose positron emission tomography (FDG-PET) in aggressive lymphoma: an early prognostic tool for predicting patient outcome. *Blood.* 2005;106(4):1376–1381.

49. Mikhaeel NG, Hutchings M, Fields PA, O'Doherty MJ, Timothy AR. FDG-PET after two to three cycles of chemotherapy predicts progression-free and overall survival in high-grade non-Hodgkin lymphoma. *Ann Oncol.* 2005;16(9):1514–1523.

50. Spaepen K, Stroobants S, Dupont P, et al. Early restaging positron emission tomography with (18) F-fluorodeoxyglucose predicts outcome in patients with aggressive non-Hodgkin's lymphoma. *Ann Oncol.* 2002;13(9):1356–1363.

51. Moskowitz CH, Schoder H, Teruya-Feldstein J, et al. Risk-adapted dose-dense immunochemotherapy determined by interim FDG-PET in Advanced-stage diffuse large B-Cell lymphoma. *J Clin Oncol.* 2010;28(11):1896–1903.

52. Terasawa T, Lau J, Bardet S, et al. Fluorine-18-fluorodeoxyglucose positron emission tomography for interim response assessment of advanced-stage Hodgkin's lymphoma and diffuse large B-cell lymphoma: a systematic review. *J Clin Oncol.* 2009; 27(11):1906–1914.

53. Hutchings M, Mikhaeel NG, Fields PA, Nunan T, Timothy AR. Prognostic value of interim FDG-PET after two or three cycles of chemotherapy in Hodgkin lymphoma. *Ann Oncol.* 2005;16(7):1160–1168.

54. Meignan M, Gallamini A, Meignan M, Gallamini A, Haioun C. Report on the first international workshop on interim-PET-scan in lymphoma. *Leuk Lymphoma.* 2009;50(8):1257–1260.

55. Meignan M, Gallamini A, Itti E, Barrington S, Haioun C, Polliack A. Report on the Third International Workshop on interim positron emission tomography in lymphoma held in Menton, France, 26–27 September 2011 and Menton 2011 consensus. *Leuk Lymphoma.* 2012;53(10):1876–81.

56. Lin C, Itti E, Haioun C, et al. Early 18F-FDG PET for prediction of prognosis in patients with diffuse large B-cell lymphoma: SUV-based assessment versus visual analysis. *J Nucl Med.* 2007;48(10):1626–1632.

57. Casasnovas RO, Meignan M, Berriolo-Riedinger A, et al. SUVmax reduction improves early prognosis value of interim positron emission tomography scans in diffuse large B-cell lymphoma. *Blood.* 2011;118(1):37–43.

58. Connors JM, Benard F, Gascoyne RD. FDG PET/CT scan guided treatment of limited stage Hodgkin lymphoma spares >80% of patients from radiotherapy while retaining excellent disease control. *Haematologica.* 2010;94(Supp 4):S15.

59. Horning SJ, Weller E, Kim K, et al. Chemotherapy with or without radiotherapy in limited-stage diffuse aggressive non-Hodgkin's lymphoma: Eastern Cooperative Oncology Group study 1484. *J Clin Oncol.* 2004;22(15):3032–3038.

60. Miller TE, LeBlanc M, Spier CM. CHOP alone compared to CHOP plus radiotherapy for early stage aggressive non-Hodgkin's lymphomas: Update of the Southwest Oncology Group (SWOG) randomized trial. *Blood.* 2001;98:Abstract 724a.

61. Straus DJ, Portlock CS, Qin J, et al. Results of a prospective randomized clinical trial of doxorubicin, bleomycin, vinblastine, and dacarbazine (ABVD) followed by radiation therapy (RT) versus ABVD alone for stages I, II, and IIIA nonbulky Hodgkin disease. *Blood.* 2004;104(12):3483–3489.

62. Meyer RM, Gospodarowicz MK, Connors JM, et al. ABVD alone versus radiation-based therapy in limited-stage Hodgkin's lymphoma. *N Engl J Med.* 2012;366(5):399–408.

63. Cerci JJ, Trindade E, Pracchia LF, et al. Cost effectiveness of positron emission tomography in patients with Hodgkin's lymphoma in unconfirmed complete remission or partial remission after first-line therapy. *J Clin Oncol.* 2010;28(8):1415–1421.

64. Kobe C, Dietlein M, Franklin J, et al. Positron emission tomography has a high negative predictive value for progression or early relapse for patients with residual disease after first-line chemotherapy in advanced-stage Hodgkin lymphoma. *Blood.* 2008;112(10):3989–3994.

65. Mikhaeel NG, Timothy AR, Hain SF, O'Doherty MJ. 18-FDG-PET for the assessment of residual masses on CT following treatment of lymphomas. *Ann Oncol.* 2000;11(Suppl 1):147–150.

66. Bangerter M, Kotzerke J, Griesshammer M, Elsner K, Reske SN, Bergmann L. Positron emission tomography with 18-fluorodeoxyglucose in the staging and follow-up of lymphoma in the chest. *Acta Oncol.* 1999;38(6):799–804.

67. Jerusalem G, Beguin Y, Fassotte MF, et al. Whole-body positron emission tomography using 18F-fluorodeoxyglucose for posttreatment evaluation in Hodgkin's disease and non-Hodgkin's lymphoma has higher diagnostic and prognostic value than classical computed tomography scan imaging. *Blood.* 1999;94(2):429–433.

68. Spaepen K, Stroobants S, Dupont P, et al. Can positron emission tomography with [(18)F]-fluorodeoxyglucose after first-line treatment distinguish Hodgkin's disease patients who need additional therapy from others in whom additional therapy would mean avoidable toxicity? *Br J Haematol.* 2001;115(2):272–278.

69. Mikhaeel NG, Timothy AR, O'Doherty MJ, Hain S, Maisey MN. 18-FDG-PET as a prognostic indicator in the treatment of aggressive Non-Hodgkin's Lymphoma-comparison with CT. *Leuk Lymphoma.* 2000;39(5–6):543–553.

70. Naumann R, Vaic A, Beuthien-Baumann B, et al. Prognostic value of positron emission tomography in the evaluation of post-treatment residual mass in patients with Hodgkin's disease and non-Hodgkin's lymphoma. *Br J Haematol.* 2001;115(4):793–800.

71. Hueltenschmidt B, Sautter-Bihl ML, Lang O, et al. Whole body positron emission tomography in the treatment of Hodgkin disease. *Cancer.* 2001;91(2):302–310.

72. Zijlstra JM, Lindauer-van der Werf G, Hoekstra OS, Hooft L, Riphagen, II, Huijgens PC. 18F-fluoro-deoxyglucose positron emission tomography for post-treatment evaluation of malignant lymphoma: a systematic review. *Haematologica.* 2006;91(4):522–529.

73. Cheson BD, Pfistner B, Juweid ME, et al. Revised response criteria for malignant lymphoma. *J Clin Oncol.* 2007;25(5):579–586.

74. Juweid ME, Stroobants S, Hoekstra OS, et al. Use of positron emission tomography for response assessment of lymphoma: consensus of the Imaging Subcommittee of International Harmonization Project in Lymphoma. *J Clin Oncol.* 2007;25(5):571–578.

75. Trotman J, Fournier M, Lamy T, et al. Positron emission tomography-computed tomography (PET-CT) after induction therapy is highly predictive of patient outcome in follicular lymphoma: analysis of PET-CT in a subset of PRIMA trial participants. *J Clin Oncol.* 2011;29(23):3194–3200.

76. Dupuis J, Meignan M, Julian A, et al. Significant prognostic impact of [18F]fluorodeoxyglucose-PET scan performed during and at the end of treatment with R-CHOP in high-tumor mass follicular lymphoma patients: A GELA-GOELAMS study. *Blood.* 2011;118:Abstract 877.

77. Bonadonna G, Bonfante V, Viviani S, Di Russo A, Villani F, Valagussa P. ABVD plus subtotal nodal versus involved-field radiotherapy in early-stage Hodgkin's disease: long-term results. *J Clin Oncol.* 2004;22(14):2835–2841.

78. Engert A, Schiller P, Josting A, et al. Involved-field radiotherapy is equally effective and less toxic compared with extended-field radiotherapy after four cycles of chemotherapy in patients with early-stage unfavorable Hodgkin's lymphoma: results of the HD8 trial of the German Hodgkin's Lymphoma Study Group. *J Clin Oncol.* 2003;21(19):3601–3608.

79. Ferme C, Eghbali H, Meerwaldt JH, et al. Chemotherapy plus involved-field radiation in early-stage Hodgkin's disease. *N Engl J Med.* 2007;357(19):1916–1927.

80. Campbell BA, Voss N, Pickles T, et al. Involved-nodal radiation therapy as a component of combination therapy for limited-stage Hodgkin's lymphoma: a question of field size. *J Clin Oncol.* 2008;26(32):5170–5174.

81. Girinsky T, Ghalibafian M, Bonniaud G, et al. Is FDG-PET scan in patients with early stage Hodgkin lymphoma of any value in the implementation of the involved-node radiotherapy concept and dose painting? *Radiother Oncol.* 2007;85(2):178–186.

82. Hutchings M, Loft A, Hansen M, Berthelsen AK, Specht L. Clinical impact of FDG-PET/CT in the planning of radiotherapy for early-stage Hodgkin lymphoma. *Eur J Haematol.* 2007;78(3):206–212.

83. Terezakis SA, Hunt MA, Kowalski A, et al. [(1)(8)F] FDG-positron emission tomography coregistration with computed tomography scans for radiation treatment planning of lymphoma and hematologic malignancies. *Int J Radiat Oncol Biol Phys.* 2011;81(3):615–622.

84. Pommier P, Dussart S, Girinsky T, et al. Impact of 18F-fluoro-2-deoxyglucose positron emission tomography on treatment strategy and radiotherapy planning for stage I-II Hodgkin disease: a prospective multicenter study. *Int J Radiat Oncol Biol Phys.* 2011;79(3):823–828.

85. Lee AI, Zuckerman DS, Van den Abbeele AD, et al. Surveillance imaging of Hodgkin lymphoma patients in first remission: a clinical and economic analysis. *Cancer.* 2010;116(16):3835–3842.

86. Mocikova H, Obrtlikova P, Vackova B, Trneny M. Positron emission tomography at the end of first-line therapy and during follow-up in patients with Hodgkin lymphoma: a retrospective study. *Ann Oncol.* 2010;21(6):1222–1227.

87. Goldschmidt N, Or O, Klein M, Savitsky B, Paltiel O. The role of routine imaging procedures in the detection of relapse of patients with Hodgkin lymphoma and aggressive non-Hodgkin lymphoma. *Ann Hematol.* 2011;90(2):165–171.

88. Petrausch U, Samaras P, Haile SR, et al. Risk-adapted FDG-PET/CT-based follow-up in patients with diffuse large B-cell lymphoma after first-line therapy. *Ann Oncol.* 2010;21(8):1694–1698.

89. Liedtke M, Hamlin PA, Moskowitz CH, Zelenetz AD. Surveillance imaging during remission identifies a group of patients with more favorable aggressive NHL at time of relapse: a retrospective analysis of a uniformly-treated patient population. *Ann Oncol.* 2006;17(6):909–913.

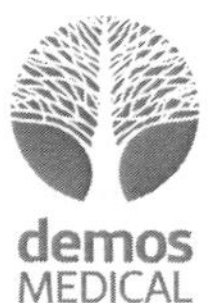

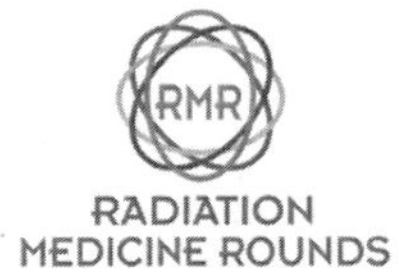

Radioimmunotherapy for Non-Hodgkin Lymphoma

Michael B. Tomblyn*

*Department of Radiation Oncology, H. Lee Moffitt Cancer Center and
Research Institute, Tampa, FL*

■ ABSTRACT

Radioimmunotherapy (RIT) is a safe and effective treatment for patients with B-cell, non-Hodgkin lymphoma. Two approved agents, ^{90}Y ibritumomab tiuxetan and ^{131}I tositumomab, target CD20 on the surface of mature B cells and B-cell malignancies. While these agents yield similar clinical outcomes, there are significant physical and chemical differences between the two radioisotopes that must be accounted for by the treating physician. Approved indications for RIT include relapsed/refractory indolent B-cell lymphomas, transformed B-cell lymphomas, and indolent lymphomas following induction therapy in the front-line setting. This paper also reviews the clinical evidence supporting the use of RIT for diffuse large B-cell lymphoma and mantle cell lymphoma, the integration of radiosensitizers with RIT, and novel RIT targets for non-Hodgkin lymphomas.

Keywords: radioimmunotherapy, B-cell lymphoma

■ INTRODUCTION

Fifteen years following the approval of the first monoclonal antibody, the use of these agents in cancer has fundamentally changed the landscape for the treatment of a number of malignancies, from B-cell non-Hodgkin lymphomas to melanoma. Rituximab, the first to gain Food and Drug Administration (FDA) approval in the United States, is a chimeric antibody directed against CD20, present on the surface of mature B cells and B cell malignancies.

The antibody exerts a direct cytotoxic effect on the target cell, primarily through induction of programmed cell death. Presence of the antibody on the surface of the cell also stimulates an antibody-dependent cell-mediated toxicity as well as complement-activated toxicity, typically leading to the recruitment of exogenous factors to elicit the lethal event. However, these processes require the direct physical association of one antibody to one cell, without significant collateral lethal effects on the surrounding unbound tumor cells. Because of this, rituximab must be given in repeat doses, either alone or with repeated cycles in conjunction with cytotoxic chemotherapy.

Most lymphomas are inherently radiosensitive, and early investigators realized the potential rationale for tagging monoclonal antibodies with radionuclides as a means of delivering potent radiotherapy directly to the surface of target tumor cells, a process referred to as radioimmunotherapy (RIT). As the labeled radionuclide moves through its predictable decay process, it releases highly energetic charged particles into the surrounding region. The radius of

---

*Corresponding author, Department of Radiation Oncology, H. Lee Moffitt Cancer Center and Research Institute, 12902 Magnolia Drive, Tampa, FL

E-mail address: michael.tomblyn@moffitt.org

Radiation Medicine Rounds 3:3 (2012) 503–512.

DOI: 10.5003/2151–4208.3.3.503

exposure is greater than the single tumor cell bound to the antibody, leading to a "cross-fire effect" where many tumor cells in the vicinity of the radionuclide have the potential to experience a lethal event (1). This negates the need for repeat dosing as with rituximab and makes RIT a particularly attractive strategy for tumor masses that are more bulky or with decreased perfusion.

Two RIT agents are currently approved by the FDA, both for the treatment of low-grade, B-cell non-Hodgkin lymphomas. The first to gain approval was ^{90}Y ibritumomab tiuxetan (Zevalin; Spectrum Pharmaceuticals, Henderson, NV). Ibritumomab is actually the parent, murine form of rituximab. The radiolabeled form carries approval for the treatment of relapsed or refractory low-grade lymphomas (2) as well as in the front-line setting following standard induction therapy (3). The other RIT agent is ^{131}I tositumomab (Bexxar; GlaxoSmithKline, Philadelphia, PA), also indicated in the relapsed/refractory setting as well as in the treatment of transformed B-cell lymphomas (4).

■ RADIONUCLIDES

While a number of different radionuclides are under investigation, ^{90}Y and ^{131}I are the two employed by the currently approved agents. These radionuclides have significantly different physical and chemical properties. [90]Y is a pure beta emitter, releasing a highly energetic electron. [131]I emits both beta and gamma radiation, which allows for patient-specific dosimetry but also comes with significant radiation exposure precautions following the infusion, including sleeping in separate beds from a partner, maintaining a six-foot distance from others for prolonged periods, and requires thyroprotection with oral iodine.

■ CHARACTERISTICS OF ^{90}Y IBRITUMOMAB TIUXETAN

[90]Y cannot be directly bound to ibritumomab but is instead held within a complex of carboxyl groups by tiuxetan, the link-chelator which is directly bound to the antibody. As ^{90}Y is a pure beta emitter, a different radioisotope must be used to perform biodosimetric studies with ibritumomab tiuxetan. [111]In, primarily a low-energy gamma emitter, is complexed to ibritumomab tiuxetan for this purpose. Patients requiring biodistribution studies initially present on Day 1 where they first receive a pre-dosing using rituximab

at 250 mg/m². They would then be infused with 5 mCi of ^{111}In ibritumomab tiuxetan. Two to three days later, the patient would return for a nuclear medicine SPECT scan to visualize the biodistribution, eligible patients having uptake in normal radiosensitive organs (lungs, kidneys, small bowel) less than hepatic uptake. Following a normal biodistribution scan, the patient returns on day 7, 8, or 9 for the therapeutic dose. Another predosing infusion of rituximab is given, followed by a ten-minute push of ^{90}Y ibritumomab tiuxetan. The specific activity for the therapeutic dose is determined solely by the patient's weight and platelet count. Those with platelets greater than 150,000/µL receive 0.4 mCi/kg body weight while those with platelets between 100,000/µL and 150,000/µL get 0.3 mCi/kg. The maximum dose infused is 32 mCi, regardless of patient weight. Because ^{90}Y is a pure beta emitter, there are no specific radiation precautions to be followed after the ^{90}Y ibritumomab tiuxetan infusion (5).

While the ^{111}In dosimetric step was required in the U.S. for nearly the first decade of approval, in nearly every other country that has approved ^{90}Y ibritumomab tiuxetan has done so without the requirement of the biodistribution scan. Very few patients exhibited true altered distribution, and a recent analysis of this drug in prospective trials revealed an altered biodistribution rate of approximately 1% on central review (6). Patients in this study with an altered biodistribution who went on to receive the therapeutic dose had clinical outcomes no different than those with a normal bioscan. Based on these data, the U.S. FDA removed the requirement of the dosimetric step in November 2011 but maintained the requirement for the Day 1 rituximab infusion.

■ CHARACTERISTICS OF ^{131}I TOSITUMOMAB

[131]I is directly and covalently linked to tositumomab, making a linker-chelator unnecessary. The isotope, emitting significant amounts of both beta and gamma radiation, can be used for both dosimetry and therapy. Unlike with ^{111}In ibritumomab tiuxetan, where the biodistribution serves only as a "go-no go decision point," [131]I tositumomab SPECT information is used to calculate clearance time. These counts from the bioscan are used to calculate the specific activity to be infused during the therapeutic step. On Day 1, patients begin with a pre-dosing infusion of unlabeled tositumomab, followed by 5 mCi ^{131}I tositumomab. The first scan is then performed to obtain

whole-body gamma counts. Patients then return for additional scans on day 2, 3, or 4 and then again on Day 6 or 7 to complete the biodosimetry process. The goal is to deliver a total body exposure of 75 cGy for patients with platelet counts of at least 150,000/µL, 65 cGy for platelets between 100,000/µL and 150,000/µL.

Because of the gamma component, ^{131}I tositumomab use requires the patient to adhere to a number of radiation precautions following the therapeutic dose (7). Patients need to sleep in separate beds for several days, maintain a distance of at least two meters during extended contact with others, and washing clothes and utensils separately. The duration of these precautions are individualized and determined by the clearance rate from the bioscans and a radiation survey performed by the radiation physicist after the infusion. Typical durations are from 7 to 10 days for most patients. Also of concern when using ^{131}I tositumomab is that radionuclide dissociation would lead to accumulation of ^{131}I within the thyroid gland. This exposure could lead to long-term complications such as hypothyroidism or malignancy. For this reason, patients are instructed to take potassium iodide or other oral iodine supplements from Day -1 for approximately 4 weeks to saturate the gland and allow dissociated ^{131}I to be excreted via the urinary system.

■ RADIOIMMUNOTHERAPY FOR RELAPSED AND REFRACTORY INDOLENT B-CELL NON-HODGKIN LYMPHOMAS

[90]Y Ibritumomab Tiuxetan

Wiseman et al. (8) reported the results of a multicenter phase II trial of 30 patients with relapsed/refractory low-grade or transformed low-grade B-cell lymphomas. All patients had platelet counts between 100,000/µL and 150,000/µL and received 0.3 mCi/kg ^{90}Y ibritumomab tiuxetan. They described overall response rate (OR) of 83%, with 37% of patients obtaining a complete response (CR). The median time to progression in this study was 9.4 months. A multicenter trial by Witzig et al. (9) treated 54 patients with rituximab-refractory disease with 0.4 mCi/kg ^{90}Y ibritumomab tiuxetan. One-half of patients obtained a CR, with an OR of 74%. The median time to progression was 6.8 months.

The pivotal study leading to approval of ^{90}Y ibritumomab tiuxetan was a randomized controlled trial (2) of the RIT agent versus rituximab in 143 patients with relapsed/refractory indolent B-cell lymphoma. The OR and CR for ^{90}Y ibritumomab tiuxetan were 80% and 30%, versus 56% and 16% for rituximab. The ability to obtain a CR was important, with a median time to progression of 24.7 months in the RIT arm versus 13.7 months for rituximab.

Evens et al. (10) reported the results of a phase I trial combining ^{90}Y ibritumomab tiuxetan with motexafin gadolinium, a known radiosensitizing agent, in 30 patients with mostly rituximab-refractory, relapsed B-cell lymphomas. Approximately two-thirds of the patients harbored follicular lymphoma, and the others had more aggressive subtypes. Standard ^{90}Y ibritumomab tiuxetan doses were given with escalating doses of motexafin gadolinium. No dose-limiting toxicities were seen. They described a 57% OR and 43% CR with a median time to progression of 10 months. The best results were seen in follicular lymphoma patients, with an OR of 86% and CR of 64% despite being rituximab-refractory. A multicenter phase II study of this novel therapeutic combination is currently open for enrollment.

While RIT is often utilized for patients who have progressed following multiple prior lines of therapy, it appears that treatment is most effective earlier in the disease process. Emmanouilides et al. (11) performed a retrospective analysis of patients with relapsed/refractory lymphoma treated with ^{90}Y ibritumomab tiuxetan. Patients treated in first relapse had a significantly higher CR rate compared to those treated in second or later relapse (51% versus 28%), along with a superior time to progression (15.4 versus 9.2 months).

[131]I Tositumomab

Kaminski et al. (12) treated 59 patients with refractory B-cell lymphomas. Patients with low-grade or transformed disease had a better OR than patients with *de novo* aggressive histologies (83% versus 44%). Approximately 50% of those with low-grade disease obtained a CR versus none of the patients with aggressive lymphomas. The ability to obtain a CR yielded a PFS of more than 20 months, versus one year for all patients.

Vose et al. (13) published a study limited to 47 patients with relapsed/refractory transformed lymphomas. Over half of the patients exhibited an objective response, with 32% in CR. In another study (4) of treatment-refractory indolent histologies, 60 patients were treated with ^{131}I tositumomab. OR and

CR rates were reported to be 65% and 20%, respectively. Another large study (14) of 273 patients with relapsed/refractory indolent lymphomas confirmed these earlier results, with a three-year PFS of 68%. Finally, Horning et al. (15) reported a study of 40 patients with rituximab-refractory disease, with an OR rate of 65% and median time to progression of 10.4 months.

■ FRONT-LINE RIT FOR INDOLENT LYMPHOMAS

While conventional wisdom had been to simply observe patients with follicular lymphoma and other indolent histologies following front-line chemotherapy, recent evidence suggests that a more aggressive consolidation approach results in superior progression-free survival, particularly for patients who can obtain a CR to therapy. A recent retrospective analysis (16) demonstrated that patients with follicular lymphoma who obtain a CR to therapy may enjoy a superior overall survival compared to patients obtaining only a PR. As only about 60% to 70% of all patients with advanced-stage indolent lymphomas are able to obtain a CR to induction chemoimmunotherapy, a novel consolidation approach could potentially improve clinical outcomes in this population.

Morschhauser et al. (3) reported the initial results of a randomized controlled trial (known as the FIT trial) of ^{90}Y ibritumomab tiuxetan versus observation in patients with advanced stage, low-grade follicular lymphoma following induction systemic therapy. The choice of front-line therapy was left to the discretion of the treating oncologist, although most received a CHOP or CHOP-like regimen. Upon the completion of induction therapy, subjects were restaged, and if they had obtained a CR or PR were eligible for randomization. Subjects randomized to receive ^{90}Y ibritumomab tiuxetan were treated with the standard 0.4 mCi/kg dose, up to a maximum of 32 mCi. After the completion of induction therapy, the CR rates were similar between the two arms, 53% for observation versus 52% for RIT consolidation. After randomization and the completion of consolidation, subjects from the RIT arm enjoyed a superior CR rate (87% versus 53%), representing a nearly 80% rate of conversion from PR to CR following RIT versus 0% conversion for those in the observation arm. The median time to progression was superior for those treated with ^{90}Y ibritumomab tiuxetan for all responders (49 versus 15 months), those who had a PR (30 versus 6 months), and those who had a CR

to therapy (92 + versus 32 months). The time to next treatment for subjects treated with ^{90}Y ibritumomab tiuxetan was more than five years longer than those undergoing observation. Given the indolent nature of follicular lymphoma and the several salvage therapies available, no differences in overall survival have been seen in relatively short follow-up. The primary critique of the FIT trial has been that only 14% of subjects were treated with rituximab-containing induction regimens. At the time the trial was written, rituximab had not been approved for use in the front-line setting.

An ongoing international randomized controlled trial (RoZetta) compares RIT consolidation with ^{90}Y ibritumomab tiuxetan to maintenance rituximab following a response to induction chemoimmunotherapy. Patients are initially treated with one of three rituximab-based regimens: R-CHOP, R-CVP, or R-bendamustine. Responders randomized to RIT are treated as per the FIT trial. Those randomized to maintenance rituximab are treated as per the PRIMA study. The primary endpoint is progression-free survival.

Several other prospective evaluations of ^{90}Y ibritumomab tiuxetan consolidation have been reported following rituximab-containing induction regimens in patients with advanced follicular lymphoma. One phase II trial (17) studied four weekly rituximab infusions, followed by three cycles of chemoimmunotherapy, prior to ^{90}Y ibritumomab tiuxetan consolidation. Complete responses rates rose from 30% following induction to 72% following RIT. After 5.5 years of follow-up, PFS was estimated to be 64%. A similar phase II trial (18) examining three cycles of induction rituximab-based therapy followed by ^{90}Y ibritumomab tiuxetan consolidation, then four infusions of maintenance rituximab improved CR rates from 46% after induction to 89% following RIT. Three additional studies (19–21) used fluadarabine-based, rituximab-containing regimens as induction therapy followed by ^{90}Y ibritumomab tiuxetan. Conversion rates from PR to CR ranged from 60% to 100% following the addition of RIT. The available evidence suggests a significant improvement in CR rates and PFS after ^{90}Y ibritumomab tiuxetan, even following induction regimens containing rituximab.

^{131}I tositumomab has also been evaluated in the setting of consolidation. SWOG recently presented the results of S0016 (22), a phase III trial comparing six cycles of R-CHOP to six cycles of CHOP plus ^{131}I tositumomab. After a median follow-up of five years, no differences in response rates or survival were seen. There were also no differences in toxicity, including secondary malignancies. While billed as a negative trial, the data seem to suggest that a single infusion of ^{131}I tositumomab is equivalent to six infusions of rituximab. The primary criticism of this trial is that both arms did not receive the same induction regimen. SWOG has recently completed the follow-up trial (S0801), examining R-CHOP induction followed by ^{131}I tositumomab consolidation and rituximab maintenance.

A number of other prospective trials (23–26) have been reported examining the role of RIT as consolidation following induction therapy, using a number of induction regimens. All seem to suggest a significant improvement in CR rates following consolidation, with promising PFS. A recent meta-analysis (27) reviewed a number of studies of RIT consolidation for patients with advanced follicular lymphoma, with two-year and five-year PFS rates of 77% and 56%, respectively.

■ RIT AS SOLE THERAPY FOR INDOLENT LYMPHOMAS

Kaminski et al. (28) performed a prospective study on 76 previously untreated patients with advanced follicular lymphoma, with ^{131}I tositumomab as sole therapy for their disease. Response rates for a single infusion of RIT were 95% OR and 75% CR. Now with over 10 years of follow-up, 40% of patients remain disease free at a decade, with a median duration of response of approximately six years. Patients obtaining a CR to RIT exhibited a median PFS of 11 years. After ten years, only a single case of myelodysplastic syndrome has been seen. Pica et al. (29) reported on 50 previously untreated patients with advanced follicular lymphoma given ^{90}Y ibritumomab tiuxetan as sole therapy. Response rates for a single infusion were 93% OR and 82% CR, with a two-year event-free survival rate of 85%.

■ REPEAT TREATMENTS WITH RIT

Illidge et al. (30) performed a study of fractionated RIT in 16 patients with relapsed follicular or transformed lymphoma. Subjects received weekly rituximab, followed by two infusions of ^{131}I rituximab to yield a cumulative total body exposure of 120 cGy. They reported a 50% CR, 94% OR, and a median time to progression of 20 months. In a phase II trial (31) of 72 follicular lymphoma patients scheduled to receive two tandem infusions of ^{90}Y ibritumomab tiuxetan, 83% of patients were able to recover blood counts quickly enough to qualify for the second infusion. The OR was 96%, with 57% CR for all patients, and 97% and 64% for those receiving both planned infusions of RIT. Despite repeat dosing, only 8 patients required any transfusional support.

Shah et al. (32) performed a retrospective analysis of patients who had received multiple infusions of ^{90}Y ibritumomab tiuxetan RIT. A total of 18 patients had been retreated, separated by a median of 16.6 months. There were no differences in response rates or toxicity following either the first or second RIT infusion. Kaminski et al. (33) have reported similar outcomes following repeat RIT with ^{131}I tositumomab.

While repeating RIT appears to be both safe and effective, the treating physician must keep in mind the possibility of the development of human anti-murine antibodies (HAMA). Patients under consideration should be tested for HAMA prior to retreatment to avoid potential serious complications. The rates of HAMA formation seem to be in the neighborhood of 5% in studies of tandem RIT (31).

■ RIT FOR MANTLE CELL LYMPHOMA

In a phase II study (34) of 34 patients with relapsed/refractory mantle cell lymphoma (MCL) treated with ^{90}Y ibritumomab tiuxetan, the OR was 31% with a 15% CR and median event-free survival of 28 months for those responding to RIT. Beaven et al. (35) performed a phase I study combining ^{90}Y ibritumomab tiuxetan with bortezomib as a radiosensitizer in patients with relapsed/refractory MCL or follicular lymphoma. No dose-limiting toxicity was observed. Response rates were reported as 50% OR and 42% CR. A phase II study of this combination in relapsed MCL recently opened for accrual.

There have been two studies examining the role of RIT in newly diagnosed MCL. Smith et al. (36) reported the results of a phase II trial in which 53 patients with a recent diagnosis of MCL were treated with four cycles of R-CHOP followed by ^{90}Y ibritumomab tiuxetan. Complete responses were seen in only 13% of patients after induction versus 55% following RIT consolidation. OR was 88% with ^{90}Y ibritumomab tiuxetan. The median PFS was 31 months. A second study (37) treated 25 newly diagnosed MCL patients, first with ^{131}I tositumomab, with 21 proceeding to CHOP consolidation. Two-year overall survival was 92%, with 67% CR and 86% OR.

RIT FOR DIFFUSE LARGE B-CELL LYMPHOMA

Morschhauser et al. (38) reported the results of a study using ^{90}Y ibritumomab tiuxetan in 104 patients with relapsed or refractory diffuse large B-cell lymphoma (DLBCL) who were not candidates for high-dose chemotherapy with autologous stem cell transplant. Overall response rates were approximately 50% for rituximab-naïve patients versus 29% for those refractory to rituximab. CR rates ranged from 12% for rituximab-refractory to 40% for rituximab-naïve disease.

There have been a number of prospective trials examining the potential role for RIT consolidation following R-CHOP induction in patients with newly diagnosed DLBCL. Hamlin et al. (39) performed a phase II study in 61 patients over the age of 60 with age-adjusted risk factors. All subjects received six cycles of R-CHOP, followed by consolidation with ^{90}Y ibritumomab tiuxetan. Complete responses were seen in 75% of patients following induction chemoimmunotherapy and in 90% after RIT. Myelosuppression was similar to that seen in previous studies with ^{90}Y ibritumomab tiuxetan. Estimated five-year overall and progression-free survival for those getting RIT were 84% and 75%, respectively.

Zinzani et al. (40) performed a similar phase II study for 20 high-risk patients with DLBCL. Subjects were treated with six cycles of CHOP followed by ^{90}Y ibritumomab tiuxetan. All patients responded to therapy, with complete responses seen in 75% of patients after CHOP and 95% following RIT consolidation. Two-year PFS was estimated to be 75%. The same investigator reported the results of another phase II trial (41) of newly diagnosed, elderly DLBCL patients who received four cycles of R-CHOP followed by ^{90}Y ibritumomab tiuxetan consolidation. The two-year PFS was 85%.

Due to these promising data, an international randomized controlled trial recently opened for elderly patients with a new diagnosis of DLBCL and one or more risk factors. All patients receive six cycles of R-CHOP induction therapy and are restaged. Those obtaining a CR by PET/CT are randomized to observation versus consolidation with a single infusion of ^{90}Y ibritumomab tiuxetan, with a primary endpoint of overall survival.

RIT FOR PRIMARY CENTRAL NERVOUS SYSTEM LYMPHOMA

Primary central nervous system lymphomas (PCNSL) were initially treated with whole brain radiotherapy (WBRT) alone, but long-term survival rates remained quite poor (42). With the addition of CNS-directed cytotoxic therapy, improvements in overall survival were seen; however, this came with increased toxicity, particularly neurocognitive effects (43). Changes in the fractionation pattern for high-dose WBRT failed to improve clinical outcomes. Recently, rituximab has been added to the systemic therapy of PCNSL, given the relatively leaky microvasculature of PCNSL suggesting a disruption of the blood-brain barrier. Iwamoto et al. (44) reported the outcomes from six patients with relapsed/refractory PCNSL who were treated with standard doses of ^{90}Y ibritumomab tiuxetan. Prior to therapy, patients underwent an ^{111}In ibritumomab tiuxetan dosimetric dose and scans to estimate dose delivered to foci of PCNSL and to normal brain. Median doses to lymphoma and normal brain were 701 cGy and 70 cGy, respectively. Objective responses were seen in half of the patients. RIT appears to be feasible for the treatment of PCNSL. The addition of low-dose WBRT below the neurotoxicity threshold and RIT following CNS-directed cytotoxic therapy may offer promising improvements in patient outcomes without the risk of significant neurocognitive defects.

RIT AND SECONDARY MALIGNANCY

One of the most cited concerns about RIT by skeptical medical oncologists is the potential for the therapy to lead to second cancers, particularly myelodysplastic syndrome (MDS). However, the available data suggest a very low potential for malignancy. From the FIT trial (3), the annualized MDS risk was a reported 0.55% per year. In the Kaminski et al. (28) trial of ^{131}I tositumomab as sole therapy for follicular lymphoma, only a single case of MDS has been seen with 10-year follow-up. In a retrospective review of nearly 750 patients treated with ^{90}Y ibritumomab tiuxetan, Czuczman et al. (45) found 19 MDS cases, occurring a median of two years after RIT, corresponding to an annualized rate of approximately 0.7%. Nearly all of those cases expressed abnormalities of chromosomes 5 and/or 7, historically linked to treatment with alkylating agents rather than to radiation. In fact, a SEER analysis (46) of chemotherapy alone for B-cell lymphomas showed the risk of developing MDS to be approximately 1%. Even with long-term follow-up, the use of RIT does not seem to increase the risk of MDS over that of using chemotherapy alone.

■ NEW TARGETS FOR RIT IN LYMPHOMA

While CD20 is the surface marker targeted by the two approved agents, it is not the only rational target specific for B-cell malignancies. CD22 is a B-cell surface marker that is rapidly internalized when bound. Epratuzumab is a humanized monoclonal antibody directed against CD22 and has shown activity against B-cell lymphomas. Labeled with ^{90}Y, the antibody is currently being evaluated in prospective clinical trials. Morschhauser et al. (47) conducted a phase I/II study of fractionated ^{90}Y epratuzumab tetraxetan in patients with relapsed B-cell lymphoma. They reported a CR rate of 56% and OR rate of 78%.

^{90}Y epratuzumab tetraxetan is currently being investigated in combination with unlabeled veltuzumab (an anti-CD20 monoclonal antibody) in patients with relapsed/refractory aggressive or transformed B-cell lymphoma. Subjects are treated with four weekly infusions of veltuzumab, and ^{90}Y epratuzumab tetraxetan is given during weeks three and four. Tomblyn et al. (48) recently presented an early interim analysis of the first ten subjects in this phase I/II trial and reported a 50% OR rate to this novel combination. Several other targets for both B-cell and T-cell lymphoma RIT have been described, including CD19, CD45, and CD74, and show evidence of efficacy in preclinical models (49–52).

■ CONCLUSIONS

Radioimmunotherapy for B-cell, non-Hodgkin lymphoma is a safe and effective therapy for a number of histologies. Its role has been demonstrated in the relapsed/refractory setting as well as front-line consolidation for indolent lymphomas. Accumulating evidence suggests a role for consolidation for DLBCL and MCL as well. Even used as sole therapy for newly diagnosed follicular lymphoma, patients have a good chance at durable disease-free survival. Several ongoing trials aim to determine the potential role for RIT in aggressive histologies or paired with radiosensitizing agents. Novel RIT agents are being developed for targets other than CD20 and may expand the indications for this treatment modality.

■ REFERENCES

1. Dixon KL. The radiation biology of radioimmunotherapy. *Nucl Med Commun.* 2003;24:951–957.

2. Witzig TE, Gordon LI, Cabanillas, et al. Randomized controlled trial of yttrium-90-labeled ibritumomab tiuxetan radioimmunotherapy versus rituximab immunotherapy for patients with relapsed or refractory low-grade, follicular, or transformed B-cell non-Hodgkin's lymphoma. *J Clin Oncol.* 2002;20:2453–2463.

3. Morschhauser F, Radford J, Van Hoof A, et al. Phase III trial of consolidation therapy with yttrium-90-ibritumomab tiuxetan compared with no additional therapy after first remission in advanced follicular lymphoma. *J Clin Oncol.* 2008;26:5156–5164.

4. Kaminski MS, Zelenetz AD, Press OW, et al. Pivotal study of iodine-131 tositumomab for chemotherapy-refractory low-grade or transformed low-grade B-cell non-Hodgkin's lymphomas. *J Clin Oncol.* 2001;19:3918–3928.

5. Wagner HN Jr., Wiseman GA, Marcus CS, et al. Administration guidelines for radioimmunotherapy of non-Hodgkin's lymphoma with (90)Y-labeled anti-CD20 monoclonal antibody. *J Nucl Med.* 2002;43:267–272.

6. Kylstra JW, Witzig TE, Huang M, et al. Discriminatory power of the indium-111 scan (111-In) in the prediction of altered biodistribution of radioimmunoconjugate in the 90-yttrium ibritumomab tiuxetan therapeutic regimen: Meta-analysis of five clinical trials and 9 years of post-approval safety data. *J Clin Oncol.* 2011;29:Abstract 8048.

7. Friedberg JW, Fisher RI. Iodine-^{131}tositumomab (Bexxar): radioimmunoconjugate therapy for indolent and transformed B-cell non-Hodgkin's lymphoma. *Expert Rev Anticancer Ther.* 2004;4:18–26.

8. Wiseman GA, Gordon LI, Multani PS, et al. Ibritumomab tiuxetan radioimmunotherapy for patients with relapsed or refractory non-Hodgkin lymphoma and mild thrombocytopenia: a phase II multicenter trial. *Blood.* 2002;99:4336–4342.

9. Witzig TE, Flinn IW, Gordon LI, et al. Treatment with ibritumomab tiuxetan radioimmunotherapy in patients with rituximab-refractory follicular non-Hodgkin's lymphoma. *J Clin Oncol.* 2002;20:3262–3269.

10. Evens AM, Spies WG, Helenowski IB, et al. The novel expanded porphyrin, motexafin gadolinium, combined with [90Y] ibritumomab tiuxetan for relapsed/refractory non-Hodgkin's lymphoma: preclinical findings and results of a phase I trial. *Clin Cancer Res.* 2009;15:6462–6471.

11. Emmanouilides C, Witzig TE, Gordon LI, et al. Treatment with yttrium 90 ibritumomab tiuxetan at early relapse is safe and effective in patients with previously treated B-cell non-Hodgkin's lymphoma. *Leuk Lymphoma.* 2006;47:629–636.

12. Kaminski MS, Estes J, Zasadny KR, et al. Radioimmunotherapy with iodine $^{(131)}$I tositumomab for relapsed or refractory B-cell non-Hodgkin lymphoma: updated results and long-term follow-up of the University of Michigan experience. *Blood.* 2000;96:1259–1266.

13. Vose JM, Wahl RL, Saleh M, et al. Multicenter phase II study of iodine-^{131} tositumomab for chemotherapy-relapsed/refractory low-grade and transformed low-grade

B-cell non-Hodgkin's lymphomas. *J Clin Oncol.* 2000; 18:1316–1323.

14. Gockerman J, Gregory S, Harwood S, et al. Interim efficacy result of Bexxar in a large multicenter expanded access study. *J Clin Oncol.* 2001;20:Abstract 1137.

15. Horning SJ, Younes A, Jain V, et al. Efficacy and safety of tositumomab and iodine-[131] tositumomab (Bexxar) in B-cell lymphoma, progressive after rituximab. *J Clin Oncol.* 2005;23:712–719.

16. Bachy E, Brice P, Delarue R, et al. Long-term follow-up of patients with newly diagnosed follicular lymphoma in the pre-rituximab era: effect of response quality on survival—A study from the groupe d'etude des lymphomes de l'adulte. *J Clin Oncol.* 2010;28:822–829.

17. Hainsworth JD, Spigel DR, Markus TM, et al. Rituximab plus short-duration chemotherapy followed by yttrium-90 ibritumomab tiuxetan as first-line treatment for patients with follicular non-Hodgkin lymphoma: a phase II trial of the Sarah Cannon Oncology Research Consortium. *Clin Lymphoma Myeloma.* 2009;9:223–228.

18. Jacobs SA, Swerdlow SH, Kant J, et al. Phase II trial of short-course CHOP-R followed by 90Y-ibritumomab tiuxetan and extended rituximab in previously untreated follicular lymphoma. *Clin Cancer Res.* 2008;14:7088–7094.

19. McLaughlin P, Neelapu S, Fanale M, et al. R-FND followed by radioimmunotherapy for high-risk follicular lymphoma. *Blood.* 2008;112(11):Abstract 3056.

20. Karmali R, Kassar M, Jimenez A, et al. Update on a prospective study evaluating the safety and efficacy of combination therapy with fludarabine, mitoxantrone and rituximab followed by yttrium-90 ibritumomab tiuxetan and maintenance rituximab as front line therapy for patients with indolent lymphomas. *Blood.* 2010;116(21):Abstract 3946.

21. Zinzani PL, Tani M, Pulsoni A, et al. A phase II trial of short course fludarabine, mitoxantrone, rituximab followed by 90Y-ibritumomab tiuxetan in untreated intermediate/high-risk follicular lymphoma. *Ann Oncol.* 2012;23(2):415–420.

22. Press OW, Unger JM, Rimsza LM, et al. A Phase III randomized intergroup trial (SWOG S0016) of CHOP chemotherapy plus rituximab versus CHOP chemotherapy plus iodine-131-tositumomab for the treatment of newly diagnosed follicular non-Hodgkin's lymphoma. *Blood.* 2011;118(Suppl. 1):Abstract 98.

23. Zinzani PL, Tani M, Fanti S, et al. A phase 2 trial of fludarabine and mitoxantrone chemotherapy followed by yttrium-90 ibritumomab tiuxetan for patients with previously untreated, indolent, nonfollicular, non-Hodgkin lymphoma. *Cancer.* 2008;112:856–862.

24. Leonard JP, Coleman M, Kostakoglu L, et al. Abbreviated chemotherapy with fludarabine followed by tositumomab and iodine I 131 tositumomab for untreated follicular lymphoma. *J Clin Oncol.* 2005;23:5696–5704.

25. Press OW, Unger JM, Braziel RM, et al. Phase II trial of CHOP chemotherapy followed by tositumomab/ iodine I-131 tositumomab for previously untreated follicular non-Hodgkin lymphoma: five-year follow-up of Southwest Oncology Group Protocol S9911. *J Clin Oncol.* 2006;24:4143–4149.

26. Fowler NH, Neelapu SS, Fanale MA, et al. Phase II study with R-FND followed by 90-Y ibritumomab tiuxetan radioimmunotherapy and rituximab maintenance for untreated high-risk follicular lymphoma. *Blood.* 2011;118(Suppl.1):Abstract 99.

27. Rose AC, Garrett G, Seward, M, et al. A systematic review and meta-analysis of radioimmunotherapy consolidation for untreated patients with follicular lymphoma (FL). *Blood.* 2011;118(Suppl.1):Abstract 101.

28. Kaminski MS, Tuck M, Estes J, et al. ^{131}I-tositumomab therapy as initial treatment for follicular lymphoma. *N Engl J Med.* 2005;352:441–449.

29. Pica G, Nati S, Vitolo U, et al. Safety and efficacy of 90Y ibritumomab tiuxetan (Zevalin) for untreated follicular non-Hodgkin's lymphoma (FL) patients, an Italian cooperative study. *Blood.* 2011;118(Suppl.1):Abstract 100.

30. Illidge TM, Bayne M, Brown MS, et al. Phase 1/2 study of fractionated (131)I-rituximab in low-grade B-cell lymphoma: the effect of prior rituximab dosing and tumor burden on subsequent radioimmunotherapy. *Blood.* 2009;113:1412–1421.

31. Illidge TM, Pettengell R, Bayne M, et al. Fractionated ^{90}Y ibritumomab tiuxetan (Zevalin) radioimmunotherapy as an initial therapy of follicular lymphoma— First results from a Phase II study in patients requiring treatment according to GELF/BNLI criteria. *Blood.* 2011;118(Suppl.1):Abstract 102.

32. Shah J, Wang W, Harrough VD, et al. Retreatment with yttrium-[90]ibritumomab tiuxetan in patients with B-cell non-Hodgkin's lymphoma. *Leuk Lymphoma.* 2007;48:1736–1744.

33. Kaminski MS, Radford JA, Gregory SA, et al. Re-treatment with I-[131] tositumomab in patients with non-Hodgkin's lymphoma who had previously responded to I-[131] tositumomab. *J Clin Oncol.* 2005;23:7985–7993.

34. Wang M, Oki Y, Pro B, et al. Phase II study of yttrium-90-ibritumomab tiuxetan in patients with relapsed or refractory mantle cell lymphoma. *J Clin Oncol.* 2009;27:5213–5218.

35. Beaven AW, Shea TC, Moore DT, et al. A phase I study evaluating ibritumomab tiuxetan (Zevalin) in combination with bortezomib (Velcade) in relapsed/refractory mantle cell and low-grade B-cell non-Hodgkin lymphoma. *Leuk Lymphoma.* 2012;53(2):254–8.

36. Smith M, Chen L, Gordon LI, et al. Phase II study of R-CHOP and ^{90}Y-ibritumomab tiuxetan in patients with previously untreated mantle cell lymphoma (E1499). *J Clin Oncol.* 2006;24:Abstract 7503.

37. Zelenetz AD, Noy A, Pandit-Taskar N, et al. Sequential radioimmunotherapy with tositumomab/iodine I[131] tositumomab followed by CHOP for mantle cell lymphoma demonstrates RIT can induce molecular remissions. *J Clin Oncol.* 2006;24:Abstract 7560.

38. Morschhauser F, Illidge T, Huglo D, et al. Efficacy and safety of yttrium-[90] ibritumomab tiuxetan in patients with relapsed or refractory diffuse large B-cell lymphoma not appropriate for autologous stem-cell transplantation. *Blood.* 2007;110:54–58.

39. Hamlin P, Moskowitz C, Wegner B, et al. Sequential RCHOP and yttrium-[90] ibritumomab tiuxetan (RIT) is a highly effective regimen for high risk elderly patients with untreated DLBCL. 10th International Conference on Malignant Lymphoma, Lugano, Switzerland, June 2008:Abstract 54.

40. Zinzani PL, Tani M, Fanti S, et al. A phase II trial of CHOP chemotherapy followed by yttrium [90] ibritumomab tiuxetan (Zevalin) for previously untreated elderly diffuse large B-cell lymphoma patients. *Ann Oncol.* 2008;19:769–773.

41. Zinzani PL, Rossi G, Franceschetti S, et al. Phase II trial of short-course R-CHOP followed by ^{90}Y-ibritumomab tiuxetan in previously untreated high-risk elderly diffuse large B-cell lymphoma patients. *Clin Cancer Res.* 2010;16:3998–4004.

42. Nelson DF, Martz KL, Bonner H, et al. Non-Hodgkin's lymphoma of the brain: can high dose, large volume radiation therapy improve survival? Report on a prospective trial by the Radiation Therapy Oncology Group (RTOG): RTOG 8315. *Int J Radiat Oncol Biol Phys.* 1992;23:9–17.

43. Glass J, Gruber ML, Cher L, et al. Pre-irradiation methotrexate chemotherapy of primary central nervous system lymphoma: long-term outcome. *J Neurosurg.* 1994;81:188–195.

44. Iwamoto FM, Scwartz J, Pandit-Taskar N, et al. Study of radiolabeled indium-111 and yttrium-[90] ibritumomab tiuxetan in primary central nervous system lymphoma. *Cancer.* 2007;110:2528–2534.

45. Czuczuman MS, Emmanouilides C, Darif M, et al. Treatment-related myelodysplastic syndrome and acute myelogenous leukemia in patients treated with ibritumomab tiuxetan radioimmunotherapy. *J Clin Oncol.* 2007;25:4285–4292.

46. Morton LM, Curtis RE, Linet MS, et al. Second malignancy risks after non-Hodgkin's lymphoma and chronic lymphocytic leukemia: differences by lymphoma subtype. *J Clin Oncol.* 2010;28:4935–4944.

47. Morschhauser F, Kraeber-Bodere F, Wegener W, et al. High rates of durable responses with anti-CD22 fractionated radioimmunotherapy: results of a multicenter, phase I/II study in non-Hodgkin's lymphoma. *J Clin Oncol.* 2010;28:3709–3716.

48. Tomblyn M, Elstrom R, Himelstein AL, et al. Novel combination of anti-CD22 radioimmunotherapy and anti-CD20 immunotherapy targeting two different antigens in non-Hodgkin lymphoma (NHL): Initial clinical experience. *J Nucl Med.* 2012;53:Abstract 500.

49. Michel RB, Rosario AV, Brechbiel MW, et al. Experimental therapy of disseminated B-cell lymphoma xenografts with 213Bi-labeled anti-CD74. *Nucl Med Biol.* 2003;30:715–723.

50. Gopal AK, Pagel JM, Fromm JR, et al. 131I anti-CD45 radioimmunotherapy effectively targets and treats T-cell non-Hodgkin lymphoma. *Blood.* 2009;113:5905–5910.

51. Vallera DA, Elson M, Brechbiel MW, et al. Radiotherapy of CD19 expressing Daudi tumors in nude mice with yttrium-90-labeled anti-CD19 antibody. *Cancer Biother Radiopharm.* 2004;19:11–23.

52. Ma D, McDevitt MR, Barendswaard E, et al. Radioimmunotherapy for model B cell malignancies using ^{90}Y-labeled anti-CD19 and anti-CD20 monoclonal antibodies. *Leukemia.* 2002;16:60–66.

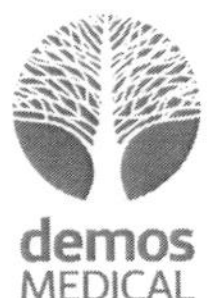

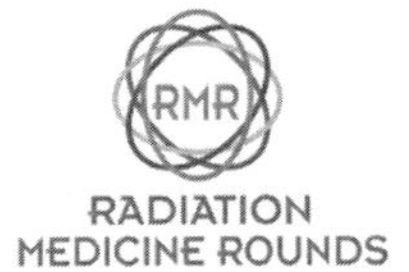

The Role of Radiotherapy in Transplantation for Lymphoma

Michael B. Tomblyn[1*] and Marcie Tomblyn[2]

[1]*Department of Radiation Oncology, H. Lee Moffitt Cancer Center and Research Institute, Tampa, FL*

[2]*Department of Blood and Marrow Transplantation, H. Lee Moffitt Cancer Center and Research Institute, Tampa, FL*

■ ABSTRACT

Hematopoietic cell transplantation is an important therapy for patients with relapsed or refractory lymphoma. Radiotherapy is often used in the peritransplant period to optimize disease control. Total body irradiation is commonly incorporated in the transplant preparative regimen, and randomized trials have suggested superiority over chemotherapy-alone regimens for some hematologic malignancies. Total lymphoid irradiation may offer similar improvements in transplant outcomes for lymphoma. Radioimmunotherapy has recently been incorporated into preparative regimens for B-cell non-Hodgkin lymphomas with promising results. External beam radiotherapy for consolidation can be targeted to areas of high risk to reduce the likelihood of post-transplant relapse. Here, we review the evidence for these uses of peritransplant radiotherapy.

Keywords: bone marrow transplant, total body irradiation, lymphoma

■ BASICS OF TRANSPLANTATION

Hematopoietic cell transplantation (HCT) is a commonly employed treatment modality for both Hodgkin lymphoma (HL) and non-Hodgkin lymphoma (NHL). For most lymphomas, this modality is utilized as a component of salvage therapy. However, for certain lymphomas such as peripheral T-cell NHL and mantle cell NHL, consideration of consolidation with upfront high-dose chemotherapy and autologous HCT is appropriate (1,2).

Over the past four decades, evolution of transplantation has occurred with newer stem cell sources and variations in conditioning regimens which allow improved targeting of disease, expansion to older populations, and increased likelihood of finding a suitable donor for allogeneic transplantation. These changes have resulted in increased numbers of both autologous and allogeneic transplants. According to data from the Center for International Blood and Marrow Transplant Research (CIBMTR), there were 3,631 transplants for NHL and 1,269 transplants for HL in the United States in 2009 (3). Autologous transplantation predominated, comprising 3,859 (79%) of these transplants (NHL = 2,754; HL = 1,105).

---

*Corresponding author, Department of Radiation Oncology, H. Lee Moffitt Cancer Center and Research Institute, 12902 Magnolia Drive, Tampa, FL

E-mail address: michael.tomblyn@moffitt.org

Radiation Medicine Rounds 3:3 (2012) 513–526.

DOI: 10.5003/2151–4208.3.3.513

Several factors must be considered when assessing a patient for potential transplant management of their disease. These include both disease and patient related issues. Lymphoma histology is crucial to determination of type of transplantation. Lymphomas with a more indolent course such as follicular NHL, small lymphocytic lymphoma, marginal zone lymphoma, and mantle cell NHL are expected to relapse following chemotherapy. Consequently, in patients with these diseases, it is highly unlikely that high-dose chemotherapy and autologous transplantation will provide a curative approach; however, there is clearly a benefit with improved duration of progression-free survival (4–7). Interestingly, these diseases show evidence of long-term disease-free survival with allogeneic transplantation with a suggestion of a plateau and potential curative effect of that approach (8–11). Therefore, assessment of patient factors such as age and comorbid conditions must be included in the decision algorithm. For other histologies such as diffuse large cell NHL and HL, it is rare to consider an allogeneic transplantation as the initial option due to evidence of potential cure with the less risky high-dose chemotherapy and autologous transplantation approach (12–14).

HCT requires a conditioning regimen which can be single agent chemotherapy, combination chemotherapy or alternatively chemotherapy with either total body irradiation (TBI) or radioimmunotherapy (RIT). The purpose of the conditioning regimen depends upon whether a patient is receiving autologous transplant or allogeneic transplantation.

Autologous Transplantation

For autologous transplantation, the conditioning regimen is the sole management of the lymphoma. Consequently, patients who are in a complete remission and those with a partial remission will have a lower likelihood of relapse than patients with chemotherapy resistant disease. The intensity of the conditioning regimen results in complete ablation of the bone marrow (myeloablation) and the reinfusion of autologous hematopoietic stem cells serve to rescue the patient from this toxicity. The role of autologous transplantation as salvage at the time of first relapse has been considered standard of care for sensitive intermediate and high-grade NHL since 1995 (14).

Outcomes following high dose chemotherapy and autologous transplantation vary based on lymphoma histology and disease status at the time of transplantation. Data published by the CIBMTR estimates a three-year overall survival (OS) of 62 ± 1% for patients with sensitive diffuse large cell NHL compared to 37±2% for those with resistant disease ($P < .0001$) for patients ($n = 6,790$) reported to the Registry and transplanted between 2000 and 2009 (3). Notably, this data likely includes many patients who never received rituximab as part of initial therapy. Data from the CORAL study suggests that prior exposure to rituximab as part of initial therapy results in a lower progression-free survival (PFS) compared to patients with no prior rituximab therapy (15). For 5,887 patients with HL transplanted between 2000 and 2009 and reported to the CIBMTR, the three-year OS is estimated at 84±1%, 71±1%, and 50±1% for patients in CR, patients not in CR but with sensitive disease, and patients with resistant disease, respectively (3).

High-dose chemotherapy and autologous HCT is an intensive approach with expected toxicities. These include damage to vital organs from the high-dose chemotherapy, risks of bleeding and transfusions, and infectious complications which are greatest in the setting of neutropenia but persist for many months following transplantation due to delayed immune reconstitution. In addition, there is a greater risk of secondary malignancies including myelodysplastic syndrome or therapy related AML (16,17). Despite all of these potential complications, the risk of dying from a toxicity of therapy is generally less than 5%. The major risk of treatment failure following autologous transplantation is relapse of the lymphoma. Attempts to decrease disease relapse rely on increased conditioning intensity or alternatively maintenance therapy for a period of time following HCT. In general, for lymphomas, there is no clear role of maintenance chemotherapy following autologous transplantation although ongoing studies with new agents may alter this treatment algorithm.

Allogeneic Transplantation

Allogeneic transplantation for the management of lymphomas treats the underlying malignancy with a two-pronged approach: (a) the conditioning regimen decreases disease burden, and (b) the introduction of a donor's immune system results in graft-versus-lymphoma effect. The approach to allogeneic transplantation is more complicated by the need for a suitable donor and decisions of conditioning intensity.

To identify a potential donor for allogeneic transplantation, the recipient must first undergo high-resolution, or allele level, human leukocyte antigen (HLA) typing at HLA-A, HLA-B, HLA-C, and HLA-DRB1. Additional HLA loci may also be considered based on transplant center preference. The optimal donor choice is an HLA identical sibling since family members are generally willing, assessable, and there is a lower risk of acute graft-versus-host disease given likely similarities between minor HLA antigens (18). Unfortunately, only about 30% of potential transplant recipients will have a suitable sibling donor. Consequently, alternative donor sources including adult volunteer unrelated donors, haploidentical (half-matched) donors, and umbilical cord blood may be used. The best data is with matched adult volunteer unrelated donors, but unfortunately, based on the recipient's ethnicity, the likelihood of finding a perfectly matched (8/8 HLA-allele) adult volunteer unrelated donor ranges from approximately 25% for African-Americans to approximately 60% for Caucasians (W. Navarro, personal communication).

After a suitable donor is identified, it is also necessary to determine the appropriate stem cell source—namely, bone marrow or peripheral blood stem cells—if umbilical cord blood units are not being used. Unfortunately, this is not clearly known. Data in related donors from a large meta-analysis suggests that there is a decreased risk of relapse for patients with late stage disease who received peripheral blood stem cells (19). However this is compounded by increased risk of chronic graft-versus-host disease (19,20). In addition, results from a large randomized phase III trial comparing marrow versus peripheral blood stem cells from unrelated donors found no impact on overall survival, but again demonstrated increased chronic graft-versus-host disease with the use of peripheral blood derived hematopoietic stem cells (21).

Choice of conditioning intensity is also important for allogeneic transplantation. As noted earlier, allogeneic transplantation can treat the disease via a graft versus lymphoma effect from the donor's immune system. Because of this, reduced intensity conditioning regimens have been developed whereby the conditioning regimen is designed to maximally immunosuppress the recipient to prevent rejection of donor cells but may not lead to myelosuppression of the recipient. This has resulted in a wide spectrum of conditioning regimens ranging from fully myeloablative conditioning to true nonmyeloablative conditioning (22,23). The choice of conditioning intensity often depends upon the disease control at the time of transplant as well as the aggressiveness of the lymphoma being treated (24). Furthermore, factors such as prior autologous transplantation, stem cell source, and donor type may also impact the choice of conditioning regimen (25,26).

The toxicities of allogeneic transplantation leading to treatment failure are greater than those following high dose chemotherapy and autologous transplantation. This is due primarily to risks of acute and chronic graft-versus-host disease (GVHD). Furthermore, the risks of infection following allogeneic transplantation are increased due to the need for ongoing immune suppressive agents to both prevent and treat GVHD. Because of these complications, the estimated treatment related mortality due to the toxicities of allogeneic transplantation range between 10% and 35% in the first year after transplant.

With all of the nuances that are incorporated into the plan for allogeneic transplantation, outcomes of this approach vary widely based on lymphoma histology. Registry analyses suggest a 3-year OS after allogeneic HCT ranging from 17±4% for chemotherapy resistant diffuse large B-cell lymphoma to 70±2% for chemotherapy sensitive follicular lymphoma (3). Furthermore, the outcomes with unrelated donors are minimally inferior to those receiving transplant from a related donor. Studies are ongoing to determine optimal conditioning intensity, timing of transplantation and specific histologies best suited to the allogeneic transplant approach.

■ TOTAL BODY IRRADIATION

TBI has been used for the treatment of advanced hematologic malignancies for over 80 years. Heublein developed a large room holding up to four patients, with a radiation source located on the opposite side of the room (27). Patients were maintained in this room until they exhibited skin erythema, and several enjoyed significant palliation of sizable lymphadenopathy. In the early 1960s, the City of Hope Medical Center created a treatment device similar to a four-poster bed, with cesium-137 sources rising from the floor at the head and foot of the bed (28). Following the first successful bone marrow transplant at the University of Minnesota, investigators postulated a role for TBI for bone marrow ablation in preparation for transplantation. In the 1970s, institutions developed multi-source techniques to deliver TBI for patients undergoing HCT (29).

There are a number of theoretical advantages of TBI over a chemotherapy-alone HCT preparative regimen (30). Most patients have relapsed disease following systemic cytotoxic therapy, likely representing the presence of clones less sensitive to such agents. Most patients have not previously received radiotherapy, and the hematologic malignancies typically treated with HCT are generally quite responsive to radiation. Unlike with systemic therapies, there are no "sanctuary sites" from radiation such as the central nervous system and testicles. Systemic therapy relies on blood flow, metabolism, and excretion to reach the intended target tissues, with significant heterogeneity both between and within patients; radiotherapy requires no metabolism or elimination and can be modulated to deliver precise doses to areas of interest and is far more reproducible.

Fractionation

The earliest TBI conditioning regimens utilized a single fraction (STBI) of 6 to 10 Gy, primarily based on murine data. However, during the 1980s, data from both animal and preclinical experience suggested that a fractionated approach (FTBI) could deliver the same biological effective dose with fewer acute and late toxicities. Since then, a number of studies have been published to support the move to FTBI. An early randomized trial from the Fred Hutchinson Cancer Research Center randomized patients with acute myelogenous leukemia (AML) in first remission to a cyclophosphamide-containing HCT regimen plus either STBI (9.2 or 10 Gy) or FTBI (12 Gy in 6 fractions). Patients receiving the FTBI regimen exhibited superior survival and less toxicity, particularly interstitial pneumonitis (IP) and veno-occlusive disease (VOD) of the liver, than patients treated with STBI (31,32). A similar trial from France randomized patients with various hematologic malignancies to cyclophosphamide plus STBI (10 Gy) versus FTBI (14.85 Gy in 11 fractions) and also found superior survival and less VOD (but no difference in IP) with the FTBI regimen (33).

In a nonrandomized study, the Minnesota group reported the results of an analysis of patients with AML in first remission undergoing HCT with cyclophosphamide plus STBI (7.5 Gy) or FTBI (13.2 Gy in 8 fractions), with a nonsignificant trend towards improved survival with FTBI but no differences in relapse rate, engraftment, or GVHD. FTBI patients did experience less nausea and vomiting, although this could have been due to the FTBI technique using a significantly lower dose rate (34). A French retrospective analysis also failed to find a significant difference between STBI (10 Gy) and FTBI (12 Gy in 6 fractions), although there was a trend for improved

disease-free survival and less treatment-related mortality (TRM) with FTBI (35). A large retrospective analysis of acute leukemia patients in first or second remission undergoing cyclophosphamide and TBI-based regimens found that FTBI resulted in no differences in survival, relapse or TRM but less IP and cataracts with fractionation and with lower instantaneous dose rates (36).

Other studies have compared two or more FTBI regimens. Clift et al. reported the results of a randomized trial of cyclophosphamide plus either 12 Gy in 6 daily fractions or 15.75 Gy in 7 daily fractions for patients with AML in first remission (37).While the risk of relapse was lower in the high-dose TBI arm, TRM was also higher, leading to identical survival between the groups. The presence of Grade 2–4 acute GVHD was also higher in the high-dose FTBI arm, but this group also received reduced GVHD prophylaxis. These outcomes persisted in long-term follow-up (38). A randomized trial in chronic myeloid leukemia (CML) patients in chronic phase using the same two regimens yielded essentially identical outcomes (39). A Swiss retrospective analysis of several six-fraction FTBI regimens (totaling 10 Gy, 12 Gy, and 13.5 Gy) described small decreases in survival with each escalation of total dose (40). However, this likely represents the differences in fraction size more so than total dose.

TBI Versus No TBI

More recently, due to the complexities of delivering TBI and the concern for late effects (particularly in children), many investigators have sought to develop multi-agent chemotherapy-alone preparative regimens for HCT. Beginning in the early 1980s, transplant groups began to replace TBI with busulfan, and early reports were promising (41,42).

Blaise et al. reported the results of the first randomized controlled trial of cyclophosphamide (Cy) plus either TBI (most got 12 Gy in 6 fractions) or oral busulfan (Bu) in AML patients in first remission (43). The Cy-TBI arm exhibited significantly superior overall survival, disease-free survival, relapse rates, and TRM compared to the Bu-Cy arm. These differences persisted in long-term follow-up (44). The Southwest Oncology Group (SWOG) performed a randomized trial in a heterogeneous group of relapsed leukemia patients receiving either TBI (13.2 Gy in 11 fractions) plus etoposide (based on the results of a prior City of Hope study (45)) or Bu-Cy (46).No differences in survival, relapse, or toxicity were seen in the overall study; however, in a subset analysis, "good risk" patients treated with TBI had a better disease-free survival than those treated with Bu-Cy. A randomized trial of Cy-TBI (12 Gy in 6 fractions) versus Bu-Cy for patients with CML in chronic phase showed no difference in transplant outcomes between the arms (47). However, there were no deaths from leukemia in the TBI arm versus three in the Bu-Cy arm. Patients in the TBI arm were more likely to have acute GVHD. A randomized trial by the Nordic Bone Marrow Transplantation Group compared Cy-TBI (both STBI and FTBI were used) with Bu-Cy in a heterogeneous group of leukemia patients (48). Overall survival and TRM was superior for Cy-TBI, while patients randomized to busulfan had significantly higher rates of VOD, hemorrhagic cystitis, and acute GVHD. In patients with advanced disease, leukemia-free survival was better with Cy-TBI. In an update with long-term follow-up, the authors confirmed the previous findings and also reported more death from GVHD, obstructive bronchiolitis, and permanent alopecia in the Bu-Cy arm (49). A French randomized trial of Cy-TBI versus Bu-CY suggested no difference in survival between the groups and possibly higher relapse with Cy-TBI; however, the TBI techniques and fractionation were not standardized and were given per local discretion in 19 different centers (50).One randomized trial comparing TBI versus no TBI has been reported in children. Bunin et al. performed a study of FTBI (12 Gy in 6 fractions) versus oral busulfan, both combined with cyclophosphamide and etoposide in pediatric patients with ALL undergoing allogeneic HCT (51). Event-free survival was superior for the TBI arm, particularly in patients undergoing an unrelated allogeneic transplant.

Two meta-analyses have been performed of trials comparing Cy-TBI to Bu-Cy (52,53). Both analyses conclude that Cy-TBI is associated with a reduction in mortality and leukemia relapse, with a significantly reduced TRM compared to Bu-Cy. Cy-TBI is associated with higher rates of cataracts, while Bu-Cy causes more VOD, hemorrhagic cystitis, and permanent alopecia. These outcome trends were confirmed with an analysis of long-term follow-up of randomized trials by Socie et al. (54) and by a large registry study (55).

While the above data support the choice of Cy-TBI over oral busulfan-based preparative regimens in leukemia patients undergoing allogeneic HCT, no randomized trials have been reported comparing TBI versus no TBI in patients undergoing autologous HCT for NHL. The Seattle group reported the results of a phase II study of FTBI plus cyclophosphamide and etoposide (TBI/Cy/E) in lymphoma patients receiving autologous HCT (56).They later compared longer-term outcomes of these patients to a cohort treated with busulfan, melphalan and thiotepa (Bu/Mel/T). Many of the Bu/Mel/T cohort had been ineligible for TBI/Cy/E due to previous irradiation for their lymphoma. No differences were seen between the groups for overall survival, event-free survival or relapse (57). Toxicities were similar in both cohorts. In a smaller Canadian retrospective analysis comparing TBI/Cy/E to carmustine, etoposide, cytarabine, and melphalan (BEAM), transplant outcomes were similar (58). Importantly, toxicities, including pneumonitis, were not higher in the TBI cohort. Dreyling et al. reported on a randomized trial of Cy-TBI (12 Gy in 6 fractions) followed by autologous HCT versus interferon maintenance in patients with advanced stage mantle cell lymphoma (59). The intensive consolidation protocol resulted in a significantly improved progression-free survival. The Stanford group reported the results of a non-randomized comparison of TBI and non-TBI conditioning regimens for patients with Hodgkin lymphoma undergoing autologous HCT (60). Three preparative regimens were utilized: FTBI (12 Gy in 10 fractions), BCNU, or CCNU, each combined with cyclophosphamide and etoposide. Transplant outcomes were similar across the treatment cohorts. Of particular interest was the absence of second malignancies in the TBI cohort, compared to four in the BCNU and two in the CCNU groups.

Reduced Intensity Conditioning

More recently, allogeneic transplants have largely shifted from a myeloablative concept to one of reduced intensity conditioning (RIC) or reduced toxicity, allowing older patients or those with poorer performance status to be considered for allogeneic HCT. Rather than relying on the cytotoxic properties of the preparative regimen, a postulated graft-versus-tumor effect could result in durable disease control (61,62).RIC transplants typically employ a preparative regimen containing either STBI (2 Gy) and/or fludarabine. An early comparison of myeloablative conditioning (MAC) versus RIC sibling transplants demonstrated a dramatic reduction in 100-day TRM (23% vs. 3%), favoring a RIC approach (63). The reduction in morbidity and mortality for the RIC cohort is even more significant considering that the RIC patients were older with more comorbidities.

The same group described similar outcomes for RIC transplants with HLA-matched unrelated donors (64). They also reported lower rates of acute but not chronic GVHD with a RIC conditioning regimen (65).Similar promising outcomes with RIC conditioning has been reported by others for various hematologic malignancies, including lymphoma (26, 66,67).

While most RIC conditioning regimens utilize 2 Gy STBI, several other RIC TBI regimens have been reported. One report of 4 Gy STBI plus cyclophosphamide and antithymocyte globulin (ATG) in patients with refractory AML described four-year overall survival and leukemia-free survival rates of 32% and 30%, respectively (68). TRM at one year was 17%. Several groups have experience with 5.5 Gy STBI-based RIC regimens, with promising transplant outcomes and low TRM rates (69–71). Stelljes et al. reported the results of 8 Gy STBI plus fludarabine for AML patients undergoing sibling or unrelated allogeneic HCT (72). For patients transplanted in remission, relapse-free survival at two years was 78% with 8% TRM. Several groups have reported their experiences using non-TBI RIC regimens (73–77), also with promising results but with a suggestion of higher relapse rates than with MAC conditioning (73,76). No studies have been published to date comparing transplant outcomes for TBI versus no TBI RIC regimens.

TBI Techniques

There are nearly as many different techniques to deliver TBI as there are institutions performing the treatment. The American Association of Physicists in Medicine published their report on TBI techniques in 1986 (78), and several novel modifications have been described since then. At the H. Lee Moffitt Cancer Center, we use an opposed lateral technique as previously described (79). Patients are seated in a semi-recumbent position on a specially-designed TBI chair. Treatment is delivered using high-energy photons (15 MV) at extended SSD (greater than 3 meters), with custom-designed aluminum compensators to allow homogeneous dose throughout the body to within +10% of the dose prescribed to the umbilicus. An acrylic beam spoiler is placed near the surface of the patient to ensure adequate skin dose. For a complete description of the opposed lateral technique, including the formalism for compensator design, Dusenbery and Gerbi provide an excellent primer (30).

The other most commonly employed TBI technique uses anterior and posterior (AP) beam arrangements (80). Patients are generally standing or reclined on a bed at extended distance. Generally, a lower photon energy (6 MV) is used for the AP technique, and lung blocks are used to limit the likelihood of developing interstitial pneumonitis. Lung shielding also reduces radiation dose to the anterior and posterior chest walls, theoretically underdosing the ribs and potentially increasing the risk of relapse, particularly for patients with acute leukemias (81). Some institutions deliver a chest wall boost using electrons, placing the 90% isodose line at the lung-chest wall interface to make up for this lost dosewhile still protecting lung tissue (82).

More recently, the desire to reduce normal tissue toxicity has led investigators to examine the potential role for intensity modulated radiation therapy to deliver total marrow irradiation (TMI). Helical tomotherapy represents an ideal solution for long fields, negating the need to match multiple fields. Hui et al. first described the technique (83) and reported the first clinical experience with TMI (84). The City of Hope group has published the results of a phase I study of TMI with helical tomotherapy, in patients undergoing autologous or allogeneic HCT for various hematologic malignancies and found the technique to be safe and associated with little toxicity (85). Other institutions have reported their attempts at TMI using helical tomotherapy or using a traditional linear accelerator (86–90).

Late Effects of TBI

There are a number of potential late complications from TBI including second malignancy, cataracts, pulmonary toxicity, and infertility. In a comprehensive review of secondary AML following autologous HCT, Hake et al. report estimates ranging from 0% to 7% for TBI regimens compared to 3% to 8.4% for non-TBI regimens in long-term follow-up (91). A number of reports have concluded that higher total dose to the lungs (92,93) and higher instantaneous dose rates (93–95) are associated with a greater risk of clinically significant pneumonitis. Use of FTBI and lower instantaneous dose rates leads to a lower incidence of cataract formation, with an incidence as low as 2% (96–100). However, the use of post-HCT steroids also significantly increases this risk, independent of the use of TBI (99,101).

■ TOTAL LYMPHOID IRRADIATION

Total lymphoid irradiation (TLI) was initially developed as a treatment for Hodgkin lymphoma with curative intent (102), encompassing the major lymphatic regions of the body including the spleen. Over the decades, as multi-agent systemic cytotoxic therapy demonstrated significant activity, radiotherapy fields and doses began to shrink. Today, TLI may still play an important role in the preparative regimen for autologous HCT for Hodgkin lymphoma. Yahalom et al. initially reported the results of accelerated TLI (20 Gy in 12 fractions delivered three times daily) plus cyclophosphamide and etoposide in patients with advanced stage, chemotherapy-refractory Hodgkin lymphoma (103). Of 17 patients treated, four died of complications of transplant. Of the remainder, 12 obtained a complete remission to this intensive HCT regimen. In a later update with 47 patients, they reported 17% TRM and a 74% complete response rate for survivors (104).

TLI is also thought to protect the allogeneic transplant recipient from GVHD by favoring regulatory T cells (105,106). In a study of 111 patients (107) with lymphoid or myeloid malignancies treated with TLI (8 Gy in 10 fractions) and rabbit ATG prior to HLA-matched sibling or unrelated allogeneic HCT, the incidence of acute GVHD was very low (2% for sibling and 10% for unrelated transplants). However, graft-versus-tumor effects appeared to remain intact, with 34 patients with measurable disease prior to transplant obtaining durable complete remissions. These results have been confirmed by other investigators (108).

■ RIT AND HCT

RIT involves the attachment of a radionuclide to a monoclonal antibody in an attempt to bypass normal tissues and deliver radiation to the surface of the target tumor cell and is reviewed extensively elsewhere in this volume. Given the perceived toxicities of TBI and the inherent radiosensitivity of B-cell NHL, there has recently been significant interest in the incorporation of RIT as part of the transplant preparative regimen. Five studies have been reported using high-dose RIT alone (without high-dose chemotherapy), using either ^{90}Y ibritumomab tiuxetan or ^{131}I tositumomab in patients with B-cell NHL undergoing autologous HCT, with promising overall and progression-free survival rates (109–113).Three studies have used high-dose RIT in conjunction with chemotherapy as part of the transplant preparative regimen (114–116). Of particular interest is the study by Winter et al. (115) which used patient-specific dosing to target up to 15 Gy to critical organs. They found that a standard weight-based calculation using twice the typical dose of ^{90}Y ibritumomab tiuxetan would have delivered a wide range of doses to individual patients from 4 Gy to 31 Gy. With individualized dosing, the authors reported a 3-year progression-free survival of 43% for patients treated at all dose levels, promising considering that two-thirds of patients entered the study with active disease at the initiation of HCT conditioning.

A number of studies have reported outcomes using standard-dose RIT plus chemotherapy for HCT conditioning prior to an autologous transplant for B-cell NHL (117–122). Three-year progression-free survival has ranged from 39% to 83% with these regimens, with overall survival ranging from 55% to 92%. One randomized controlled trial of standard-dose RIT plus high-dose chemotherapy as an HCT preparative regimen was recently reported (123). The study by the Blood and Marrow Transplant Clinical Trials Network compared ^{131}I tositumomab to rituximab in patients with relapsed aggressive NHL undergoing autologous HCT with carmustine, etoposide, cytarabine and melphalan (BEAM) conditioning. Standard dosing of ^{131}I tositumomab (75 cGy total body exposure) was used in the RIT arm. No significant differences were seen between the arms for overall or progression-free survival. However, the study has been criticized for using only standard RIT doses and for using large amounts of rituximab which may have led to inefficient targeting of lymphoma cells by ^{131}I tositumomab.

■ PERITRANSPLANT CONSOLIDATIVE RADIOTHERAPY

While high-dose chemotherapy and autologous HCT can offer a majority of relapsed aggressive lymphoma patients long-term disease-free survival, the major cause of death following transplant remains relapse. As in the front-line setting, the most likely sites of relapse of lymphoma following HCT are those with involvement prior to treatment, particularly in sites of previous bulk disease (124,125).Several retrospective series support consolidation radiotherapy in autologous HCT patients (124–130). These studies demonstrate improvements in local control (125,128–130), progression-free survival (124,130), and even overall survival (126,127).However, other retrospective analyses failed to find these effects (131–133). Of interest, the positive series largely used post-HCT radiotherapy while the negative series were primarily pre-HCT.

■ CONCLUSIONS

Radiotherapy plays an important role in the HCT process. TBI has long been used as part of the transplant preparative regimen. While many institutions have moved to chemotherapy-alone regimens, the randomized data suggest a clear benefit for Cy-TBI over Bu-Cy conditioning for several hematologic disorders. Improvements in radiotherapy delivery and supportive care have significantly improved transplant outcomes. Novel TBI delivery methods such as helical tomotherapy can dose escalate to marrow spaces while reducing dose to radiosensitive organs. Incorporation of TLI can yield similar improvements in outcomes for lymphoma patients undergoing autologous HCT. Several studies suggest a benefit to the incorporation of RIT into conditioning regimens for B-cell lymphomas, and patient-specific dosing may allow for RIT dose escalation and improved disease control following HCT. Finally, peritransplant radiotherapy to areas of previous lymphoma bulk likely reduces the risk of relapse following autologous HCT. Post-HCT radiotherapy may be of greater benefit than delivering radiation prior to transplant.

■ REFERENCES

1. Damon LE, Johnson JL, Niedzwiecki D, et al. Immunochemotherapy and autologous stem-cell transplantation for untreated patients with mantle-cell lymphoma: CALGB 59909. *J Clin Oncol.* 2009;27:6101–6108.

2. Prochazka V, Faber E, Raida L, et al. Long-term outcome of patients with peripheral T-cell lymphoma treated with first-line intensive chemotherapy followed by autologous stem cell transplantation. *Biomed Pap Med Fac Univ Palacky Olomouc Czech Repub.* 2011;155:63–69.

3. Pasquini, MC, Wang Z. Current use and outcome of hematopoietic stem cell transplantation: CIBMTR Summary Slides, 2011. (Available at http://www.cibmtr.org.)

4. Dreyling M, Lenz G, Hoster E, et al. Early consolidation by myeloablative radiochemotherapy followed by autologous stem cell transplantation in first remission significantly prolongs progression-free survival in mantle-cell lymphoma: results of a prospective randomized trial of the European MCL Network. *Blood.* 2005;105:2677–2684.

5. Ladetto M, Vallet S, Benedetti F, et al. Prolonged survival and low incidence of late toxic sequelae in advanced follicular lymphoma treated with a TBI-free autografting program: updated results of the multicenter consecutive GITMO trial. *Leukemia.* 2006;20:1840–1847.

6. Lenz G, Dreyling M, Schiegnitz E, et al. Myeloablative radiochemotherapy followed by autologous stem cell transplantation in first remission prolongs progression-free survival in follicular lymphoma: results of a prospective, randomized trial of the German Low-Grade Lymphoma Study Group. *Blood.* 2004;104:2667–2674.

7. Schouten HC, Qian W, Kvaloy S, et al. High-dose therapy improves progression-free survival and survival in relapsed follicular non-Hodgkin's lymphoma: results from the randomized European CUP trial. *J Clin Oncol.* 2003;21:3918–3927.

8. Khouri IF, Lee MS, Saliba RM, et al. Nonablative allogeneic stem-cell transplantation for advanced/recurrent mantle-cell lymphoma. *J Clin Oncol.* 2003;21:4407–4412.

9. Khouri IF, Saliba RM, Erwin WD, et al. Nonmyeloablative allogeneic transplantation with or without ^{90}yttrium ibritumomab tiuxetan is potentially curative for relapsed follicular lymphoma: 12-year results. *Blood.* 2012;119:6373–6378.

10. Maris MB, Sandmaier BM, Storer BE, et al. Allogeneic hematopoietic cell transplantation after fludarabine and 2 Gy total body irradiation for relapsed and refractory mantle cell lymphoma. *Blood.* 2004;104:3535–3542.

11. Tomblyn MR, Ewell M, Bredeson C, et al. Autologous versus reduced-intensity allogeneic hematopoietic cell transplantation for patients with chemosensitive follicular non-Hodgkin lymphoma beyond first complete response or first partial response. *Biol Blood Marrow Transplant.* 2011;17:1051–1057.

12. Linch DC, Winfield D, Goldstone AH, et al. Dose intensification with autologous bone-marrow transplantation in relapsed and resistant Hodgkin's disease: results of a BNLI randomised trial. *Lancet.* 1993;341:1051–1054.

13. Majhail NS, Bajorunaite R, Lazarus HM, et al. Long-term survival and late relapse in 2-year survivors of autologous haematopoietic cell transplantation for Hodgkin and non-Hodgkin lymphoma. *Br J Haematol.* 2009;147:129–139.

14. Philip T, Guglielmi C, Hagenbeek A, et al. Autologous bone marrow transplantation as compared with salvage chemotherapy in relapses of chemotherapy-sensitive non-Hodgkin's lymphoma. *N Engl J Med.* 1995;333:1540–1545.

15. Gisselbrecht C, Glass B, Mounier N, et al. Salvage regimens with autologous transplantation for relapsed large B-cell lymphoma in the rituximab era. *J Clin Oncol.* 2010;28:4184–4190.

16. Bhatia S, Louie AD, Bhatia R, et al. Solid cancers after bone marrow transplantation. *J Clin Oncol.* 2001;19:464–471.

17. Sureda A, Arranz R, Iriondo A, et al. Autologous stem-cell transplantation for hodgkin's disease: results and prognostic factors in 494 patients from the Grupo Español de

Linfomas/Transplante Autólogo de Médula Ósea Spanish Cooperative Group. *J Clin Oncol.* 2001;19:1395–1404.

18. Tomblyn M, Weisdorf D. *Optimal Donor Selection for Allogeneic Hematopoietic Stem Cell Transplantation.* Bethesda, MD: AABB; 2009.

19. Group SCTC. Allogeneic peripheral blood stem-cell compared with bone marrow transplantation in the management of hematologic malignancies: an individual patient data meta-analysis of nine randomized trials. *J Clin Oncol.* 2005;23:5074–5087.

20. Cutler C, Giri S, Jeyapalan S, Paniagua D, Viswanathan A, Antin JH. Acute and chronic graft-versus-host disease after allogeneic peripheral-blood stem-cell and bone marrow transplantation: A meta-analysis. *J Clin Oncol.* 2001;19:3685–3691.

21. Anasetti C, Logan BR, Lee SJ, et al. Increased incidence of chronic graft-versus-host disease (GVHD) and no survival advantage with filgrastim-mobilized peripheral blood stem cells (PBSC) compared to bone marrow (BM) transplants from unrelated donors: results of blood and marrow transplant clinical trials network (BMT CTN) protocol 0201, a phase III, prospective, randomized trial. *Blood.* 2011;118:Abstract 1.

22. Bacigalupo A, Ballen K, Rizzo D, et al. Defining the intensity of conditioning regimens: working definitions. *Biol Blood Marrow Transplant.* 2009;15:1628–1633.

23. Giralt S, Ballen K, Rizzo D, et al. Reduced-intensity conditioning regimen workshop: defining the dose spectrum. Report of a workshop convened by the center for international blood and marrow transplant research. *Biol Blood Marrow Transplant.* 2009;15:367–369.

24. Armand P, Kim HT, Ho VT, et al. Allogeneic transplantation with reduced-intensity conditioning for Hodgkin and non-Hodgkin lymphoma: importance of histology for outcome. *Biol Blood Marrow Transplant.* 2008;14:418–425.

25. Rodriguez R, Nademanee A, Ruel N, et al. Comparison of reduced-intensity and conventional myeloablative regimens for allogeneic transplantation in non-Hodgkin's lymphoma. *Biol Blood Marrow Transplant.* 2006;12:1326–1334.

26. Tomblyn M, Brunstein C, Burns LJ, et al. Similar and promising outcomes in lymphoma patients treated with myeloablative or nonmyeloablative conditioning and allogeneic hematopoietic cell transplantation. *Biol Blood Marrow Transplant.* 2008;14:538–545.

27. Heublein AC. Preliminary report of continuous irradiation of the entire body. *Radiol.* 1932;18:1051–1062.

28. Jacobs ML, Pape L. A total body irradiation chamber and its uses. *Int J App Radiat Isotopes.* 1960;9:141–143.

29. Thomas ED, Storb R, Buckner CD. Total body irradiation in preparation for marrow engraftment. *Transplant Proc.* 1976;8:591–593.

30. Dusenbery KE, Gerbi BJ. Total body irradiation conditioning regimens in stem cell transplantation. In: Levitt SH, Purdy JA, Perez CA, Vijayakumar S, (Eds.). *Technical Basis of Radiation Therapy: Practical Clinical Applications,* 4th rev ed. Heidelberg, Germany: Springer; 2008:785–804.

31. Thomas ED, Clift RA, Hersman J, et al. Marrow transplantation for acute nonlymphoblastic leukemia in first remission using fractionated or single-dose irradiation. *Int J Radiat Oncol Biol Phys.* 1982;8:817–821.

32. Deeg HJ, Sullivan KM, Buckner CD, et al. Marrow transplantation for acute nonlymphoblastic leukemia in first remission: toxicity and long-term follow-up of patients conditioned with single-dose or fractionated total body irradiation. *Bone Marrow Transplant.* 1986;1:151–157.

33. Girinsky T, Benhamou E, Bourhis J-H, et al. Prospective randomized comparison of single-dose versus hyperfractionated total-body irradiation in patients with hematologic malignancies. *J Clin Oncol.* 2000;18:981–986.

34. Kim TH, McGlave PB, Ramsay N, et al. Comparison of two total body irradiation regimens in allogeneic bone marrow transplantation for acute non-lymphoblastic leukemia in first remission. *Int J Radiat Oncol Biol Phys.* 1990;19:889–897.

35. Resbeut M, Altschuler C, Blaise D, et al. Fractionated or single-dose total body irradiation in 171 acute myeloblastic leukemias in first complete remission: is there a best choice? *Int J Radiat Oncol Biol Phys.* 1995;31:509–517.

36. Belkacemi Y, Pene F, Touboul E, et al. Total-body irradiation before bone marrow transplantation for acute leukemia in first or second complete remission. Results and prognostic factors in 326 consecutive patients. *StrahlentherOnkol.* 1998;174:92–104.

37. Clift RA, Buckner CD, Appelbaum FR, et al. Allogeneic marrow transplantation in patients with acute myeloid leukemia in first remission: a randomized trial of two irradiation regimens. *Blood.* 1990;76:1867–1871.

38. Clift RA, Buckner CD, Appelbaum FR, et al. Long-term follow-up of a randomized trial of two irradiation regimens for patients receiving allogeneic marrow transplants during first remission of acute myeloid leukemia. *Blood.* 1998;15:1455–1456.

39. Clift RA, Buckner CD, Appelbaum FR, et al. Allogeneic marrow transplantation in patients with chronic myeloid leukemia in the chronic phase: a randomized trial of two irradiation regimens. *Blood.* 1991;77:1660–1665.

40. Bieri S, Helg C, Chapuis B, et al. Total body irradiation before allogeneic bone marrow transplantation: is more dose better? *Int J Radiat Oncol Biol Phys.* 2001;49:1071–1077.

41. Santos GW, Tutschka PJ, Brookmeyer R, et al. Marrow transplantation for acute nonlymphocytic leukemia after treatment with busulfan and cyclophosphamide. *N Engl J Med.* 1983;309:1347–1353.

42. Tutschka PJ, Copelan EA, Klein JP. Bone marrow transplantation for leukemia following a new busulfan and cyclophosphamide regimen. *Blood.* 1987;70:1382–1388.

43. Blaise D, Maraninchi D, Archimbaud E, et al. Allogeneic bone marrow transplantation for acute myeloid leukemia in first remission: a randomized trial of a busulfan-Cytoxan versus Cytoxan-total body irradiation as

preparative regimen: a report from the Group d'Etudes de la Greffe de MoelleOsseuse. *Blood*. 1992;10:2578–2582.

44. Blaise D, Maraninchi D, Michallet M, et al. Long-term follow-up of a randomized trial comparing the combination of cyclophosphamide with total body irradiation or busulfan as conditioning regimen for patients receiving HLA-identical marrow grafts for acute myeloblastic leukemia in first complete remission. *Blood*. 2001;97:3669–3671.

45. Blume KG, Forman SJ, O'Donnell MR, et al. Total body irradiation and high-dose etoposide: a new preparatory regimen for bone marrow transplantation in patients with advanced hematologic malignancies. *Blood*. 1987;69:1015–1020.

46. Blume KG, Kopecky KJ, Henslee-Downey JP, et al. A prospective randomized comparison of total body irradiation-etoposide versus busulfan-cyclophosphamide as preparatory regimens for bone marrow transplantation in patients with leukemia who were not in first remission: a Southwest Oncology Group study. *Blood*. 1993;81:2187–2193.

47. Clift RA, Buckner CD, Thomas ED, et al. Marrow transplantation for chronic myeloid leukemia: a randomized study comparing cyclophosphamide and total body irradiation with busulfan and cyclophosphamide. *Blood*. 1994;84:2036–2043.

48. Ringden O, Ruutu T, Remberger M, et al. A randomized trial comparing busulfan with total body irradiation as conditioning in allogeneic marrow transplant receipients with leukemia: a report from the Nordic Bone Marrow Transplantation Group. *Blood*. 1994;83:2723–2730.

49. Ringden O, Remberger M, Ruutu T, et al. Increased risk of chronic graft-versus-host disease, obstructive bronchiolitis, and alopecia with busulfan versus total body irradiation: long-term results of a randomized trial in allogeneic marrow recipients with leukemia. *Blood*. 1999;93:2196–2201.

50. Devergie A, Blaise D, Attal M, et al. Allogeneic bone marrow transplantation for chronic myeloid leukemia in first chronic phase: a randomized trial of busulfan-cytoxan versus cytoxan-total body irradiation as preparative regimen: a report from the French Society of Bone Marrow Graft (SFGM). *Blood*. 1995;85:2263–2268.

51. Bunin N, Aplenc R, Kamani N, et al. Randomized trial of busulfan vs total body irradiation containing conditioning regimens for children with acute lymphoblastic leukemia: a Pediatric Blood and Marrow Transplant Consortium study. *Bone Marrow Transplant*. 2003;32:543–548.

52. Shi-Xia X, Xian-Hua T, Hai-Qin X, et al. Total body irradiation plus cyclophosphamide versus busulphan with cyclophosphamide as conditioning regimen for patients with leukemia undergoing allogeneic stem cell transplantation: a meta-analysis. *Leukemia Lymphoma*. 2010;51:50–60.

53. Gupta T, Kannan S, Dantkale V, et al. Cyclophosphamide plus total body irradiation compared with busulfan plus cyclophosphamide as a conditioning regimen prior to hematopoietic stem cell transplantation in patients with leukemia: a systematic review and meta-analysis. *Hematol Oncol Stem Cell Ther*. 2011;4:17–29.

54. Socie G, Clift RA, Blaise D, et al. Busulfan plus cyclophosphamide compared with total-body irradiation plus cyclophosphamide before marrow transplantation for myeloid leukemia: long-term follow-up of 4 randomized studies. *Blood*. 2001;98:3569–3574.

55. Litzow MR, Perez WS, Klein JP, et al. Comparison of outcome following allogeneic bone marrow transplantation with cyclophosphamide-total body irradiation versus busulphan-cyclophosphamide conditioning regimens for acute myelogenous leukaemia in first remission. *Br J Haematol*. 2002;119:1115–1124.

56. Weaver CH, Petersen FB, Appelbaum FR, et al. High-dose fractionated total-body irradiation, etoposide, and cyclophosphamide followed by autologous stem-cell support in patients with malignant lymphoma. *J Clin Oncol*. 1994;12:2559–2566.

57. Gutierrez-Delgado F, Maloney DG, Press OW, et al. Autologous stem cell transplantation for non-Hodgkin's lymphoma: comparison of radiation-based and chemotherapy-only preparative regimens. *Bone Marrow Transplant*. 2001;28:455–461.

58. Liu HW, Seftel MD, Rubinger M, et al. Total body irradiation compared with BEAM: long-term outcomes of peripheral blood autologous stem cell transplantation for non-Hodgkin's lymphoma. *Int J Radiat Oncol Biol Phys*. 2010;78:513–520.

59. Dreyling M, Lenz G, Hoster E, et al. Early consolidation by myeloablative radiochemotherapy followed by autologous stem cell transplantation in first remission significantly prolongs progression-free survival in mantle-cell lymphoma: results of a prospective randomized trial of the European MCL Network. *Blood*. 2005;105:2677–2684.

60. Horning SJ, Chao NJ, Negrin RS, et al. High-dose therapy and autologous hematopoietic progenitor cell transplantation for recurrent or refractory Hodgkin's disease: analysis of the Stanford University results and prognostic indices. *Blood*. 1997;89:801–813.

61. Giralt S, Estey E, Albitar M, et al. Engraftment of allogeneic hematopoietic progenitor cells with purine analog-containing chemotherapy: harnessing graft-versus-leukemia without myeloablative therapy. *Blood*. 1997;89:4531–4536.

62. McSweeney PA, Niederwieser D, Shizuru JA, et al. Hematopoietic cell transplantation in older patients with hematologic malignancies: replacing high-dose cytotoxic therapy with graft-versus-tumor effects. *Blood*. 2001;97:3390–3400.

63. Diaconescu R, Flowers CR, Storer B, et al. Morbidity and mortality with nonmyeloablative compared with myeloablative conditioning before hematopoietic cell transplantation from HLA-matched related donors. *Blood*. 2004;104:1550–1558.

64. Sorror ML, Maris MB, Storer B, et al. Comparing morbidity and mortality of HLA-matched unrelated donor hematopoietic cell transplantation after non-myeloablative and myeloablative conditioning:

influence of pretransplantation comorbidities. *Blood.* 2004;104:961–968.

65. Mielcarek M, Martin PJ, Leisenring W, et al. Graft-versus-host disease after nonmyeloablative versus conventional hematopoietic stem cell transplantation. *Blood.* 2003;102:756–762.

66. Kahl C, Storer BE, Sandmaier BM, et al. Relapse risk in patients with malignant diseases given allogeneic hematopoietic cell transplantation after nonmyeloablative conditioning. *Blood.* 2007;110:2744–2748.

67. Laport GG, Sandmaier BM, Storer BE, et al. Reduced-intensity conditioning followed by allogeneic hematopoietic cell transplantation for adult patients with myelodysplastic syndrome and myeloproliferative disorders. *Biol Blood Marrow Transplant.* 2008;14:246–255.

68. Schmid C, Schleuning M, Schwerdtfeger R, et al. Long-term survival in refractory acute myeloid leukemia after sequential treatment with chemotherapy and reduced-intensity conditioning for allogeneic stem cell transplantation. *Blood.* 2006;108:1092–1099.

69. Blum W, Brown R, Lin HS, et al. Low-dose (550 cGy), single-exposure total body irradiation and cyclophosphamide: consistent, durable engraftment of related-donor peripheral blood stem cells with low treatment-related mortality and fatal organ toxicity. *Biol Blood Marrow Transplant.* 2002;8:608–618.

70. Khoury H, Adkins D, Brown R, et al. Low incidence of transplantation-related acute complications in patients with chronic myeloid leukemia undergoing allogeneic stem cell transplantation with a low-dose (500 cGy) total body irradiation conditioning regimen. *Biol Blood Marrow Transplant.* 2001;7:352–358.

71. Hallemeier C, Grigis M, Blum W, et al. Outcomes of adults with acute myelogenous leukemia in remission given 500 cGy of single-exposure total body irradiation, cyclophosphamide, and unrelated donor bone marrow transplants. *Biol Blood Marrow Transplant.* 2004;10:310–319.

72. Stelljes M, Bornhauser M, Kroger M, et al. Conditioning with 8-Gy total body irradiation and fludarabine for allogeneic hematopoietic stem cell transplantation in acute myeloid leukemia. *Blood.* 2005;106:3314–3321.

73. Hari P, Carreras J, Zhang MJ, et al. Allogeneic transplants in follicular lymphoma: higher risk of disease progression after reduced-intensity compared to myeloablative conditioning. *Biol Blood Marrow Transplant.* 2008;14:236–245.

74. Rodriguez R, Nademanee A, Ruel N, et al. Comparison of reduced-intensity and conventional myeloablative regimens for allogeneic transplantation in non-Hodgkin's lymphoma. *Biol Blood Marrow Transplant.* 2006;12:1326–1334.

75. Martino R, Iacobelli S, Brand R, et al. Retrospective comparison of reduced-intensity conditioning and conventional high-dose conditioning for allogeneic hematopoietic stem cell transplantation using HLA-identical sibling donors in myelodysplastic syndromes. *Blood.* 2006;108:836–846.

76. Alyea EP, Kim HT, Ho V, et al. Comparative outcome of nonmyeloablative and myeloablative allogeneic hematopoietic cell transplantation for patients older than 50 years of age. *Blood.* 2005;105:1810–1814.

77. Valcarcel D, Martino R, Caballero D, et al. Sustained remissions of high-risk acute myeloid leukemia and myelodysplastic syndrome after reduced-intensity conditioning allogeneic hematopoietic transplantation: chronic graft-versus-host disease is the strongest factor improving survival. *J Clin Oncol.* 2008;26:577–584.

78. Van Dyk J, Galvin JM, Glasgow GP, et al. The physical aspects of total and half body photon irradiation. A report of Task Group 29 Radiation Therapy Committee, American Association of Physicists in Medicine. *AAPM Report No. 17* 1986.

79. Khan FM, Williamson JF, Sewchand W, et al. Basic data for dosage calculation and compensation. *Int J Radiat Oncol Biol Phys.* 1980;6:745–751.

80. Shank B, Chu FC, Dinsmore R, et al. Hyperfractionated totalbody irradiation for bone marrow transplantation. Results in seventy leukemia patients with allogeneic transplants. *Int J Radiat Oncol Biol Phys.* 1983;9:1607–1611.

81. Girinsky T, Socie G, Ammarguellat H, et al. Consequences of two different doses to the lungs during a single dose of total body irradiation: results of a randomized study on 85 patients. *Int J Radiat Oncol Biol Phys.* 1994;30:821–824.

82. Shank B, O'Reilly RJ, Cunningham I, et al. Total body irradiation for bone marrow transplantation: the Memorial Sloan-Kettering Cancer Center experience. *Radiother Oncol.* 1990;18(Suppl. 1):68–81.

83. Hui SK, Kapatoes J, Fowler J, et al. Feasibility study of helical tomotherapy for total body or totalmarrow irradiation. *Med Phys.* 2005;32:3214–3224.

84. Hui S, Verneris M, Higgins P, et al. Helical tomotherapy targeting total bone marrow—Initial clinical experience at the University of Minnesota. *Med Phys.* 2006; 33:2215.

85. Wong JY, Rosenthal J, Liu A, et al. Image-guided total-marrow irradiation using helical Tomotherapy in patients with multiple myeloma and acute leukemia undergoing hematopoietic cell transplantation. *Int J Radiat Oncol Biol Phys.* 2009;73:273–279.

86. Corvo R, Zeverino M, Vagge S, et al. Helical Tomotherapy targeting total bone marrow after total body irradiation for patients with relapsed acute leukemia undergoing an allogeneic stem cell transplant. *Radiother Oncol.* 2011;98:382–386.

87. Yeginer M, Roeske JC, Radosevich JA, et al. Linear accelerator-based intentisty-modulated total marrow irradiation technique for treatment of hematologic malignancies: a dosimetric feasibility study. *Int J Radiat Oncol Biol Phys.* 2011;79:1256–1265.

88. Shueng PW, Lin SC, Chong NS, et al. Totalmarrow irradiation with helical tomotherapy for bone marrow transplantation of multiple myeloma: first experience in Asia. *Technol Cancer Res Treat.* 2009;8:29–38.

89. Aydogan B, Yeginer M, Kavak GO, et al. Totalmarrow irradiation with RapidArc volumetric arc therapy. *Int J Radiat Oncol Biol Phys.* 2011;81:592–599.

90. Zeverino M, Agostinelli S, Taccini G, et al. Advances in the implementation of helical tomotherapy-based total-marrow irradiation with a novel field junction technique. *Med Dosim.* 2012;37:314–320.

91. Hake CR, Garubert TA, Fenske TS. Does autologous transplantation directly increase the risk of secondary leukemia in lymphoma patients? *Bone Marrow Transplant.* 2007;39:59–70.

92. Sampath S, Schultheiss TE, Wong, J. Dose response and factors related to interstitial pneumonitis after bone marrow transplant. *Int J Radiat Oncol Biol Phys.* 2005;63:876–884.

93. Girinsky T, Benhamou E, Bourhis JH, et al. Prospective randomized comparison of single-dose versus hyperfractionated total-body irradiation in patients with hematologic malignancies. *J Clin Oncol.* 2000;18:981–986.

94. Ozsahin M, Belkacemi Y, Pene F, et al. Interstitial pneumonitis following autologous bone-marrow transplantation conditioned with cyclophosphamide and total-body irradiation. *Int J Radiat Oncol Biol Phys.* 1996;34:71–77.

95. Weiner RS, Bortin MM, Gale RP, et al. Interstitial pneumonitis after bone marrow transplantation. Assessment of risk factors. *Ann Intern Med.* 1986;104:168–175.

96. Ozsahin M, Belkacemi Y, Pene F, et al. Total-body irradiation and cataract incidence: a randomized comparison of two instantaneous dose rates. *Int J Radiat Oncol Biol Phys.* 1994;28:343–347.

97. Benvunes MC, Sullivan KM, Deeg HJ, et al. Cataracts after bone marrow transplantation: long-term follow-up of adults treated with fractionated total body irradiation. *Int J Radiat Oncol Biol Phys.* 1995;32:661–670.

98. Belkacemi Y, Ozsahin M, Pene F, et al. Cataractogenesis after total body irradiation. *Int J Radiat Oncol Biol Phys.* 1996;35:53–60.

99. vanKempen-Harteveld ML, Struikmans H, Kal HB, et al. Cataract-free interval and severity of cataract after total body irradiation and bone marrow transplantation: influence of treatment parameters. *Int J Radiat Oncol Biol Phys.* 2000;48:807–815.

100. Aristei C, Alessandro M, Santucci A, et al. Cataracts in patients receiving stem cell transplantation after conditioning with total body irradiation. *Bone Marrow Transplant.* 2002;29:503–507.

101. Hamon MD, Gale RF, Macdonald ID, et al. Incidence of cataracts after single fraction total body irradiation: the role of steroids and graft versus host disease. *Bone Marrow Transplant.* 1993;12:233–236.

102. Kaplan HS, Rosenberg SA. Extended field radical radiotherapy in advanced Hodgkin's disease: short term results of 2 randomized clinical trials. *Cancer Res.* 1966;26:1268–1276.

103. Yahalom J, Gulati S, Shank B, et al. Total lymphoid irradiation, high-dose chemotherapy and autologous bone marrow transplantation for chemotherapy-resistant Hodgkin's disease. *Int J Radiat Oncol Biol Phys.* 1989;17:915–922.

104. Yahalom J, Gulati SC, Toia M, et al. Accelerated hyperfractionated total-lymphoid irradiation, high-dose chemotherapy, and autologous bone marrow transplantation for refractory and relapsing patients with Hodgkin's disease. *J Clin Oncol.* 1993;11:1062–1070.

105. Slavin S, Fuks Z, Kaplan HS, et al. Transplantation of allogeneic bone marrow without graft-versus-host disease using total lymphoid irradiation. *J Exp Med.* 1978;147:963–972.

106. Lan F, Zeng D, Higuchi M, et al. Predominance of NK1.1+TCR alpha beta+ or DX5+TCR alpha beta+ T cells in mice conditioned with fractionated lymphoid irradiation protects against graft-versus-host disease: "natural suppressor" cells. *J Immunol.* 2001;167:2087–2096.

107. Kohrt HE, Turnbull BB, Hevdari K, et al. TLI and ATG conditioning with low risk of graft-versus-host disease retains antitumor reactions after allogeneic hematopoietic cell transplantation from related and unrelated donors. *Blood.* 2009;114:1099–1109.

108. Messina G, Giaccone L, Festuccia M, et al. Multicenter experience using total lymphoid irradiation and antithymocyte globulin as conditioning for allografting in hematological malignancies. *Biol Bone Marrow Transplant.* 2012;18(10):1600–1607.

109. Devizzi L, Guidetti A, Tarella C, et al. High-dose yttrium-90-ibritumomab tiuxetan with tandem stem-cell reinfusion: an outpatient preparative regimen for autologous hematopoietic cell transplantation. *J Clin Oncol.* 2008;26:5175–5182.

110. Gopal AK, Rajendran JG, Gooley TA, et al. High-dose ^{131}I tositumomab (anti-CD20) radioimmunotherapy and autologous hematopoietic stem-cell transplantation for adults > 60 years old with relapsed or refractory B-cell lymphoma. *J Clin Oncol.* 2007;25:1396–1402.

111. Liu SY, Eary JF, Petersdorf SH, et al. Follow-up of relapsed B-cell lymphoma patients treated with iodine-131-labeled anti-CD20 antibody and autologous stem-cell rescue. *J Clin Oncol.* 1998;16:3270–3278.

112. Vanazzi A, Ferrucci P, Grana C, et al. High dose [90]yttrium ibritumomab tiuxetan with PBSC support in refractory-resistant NHL patients. *Blood.* 2008;112:Abstract 1890.

113. Swinnen LJ, Flinn IW, Kahl B, et al. Phase I trial of yttrium 90 ibritumomab tiuxetan ^{90}Y-RIT with autologous stem cell transplantation (ASCT) in patients with relapsed or refractory B-cell non-Hodgkin's lymphoma (NHL). *J Clin Oncol.* 2008;26(15 Suppl):Abstract 8565.

114. Nademanee A, Raubitschek A, Molina A, et al. Updated results of high-dose yttrium 90 (^{90}Y) ibritumomab tiuxetan with high-dose etoposide (VP-16) and cyclophosphamide (CY) followed by autologous hematopoietic stem cell transplant (AHSCT) for poor-risk or refractory B-cell non-Hodgkin's lymphoma. *Blood.* 2007;110:Abstract 1891.

115. Winter JN, Inwards DJ, Spies S, et al. Yttrium-90 ibritumomab tiuxetan doses calculated to deliver up to 15 Gy

to critical organs may be safely combined with high-dose BEAM and autologous transplantation in relapsed or refractory B-cell non-Hodkin's lymphoma. *J Clin Oncol.* 2009;27:1653–1659.

116. Press OW, Eary JF, Cooley T, et al. A phase I/II trial of iodine-131-tositumomab (anti-CD20), etoposide, cyclophosphamide, and autologous stem cell transplantation for relapsed B-cell lymphomas. *Blood.* 2000;96:2934–2942.

117. Khouri IF, Saliba RM, Hosing C, et al. Efficacy and safety of yttrium 90 (^{90}Y) ibritumomab tiuxetan in autologous and nonmyeloablative stem cell transplantation (NST) for relapsed non-Hodgkin's lymphoma (NHL). *Blood.* 2006;108: Abstract 315.

118. Shimoni A, Zwas ST, Oksman Y, et al. Yttrium-90-ibritumomab tiuxetan (Zevalin) compared with high-dose BEAM chemotherapy and autologous stem cell transplantation for chemo-refractory aggressive non-Hodgkin's lymphoma. *ExpHematol.* 2007;35:534–540.

119. Krishnan A, Nademanee A, Fung HC, et al. Phase II trial of a transplantation regimen of yttrium-90 ibritumomab tiuxetan and high-dose chemotherapy in patients with non-Hodgkin's lymphoma. *J Clin Oncol.* 2008;26:90–95.

120. Shimabukuro-Vornhagen A, Josting A, Hubel K, et al. Yttrium-90 ibritumomab tiuxetan combined with high-dose BEAM chemotherapy and autologous stem cell transplantation for relapsed/refractory B-cell non-Hodgkin's lymphoma. *J Clin Oncol.* 2008;26(15 Suppl):Abstract 8615.

121. Vose JM, Bierman PJ, Enke C, et al. Phase I trial of iodine-131 tositumomab with high-dose chemotherapy and autologous stem-cell transplantation for relapsed non-Hodgkin's lymphoma. *J Clin Oncol.* 2005;23:461–467.

122. Vose J, Bierman P, Bociek G, et al. Radioimmunotherapy with 131-I-tositumomab enhanced survival in good prognosis relapsed and high-risk diffuse large B-cell lymphoma (DLBCL) patients receiving high-dose chemotherapy and autologous stem cell transplantation. *J Clin Oncol.* 2007;25 (18 Suppl):Abstract 8013.

123. Vose JM, Carter SL, Burns LJ, et al. Randomized phase III trial of ^{131}iodine-tositumomab (bexxar)/carmustine, etoposide, cytarabine, melphalan (BEAM) vs. Rituximab/BEAM and autologous stem cell transplantation for relapsed diffuse large B-cell lymphoma (DLBCL): no difference in progression-free (PFS) or overall survival (OS). *Blood.* 2011;118: Abstract 661.

124. Rapoport AP, Lifton R, Constine LS, et al. Autotransplantation for relapsed or refractory non-Hodgkin's lymphoma (NHL): long-term follow-up and analysis of prognostic factors. *Bone Marrow Transplant.* 1997;19:883–890.

125. Oehler-Janne C, Taverna C, Stanek N, et al. Consolidative involved field radiotherapy after high dose chemotherapy and autologous stem cell transplantation for non-Hodgkin's lymphoma: a case-control study. *Hematol Oncol.* 2008;26:82–90.

126. Vose JM, Zhang MJ, Rowlings PA, et al. Autologous transplantation for diffuse aggressive non-Hodgkin's lymphoma in patients never achieving remission: a report from the Autologous Blood and Marrow Transplant Registry. *J Clin Oncol.* 2001;19:406–13.

127. Biswas T, Dhakal S, Chen R, et al. Involved field radiation after autologous stem cell transplant for diffuse large B-cell lymphoma in the rituximab era. *Int J Radiat Oncol Biol Phys.* 2010;77:79–85.

128. Hoppe BS, Moskowitz CH, Zhang Z, et al. The role of FDG-PET imaging and involved field radiotherapy in relapsed or refractory diffuse large B-cell lymphoma. *Bone Marrow Transplant.* 2009;43:941–948.

129. Mundt AJ, Williams SF, Hallahan D. High dose chemotherapy and stem cell rescue for aggressive non-Hodgkin's lymphoma: pattern of failure and implications for involved-field radiotherapy. *Int J Radiat Oncol Biol Phys.* 1997;39:617–625.

130. Kahn S, Flowers C, Xu Z, Esiashvili N. Does the addition of involved field radiotherapy to high-dose chemotherapy and stem cell transplantation improve outcomes for patients with relapsed/refractory Hodgkin lymphoma? *Int J Radiat Oncol Biol Phys.* 2011;81:175–180.

131. Friedberg JW, Neuberg D, Monson E, et al. The impact of external beam radiation therapy prior to autologous bone marrow transplantation in patients with non-Hodgkin's lymphoma. *Biol Blood Marrow Transplant.* 2001;7:446–453.

132. Wendland MM, Smith DC, Boucher KM, et al. The impact of involved field radiation therapy in the treatment of relapsed or refractory non-Hodgkin lymphoma with high-dose chemotherapy followed by hematopoietic progenitor cell transplant. *Am J Clin Oncol.* 2007;30:156–162.

133. Kewalramani T, Zelenetz AD, Hedrick EE, et al. High-dose chemoradiotherapy and autologous stem cell transplantation for patients with primary refractory aggressive non-Hodgkin lymphoma: an intention-to-treat analysis. *Blood.* 2000;96:2399–2404.

Index

Note: Page numbers in **bold** and *italics* refer to figures and tables, respectively.